Oxford
Handbook of
Oncology

Dose schedules are being continually revised and new side effects recognized. Oxford University Press makes no representation, express or implied, that the drug dosages in this book are correct. For these reasons the reader is strongly urged to consult the pharmaceutical company's printed instructions before administering any of the drugs recommended in this book.

Oxford Handbook of Oncology

Jim Cassidy
Professor of Oncology,
Institute of Medical Sciences,
Aberdeen

Donald Bissett
Consultant Clinical Oncologist,
Aberdeen Royal Infirmary,
Aberdeen

and

Roy AJ Spence OBE
Consultant Surgeon,
Belfast City Hospital;
Honorary Professor,
Queen's University, Belfast;
Honorary Professor
University of Ulster

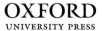

OXFORD
UNIVERSITY PRESS

OXFORD
UNIVERSITY PRESS

Great Clarendon Street, Oxford OX2 6DP

Oxford University Press is a department of the University of Oxford.
It furthers the University's objective of excellence in research, scholarship,
and education by publishing worldwide in

Oxford New York

Athens Auckland Bangkok Buenos Aires Cape Town Chennai
Dar es Salaam Delhi Hong Kong Istanbul Karachi Kolkata
Kuala Lumpur Madrid Melbourne Mexico City Mumbai
Nairobi São Paulo Shanghai Taipei Tokyo Toronto
and an associated company in Berlin

Oxford is a registered trade mark of Oxford University Press
in the UK and in certain other countries

Published in the United States
by Oxford University Press Inc., New York

A catalogue record for this title is available from the British Library

Library of Congress Cataloguing in Publication Data
(Data available)

ISBN 0 19 263035 0

10 9 8 7 6 5 4 3 2 1

Typeset by EXPO Holdings, Malaysia
Printed in Great Britain
on acid-free paper by The Bath Press, Avon

Preface

Cancer is a word that describes a large number of related diseases. It will affect about one in three of the Western population. The disease requires expertise from many disciplines if it is to be cured or adequately palliated. Much has been written about cancer. This is daunting for the student, trainee, or other professional involved with cancer patients.

This book is designed as a primer for those who are involved with cancer patients or the study of cancer. It is intended to supply sufficient background knowledge to allow the reader to seek more detailed information from the numerous textbooks and web resources in oncology. As such, it is deliberately not all-inclusive. It does cover the principles of oncology and the common cancers as well as the complex clinical pictures that cancer can produce.

We are very grateful to the long list of contributors who took time to give insight into their own specialist areas. Special thanks should to go to Roy Spence – who, in football terms, 'came into the team from the bench and scored the winning goal!'.

I hope you enjoy this Handbook and it inspires you to learn more about this most fascinating disease.

J.C.

Contents

List of contributors

Dr F. Ahmed Aberdeen Royal Infirmary, Aberdeen, UK

J. W. Arndt Department of Diagnostic Radiology, Leiden University Hospital, Leiden, The Netherlands

Dr Ahmed Awada Chemotherapy Unit, Jules Bardet Institute, Brussels, Belgium

Professor Anne Barrett Professor of Radiation Oncology, Glasgow University and Beatson Oncology Centre, Western Infirmary, Glasgow, UK

Professor H. Bartelink The Netherlands Cancer Institute, The Netherlands

Professor H. Bismuth University of South Paris, Paris, France

Dr Bissett Aberdeen Royal Infirmary, Aberdeen, UK

Professor A. K. Burnett Department of Haematology, University Hospital of Wales, Cardiff Royal Infirmary, Cardiff, UK

Dr Sally Burtles Cancer Research Campaign, London, UK

Professor Hilary Calvert Director of Oncology Research Unit, University of Newcastle-upon Tyne, Newcastle, UK

Dr David Cameron Senior Lecturer in Medical Oncology, Edinburgh University, Edinburgh, UK

Dr Etienne Chatelut Pharmacology Laboratory, Institute Claudis Regard, Toulouse, France

Dr John Chester ICRF Cancer Medical Research Unit, University of Leeds, Leeds, UK

Dr John S. Cockburn Consultant Cardiothoracic Surgeon, Department of Cardiothoracic Surgery, Aberdeen Royal Infirmary, Aberdeen, UK

Professor Robert Coleman Cancer Research Centre, YCR Department of Clinical Oncology, Western Park Hospital, Sheffield UK

Professor Tim Cooke Department of Surgery, Royal Infirmary, Glasgow, UK

Professor Alan Craft Head of Department of Child Health, The Royal Victoria Infirmary, Newcastle-upon-Tyne, Newcastle, UK

Dr John Crown Department of Medical Oncology, St Vincent's Hospital, Dublin, Ireland

Dr Dominic Culligan Consultant Haematologist and Honorary Senior Lecturer, Aberdeen Royal Infirmary, Aberdeen, UK

Dr David Cunningham Royal Marsden NHS Trust, Institute for Cancer Research, Sutton, Surrey, UK

Dr Rosie Daniel Medical Director, Bristol Cancer Help Centre, Clifton, Bristol, UK

Dr Gedeske Daugaard Department of Oncology, Rigshospitalet, Blegdamsvejq, National University Hospital, Copenhagen, Denmark

Dr Carol Davies Southampton General Hospital, Southampton, UK

R. H. deBoer Royal Marsden Hospital, Sutton, Surrey, UK

Dr John Dewar Dundee University, Dundee, UK

Professor S. Dische Centre for Cancer Treatment, Mount Vernon Hospital, Northwood, Middlesex, UK

Dr David Dodds Beatson Oncology Centre, Western Infirmary, Glasgow, UK

Dr. Sinead Donnelly Marie Curie Centre, Glasgow, UK

J. Doughty Department of Surgery, Glasgow University, Glasgow, UK

Dr. David Dunlop Beatson Oncology Centre, Western Infirmary, Glasgow, UK

Professor L. Fallowfield Royal Free and UCL Medical School, London, UK

Dr T. A. F. El-Maghraby Leiden University Hospital, Leiden, Netherlands

Dr Marie Fallon Senior Lecturer in Palliative Care, Beatson Oncology Centre, Western Infirmary, Glasgow, UK; Senior Lecturer in Palliative Medicine, University of Glasgow, Glasgow, UK

Paula Ganeh Department of Oncology, University of Birmingham, Birmingham, UK

Professor Andrew Gesher MRC Toxicology Unit, University of Leicester, Leicester, UK

Professor O. J. Garden University Department of Surgery, Edinburgh Royal Infirmary, Edinburgh University, Edinburgh, UK

Professor Fiona Gilbert Department of Radiology, Foresterhill House Annexe, Foresterhill, Aberdeen, UK

Professor A. Goldstone Department of Haematology, University College Hospital, London, UK

Dr Martin Gore Consultant in Medical Oncology, Royal Marsden Hospital, South Kensington, London, UK

Dr John Graham Consultant in Clinical Oncology, Bristol Oncology Centre, Bristol, UK

Professor M. Greaves Department of Medicine and Therapeutics, University of Aberdeen, Aberdeen, UK

Dr Anna Gregor Consultant in Clinical Oncology, Macmillan Lead Cancer Clinician, Western General Hospital, Edinburgh, UK

Professor Neva Haites Department of Medical Genetics, University of Aberdeen, Aberdeen, UK

Dr Adrian Harnett Consultant in Clinical Oncology, Beatson Oncology Centre, Western Infirmary, Glasgow, UK

Dr Mark Harrison Consultant Oncologist, Mount Vernon Cancer Centre, Middlesex, UK

Professor G. Hawksworth Department of Medicine and Therapeutics, University of Aberdeen, Aberdeen, UK

Professor Alan Horwich Head of Clinical Laboratories, Royal Marsden NHS Trust, Institute for Cancer Research, Sutton, Surrey, UK

Dr Grahame Howard Honorary Senior Lecturer, Directorate of Clinical Oncology and Haematology, Western General Hospital, Edinburgh, UK

Dr Robin Hunter Christie Hospital, National Health Service Trust, Manchester, UK

Dr N. D. James Institute for Cancer Studies, Birmingham University, Birmingham, UK

Dr Roger James Kent Cancer Centre, Maidstone, Kent, UK

Dr Anthony Jeliffe 152 Harley Street, London, UK

Dr Jonathan Joffee Macmillan Consultant in Medical Oncology, Greenlea Oncology Unit, Huddersfield Royal Infirmary, Huddersfield, UK

Lucie Jones Department of Oncology, University of Birmingham, Birmingham, UK

Dr Ian Judson Reader in Clinical Pharmacology, Royal Marsden NHS Trust, Institute for Cancer Research, Sutton, Surrey, UK

Dr Nicol Keith CRC Department of Medical Oncology, Beatson Oncology Centre, Western Infirmary, Glasgow, UK

Professor David Kerr Professor of Clinical Oncology, CRC Institute for Cancer Studies, University of Birmingham, Birmingham, UK

Professor Henry Kitchener Academic Unit of Obstetrics, Gynaecology & Reproductive Health, St Mary's Hospital, Manchester, UK

Dr Robin Leake Division of Biochemistry and Molecular Biology, University of Glasgow, Glasgow, UK

Dr Mike Lind The University of Hull School of Medicine, Academic Department of Oncology, Princess Royal Hospital, Hull, UK

Professor Julian Little Department of Epidemiology, Aberdeen University, Aberdeen, UK

Professor Valerie Lund Professor Rhinology, University College London Medical School and Royal National ENT Hospital, London, UK

Dr Fergus Macbeth Clinical Effectiveness Support Unit, University Hospital of Wales and Llandough Hospital NHS Trust, Penarth, UK

Dr A. McDonald Aberdeen Royal Infirmary, Aberdeen, UK

Dr D. Machin MRC Cancer Trials Office, Cambridge, UK

Professor Rona MacKie Department of Dermatology, University of Glasgow, Glasgow, UK

Professor J. MacVie Cancer Research Campaign, London, UK

Mr Pietro E. Majno Department of Surgery, Hôpital Cantonal, Geneva, Switzerland

Dr S. G. Martin University of Nottingham, CRC Department of Clinical Oncology, City Hospital, Nottingham, UK

Dr Dynes McConnell Aberdeen Royal Infirmary, Aberdeen, UK

Dr John McLelland, Department of Radiotherapy, Aberdeen Royal Infirmary, Aberdeen, UK

Dr Howard McLeod Washington University, St Louis, USA

Dr Stuart McNee Radiotherapy Physics Department, Beatson Oncology Centre, Western Infirmary, Glasgow, UK

Professor W. R. Miller Professor of Experimental Oncology, Edinburgh Breast Unit Research Group, The University of Edinburgh, The Paderewski Building, Western General Hospital, Edinburgh, UK

Dr Christopher Mitchell The John Radcliffe Hospital, Oxford, UK

Dr Nicole Moreland London, UK

Dr Graeme Murray Department of Pathology, University of Aberdeen, Aberdeen, UK

Professor J. P. Neoptolemos Department of Surgery, Royal Liverpool University Hospital, Liverpool, UK

Dr Don Newling Academisch Ziekenhuis, Vrije Universiteit, The Netherlands

Dr M. C. Nicolson Aberdeen Royal Infirmary, Aberdeen, UK

Professor John Northover Consultant Surgeon, St Mark's Hospital, Harrow, Middlesex, London, UK

Professor P. J. O'Dwyer Department of Surgery, Western Infirmary, Glasgow, UK

Dr. K. Oberg Department of Internal Medicine, University Hospital, Uppsala, Sweden

Professor Jan Olofsson Department of Otolaryngology, University of Bergen, Haukeland University Hospital, Bergen, Norway

Dr. Daniel Palmer Department of Oncology, University of Birmingham, Birmingham UK

Dr H. Pandha Department of Cellular and Molecular Sciences, Division of Oncology, St George's Hospital Medical School, London, UK

M. K. B. Parmar Cancer Division, MRC Clinical Trials Unit, Cambridge, UK

Professor Pauwels Department of Diagnostic Radiology, Leiden University Hospital, Leiden, Netherlands

Dr Martine Piccart Head, Chemotherapy Uni, Institute Jules Bordet, Brussels, Belgium

Professor Ross Pinkerton CRC Professor of Paediatric Oncology, Children's Department, Institute of Cancer Research and The Royal Marsden Hospital, Sutton, Surrey, UK

Dr P. N. Plowman Radiotherapy and Clinical Oncology Department, St Bartholomew's Hospital, London, UK

Professor B. Ponder Department of Oncology, University of Cambridge, Cambridge, UK

Dr Graeme Poston Consultant Surgical Oncologist, The Royal Liverpool University Hospitals, Liverpool, UK

Professor Allan Price Western General Hospital, Edinburgh, UK

Dr Pat Price Cancer Centre, Hammersmith Hospital, London, UK; Reader in Clinical Oncology, Head of Cancer Therapeutics, Imperial College School of Medicine, London, UK

Dr Roy Rampling Reader and Honorary Consultant in Clinical Oncology, University of Glasgow, Glasgow, UK; Neuro-oncology unit, Beatson Oncology Centre, Western Infirmary, Glasgow, UK

Dr A. T. Redpath Head of Radiotherapy Physics, Radiation Physics Department, Western General Hospital, Edinburgh, UK

Dr N. S. Reed Consultant Clinical Oncologist, Beatson Oncology Centre, Western Infirmary, Glasgow, UK

Professor F Rilke Instituto Nazionale per lo Studio e la Cura dei Tumori, Milan, Italy

Dr J. Trevor Roberts Consultant Clinical Oncologist and Clinical Director, Northern Centre for Cancer Treatment, Newcastle General Hospital, Newcastle-upon-Tyne

Professor Mikael Rorth Department of Oncology, Rigshospitalet, Blegdamsvejq, National University Hospital, Copenhagen, Denmark

Dr Paul Ross Royal Marsden NHS Trust, Institute for Cancer Research, Sutton, Surrey, UK

Dr G. J. S Rustin Director of Medical Oncology, Centre for Cancer Treatment, Mount Vernon Hospital, Northwood, Middlesex, UK

Professor M. I. Saunders Consultant, Centre for Cancer Treatment, Mount Vernon Hospital, Northwood, Middlesex, UK

Dr. Schoefield Reader in Surgery, University Hospital Nottingham, Nottingham, UK

Dr Michael Seckl Senior Lecturer, Department of Medical Oncology, Imperial College, London, UK; Trophoblastic Tumour Screening and Treatment Centre, Department of Cancer Medicine, Charing Cross Hospital, London, UK

Dr Matt Seymour ICRF Cancer Medical Research Unit, University of Leeds, Leeds, UK

Dr Duncan Shaw Professor in Genetics, Department of Molecular and Cell Biology, University of Aberdeen

Professor Karol Sikora Imperial College School of Medicine, London, UK

Dr C. R. J. Singer Department of Haematology, Royal United Hospital, Bath

Dr Ian Smith Head of Section of Medicine, Royal Marsden Hospital, Sutton, Surrey, UK

Professor John Smyth Department of Oncology, Western General Hospital, Edinburgh, UK

Dr Margaret Spittle Clinical Consultant Oncologist, Meyerstein Institute of Oncology, Middlesex Hospital, London

Dr Davis Spooner Department of Oncology, Queen Elizabeth Hospital, Birmingham

Karen Steadman Senior Registrar in Palliative Medicine, Countess Mountbatten House, Southampton

Professor Gordon Steel Radiotherapy Research Unit, Institute of Cancer Research, Sutton, Surrey, UK

Professor R. J. C. Steele Professor of Surgical Oncology, University of Dundee; Department of Surgery and Molecular Oncology, Ninewells Hospital and Medical School, Dundee, UK

Dr David Stevenson Department of Medical Genetics, Aberdeen University, Aberdeen, UK

Professor W. P. Steward Professor of Oncology, University Department of Oncology, Leicester Royal Infirmary, Leicester, UK

Dr D. J. Sugarbaker Associate Professor of Surgery, Brigham and Women's Hospital, Harvard Medical School, USA

Dr John Sweetenham University of Southampton, Southampton, UK

Dr Paul Symonds Department of Oncology, Leicester Royal Infirmary, Leicester, UK

Professor Kostas Syrigos Head, Oncology Unit, Athens Medical School, Athens, Greece

Professor Nick Thatcher Department of Medical Oncology, Christie Hospital, Manchester, UK

Dr Eoin Tiernan Tor-na-dee Hospital, Aberdeen, UK

Dr Chris Twelves Senior Lecturer in Medical Oncology, CRC Department, Beatson Oncology Centre, Western Infirmary, Glasgow

R. Valkema Department of Diagnostic Radiology, Leiden University Hospital, Leiden, Netherlands

Professor A. J. van der Kogel Professor of Clinical Radiobiology, Institute of Radiotherapy, University Hospital Niymegen, The Netherlands

Professor Veronesi Scientific Director, Instituto Europeo di Oncologia, Milan, Italy

Dr Jaap Verweij Rotterdam Cancer Institute (Daniel den hoed Kliniek), University Hospital, Rotterdam, The Netherlands

Professor Jamie Weir Consultant Radiologist, Academic Department of Radiology, Aberdeen Royal Infirmary, Aberdeen, UK

Professor John Welsh Department of Palliative Medicine, Beatson Oncology Centre, Western Infirmary, Glasgow, UK

Dr Tom Wheldon Department of Radiation Oncology, Cancer Research UK Beatson Laboratories, Glasgow, UK

Mr S. J. Wigmore Department of Surgery, University of Edinburgh, Edinburgh, UK

Professor P. Workman Centre Director, CRC Centre for Cancer Therapeutics, Institute of Cancer Research, Sutton, Surrey, UK

Dr P. Wou CRC Department of Clinical Oncology, City Hospital, Nottingham, UK

Abbreviations

CH$_2$-FH$_4$	5-10-methylene-tetrahydrofolate
dUMP	2′-deoxyuridine-5′ monophosphate
dTTP	2′-deoxythymidine-5′ monophosphate
10-CHO-FH$_4$	10-formyl-tetrahydrofolate
FudR	5-fluoro-2-deoxyuridine
DHPD	dihydropyrimidine dehydrogenase
FdUMP	5-fluoro-2-deoxyuridine-5-monophosphate
PALA	N-(phosphonacetyl)-L-aspartate
HGPRT	hypoxanthine-guanine phosphoribosyltransferase
PRPP	5-phosphoribosylpyrophsophate
CDHP	5-chloro-2, 4-dihydroxypyridine

Part 1
Background

Chapter 1
Multidisciplinary approach to cancer

Management of cancer involves a number of clinical disciplines. A straightforward presentation of a cancer can (and should) draw on these and other health care professionals.

With the development of more effective additional therapies for cancer (radiotherapy, chemotherapy), the management of cancer has become increasingly complex. No single clinician has all the skills needed to treat all cancers. This has led to the development of multidisciplinary teams that deal with certain types of cancer. Many professions allied to medicine have major roles to play in these teams (e.g. physiotherapists, stoma nurses, counsellors). The team may include individuals who are not directly involved in the treatment at presentation but have adjunctive roles at some stage in the course of the illness (e.g. palliative care). The composition of the team will vary considerably between institutions—and disease states. There must be a sufficient range of expertise to allow for informed discussion of the management policy for individual patients. The team's various roles include:

- To plan diagnostic and staging procedures, primary treatment approach, and any adjuvant therapy to be delivered pre- or post-operatively.

- To prepare patients physically and psychologically for anti-cancer therapy and subsequent follow-up.

- To provide information on treatment, prognosis, side-effects, and any other pertinent matters (e.g. stoma care).

- To efficiently plan and deliver surgery, radiotherapy, and chemotherapy as appropriate.

- To aid rehabilitation from the illness.

- To provide appropriate follow-up care.

- To ensure the transition from curative to palliative care is appropriately managed.

Management within such a team structure results in better outcomes for patients. Studies demonstrate survival advantages but, equally importantly, patients also have functional, psychological, cosmetic, and quality of life benefits.

Chapter 2
Epidemiology of cancer

Approximately 7.8 million cases of cancer were diagnosed worldwide in 1990. The number of new cases doubled between 1970 and 2001. Factors involved in the causation of cancer include the following.

Genetic factors

The majority of recognized carcinogens cause genetic mutations. Changes in gene expression in somatic cells, mostly due to mutation, are thought to be the basis for malignant transformation; there may be one or more, rare, dominantly inherited susceptibilities to every type of cancer. The contribution made by these highly penetrant, dominant susceptibilities to the total incidence of cancer has been estimated at 2–5% of fatal cancers. Genetic variation in susceptibility to cancer may also arise because of genetic polymorphism affecting the absorption, transport, metabolic activation, or detoxification of environmental carcinogens. A number of studies have suggested an interaction between some genetic polymorphisms and environmental carcinogens.

Environmental factors

The incidence of many types of cancer varies greatly between geographical areas. There are changes of rates following migration between areas of contrasting incidence, changes in incidence over time, and variation within populations according to socio-economic status. Thus environmental factors appear to have a major role in the aetiology of most types of cancer, accounting for over 80% of human cancer. Identification of the precise causes depends on multidisciplinary research, with analytical epidemiological studies an essential component. Based on evidence from analytical studies, a number of estimates of the proportion of cancer attributable to specific exposures have been made[1,2].

Smoking

Tobacco smoking is the largest single avoidable cause of premature death and the most important known carcinogen. Based on proportions of cancers of lung, larynx, oral cavity and pharynx, oesophagus, pancreas, kidney, and bladder due to smoking, 15% (1.1 million new cases per year) of all cancer cases worldwide are attributed to smoking (25% of cases worldwide in men, 4% in women).

Recent cohort studies show that smoking for 30 years or more increases the risk of colon cancer, with about 25% of cases being attributable to smoking. In addition, passive smoking may account for a small proportion of the cancer burden. In men from developed countries, the tobacco burden has been estimated as 32% of all annual incident cases, whereas in those from developing countries, it has been estimated as 19%. In regions where men have smoked for several decades, 30–40% of all cancers are attributable to tobacco. In women from developed countries, 6% of all annual incident cases are accounted for by tobacco, in contrast with 2% in those from developing countries.

As a consequence of the massive rise in cigarette consumption over the last few decades in women and in developing countries, a substantial increase in the cancer burden is to be expected unless measures to control consumption are strengthened. Smoking cessation reduces the risk of cancer, but there has only been limited success in programmes promoting cessation.

Alcohol

The main effect of alcohol is a joint effect with tobacco smoking in cancers of the oral cavity, pharynx, larynx, and oesophagus. Alcohol alone is implicated in cirrhosis (liver cancer) and may contribute to some cancers of the breast and large bowel.

Diet

High intake of vegetables and fruit show a consistent inverse relationship with cancer of the larynx, lung, oesophagus, and stomach, and there is weaker evidence that this is the case also for cancer of the mouth and pharynx, pancreas, and cervix. High levels of vegetable consumption are associated with a reduced risk of colon cancer; high levels of meat consumption appear to increase the risk of colon cancer. Obesity in adult life is considered to be the main factor in endometrial cancer, probably increases the risk of post-menopausal breast cancer, and is associated with cancer of the kidney. Regular physical activity is consistently associated with a reduced risk of colon cancer.

Low levels of consumption of fruit and vegetables, high levels of meat consumption, obesity, and lack of regular physical activity tend to be aspects of a lifestyle more typical of developed than of developing countries.

In developing countries it has been estimated that 33–50% of nasopharyngeal cancer cases could be prevented by avoiding regular consumption of salt fish. Generalized dietary deficiencies are associated with increased risk of oesophageal cancer in areas of high incidence in developing countries. In randomized controlled trials in Linxian, China, a combination of carotene, tocopherol, and selenium reduced mortality from cancer of all types and mortality from stomach cancer in particular[3]. Contamination of foods with aflatoxins increases the risk of hepatocellular cancer; halving the median daily intake of aflatoxin might reduce its incidence by 40% in Africa and Asia.

Infections

16% of the worldwide incidence of cancer is due to infection. For developed countries, the proportion is 9%, and for developing countries, 21%. Human papillomavirus (HPV) of any type accounts for 82% of cervical cancers in developed countries and 91% in developing countries. The human papillomaviruses occur in 70 different types. The strongest evidence for carcinogeneity is for HPV types 16 and 18. 81% of cases of liver cancer are attributable to chronic infection with hepatitis B or hepatitis C.

Strong evidence supports a causal relationship between chronic infection with the bacterium *Helicobacter pylori* and the development of gastric adenocarcinoma, and there is some evidence for gastric lymphoma. 60% of cases of gastric cancer in developed countries, and 53% in developing countries, may be attributable to *Helicobacter pylori*.

Epstein–Barr virus may account for up to 60% of Hodgkin's disease in developed countries, and 80% in developing countries. The virus accounts for over 90% of cases of Burkitt's lymphoma in sub-Saharan Africa, just over 80% in north Africa and the Middle East, just under 50% in Latin America and the Caribbean, and less than a quarter of cases elsewhere. There is greater uncertainty about the role of the virus in other types of non-Hodgkin's lymphoma and nasopharyngeal carcinoma.

Other infections considered to be carcinogenic include:

- *Schistosomiasis haematobium* and bladder cancer (attributable proportion in developing countries 8%, in developed countries 0%).

- Human T-cell lymphotrophic virus and acute T-cell leukaemia/ lymphoma (attributable proportion worldwide 1%).
- HIV and Kaposi's sarcoma.
- HIV and non-Hodgkin's lymphomas.
- *Opisthorchis viverrini* and *Clonorchis sinensis* and cholangio- carcinoma.

Solar exposure

The 1996 Harvard Report on Cancer Prevention concluded that over 90% of malignant melanoma is attributable to solar radiation. Malignant melanoma accounted for just over 1% of the world cancer burden in 1985. Uncertainties remain, even though it is widely assumed that exposure to solar radiation also accounts for the great majority of cases of basal cell and squamous cell carcinoma.

Other exposures

Other exposures account for 5% or less of the cancer burden. Occupational exposures have been linked with lung, bladder, and haematopoietic malignancies. Breast cancer has consistently been associated with early age at menarche, late age at first birth, and late age at menopause with relative risks of the order of 2.0 or less. Parity is associated inversely with endometrial and ovarian cancer.

Although most types of cancer are more common in urban than in rural areas, few causal links with environmental pollutants have been firmly established. It has been estimated that 1% of lung cancer deaths in the US are attributable to air pollution. While exposure to ionizing radiation at doses of 500–2000 mSv is known to be carcinogenic, exposures of this magnitude are unusual—about 1% of the deaths of the Japanese atomic bomb survivors could be attributed to radiation. The average per capita dose from all sources of ionizing radiation is about 3.4 mSv per year, of which about 88% is from natural sources and the remainder primarily from medical exposures. Extrapolation from data on people exposed to doses of 500 mSv or more suggests that 1–3% of all cancers might be attributable to radiation arising largely from natural sources. No clear association with exposure to extremely low frequency magnetic fields has been established.

Table 2.1 Estimates of the proportion of cancer attributable to specific exposures

Exposure	USA		Estimates (%) USA	Nordic countries Men	Nordic countries Women	Worldwide
	Best estimate	Range				
Tobacco	30	(25–40)	30	19	9	15
Passive smoking				<1	<1	
Alcohol consumption	3	(2–4)	3	2	2	
Diet	35	(10–70)	30	?	?	
Obesity	<1	(–5ᵃ–2)	<1	<1	1	30–40
Food additives			1			
Sedentary lifestyle			5			
Infections	10	(1–?)	5	2ᵇ	3ᵇ	16
Sexual behaviour	1	(1)				
Occupation	4	(2–8)	5	3	<1	
Perinatal factors/growth			5			
Reproductive factors	6	(0–12)	3			
Environmental pollution	2	(1–5)	2			
Industrial products	<1	(<1–2)				
Man-made ionizing radiation				2	2	
Random			2	<1	<1	
Solar and ultraviolet radiation				4	5	
Medicines and procedures	1	(0.5–3)	1			
Socio-economic status			3			
Geographical factors	3	(2–4)	5			
Family history of cancer			1			

ᵃ Allows for protective effect of preservatives
ᵇ Infection with human papillomavirus or *Helicobacter pylori*
? No precise data available

Some pharmaceutical agents (e.g. immunosuppressive agents, anti-neoplastic drugs, and hormonal preparations) are human carcinogens.

1   Doll, R. and Peto, R. (1981) The causes of cancer: quantitative
    estimates of avoidable risks of cancer in the United States today. *Journal of
    the National Cancer Institute* **66**, 1191–308.

2   Parkin, D.M., Pisani, P., Lopez, A.D., and Masuyer, E. (1994) At least one in
    seven cases of cancer is caused by smoking. Global estimates for 1985.
    International Journal of Cancer **59**, 494–504.

3   Blot, W.J., Li, J.Y., Taylor, P.R., Guo, W., Dawsey, S., Wang, G.Q., *et al.* (1993)
    Nutrition intervention trials in Linxian, China: supplementation with
    specific vitamin/mineral combinations, cancer incidence, and
    disease-specific mortality in the general population. *Journal of the National
    Cancer Institute* **85**, 1483–92.

Chapter 3
Biology of cancer

Molecular biology is an approach to understanding how organisms work by studying the molecules—in particular nucleic acids that encode genetic information and proteins that process this information and carry out activities in cells. It is grounded in other scientific fields, particularly biochemistry, chemistry, microbiology, genetics, and maths/computer science.

Molecular biology is a development of biochemistry, with less emphasis on the chemistry of biological molecules and more on how they function within cells and organisms. To study this, convenient biological systems are needed and microbiology plays a crucial role. Yeast and bacteria are often used in experiments because they are simple, cheap, and ethically acceptable. In cancer, there are two excellent recent examples of this:

- Understanding of the cell cycle (work with yeast).
- Repair of damaged DNA (using the bacterium *Escherichia coli*).

Although humans and micro-organisms are a long way apart in evolutionary terms, their fundamental cellular processes are remarkably similar.

The role of genetics

Molecular biology relies heavily on genetics; traditionally many interesting properties of organisms have been studied via their inheritance, so identifying the genes responsible. Once the genes are found, how they work can be investigated using molecular biology. In human genetics, much emphasis has been on what goes wrong—i.e. the genetics of inherited disease. The full implications of this for cancer are now becoming clear, since most of these diseases carry a genetic predisposition of some kind. If these predisposing genes are identified, we have a new handle on some crucial aspects of the disease process; recently several cancer susceptibility genes have been isolated.

The Human Genome Project (a multi-laboratory collaboration to identify the DNA sequence of all the genes in an organism) is now complete; the task of identifying genes will become routine. Linking these genes with certainty to the risk of diseases such as cancer is still problematic: there are many other factors involved (e.g. environmental).

The Human Genome Project has shown the DNA sequence for 30 000 genes. Most are novel with no resemblance to a gene of known function. The amino-acid sequence of the protein product is predictable, but current methods do not lead to a prediction of the three-dimensional structure of the protein. Once possible, there will still be great difficulties in defining the role of novel gene products in the organism's biology.

Applications to health care

- Using genetically engineered vaccines, therapeutic proteins and hormones, antibodies, etc.—essentially existing therapies with improved products.

- Identifying new drug targets and therapeutic strategies. These will come from research into identification of genetic factors in disease and the development of methods for relating protein sequence (deduced from the DNA sequence) to the function of the protein and its role in pathology.

- Developing DNA (or derivatives) as drugs i.e. gene therapy. There have been promising preliminary results with diseases such as cystic fibrosis, but there is still a long way to go before this becomes a general therapeutic method. The question of individual risk modification according to genotype and attendant issues of privacy, right to know, consequences for those with a financial stake in the individual's health, are important. Because genetic risk factors are already being identified, these are pressing issues which can only be resolved by full and informed debate between the public, lawmakers, scientists, and clinicians.

Molecular biology techniques

Scientific advances

All cancers arise as a result of changes in genes that regulate cell growth and behaviour; DNA research now offers the greatest potential for the development of new cancer diagnostics and therapies. Molecular medicine is thus concerned with turning genes into new therapeutic targets. Developing and applying molecular technologies is the key to a new understanding of cancer.

Molecular techniques comprise two groups: lysate and analysis and *in situ* analysis.

* With lysate methods, tumour biopsies are homogenized and spatial relationships between tumour cells are destroyed (Southern blot analysis and PCR). This leads to loss of information on heterogeneity and small subpopulations and an averaging of changes. However, quantitation can be simpler and more accurate than *in situ* approaches.

* *In situ* techniques such as fluorescence *in situ* hybridization (FISH) allow the genetic make-up of individual cells within their histological context to be visualized.

Genetic analysis

Southern blot analysis

Loss of genetic material from cancer cells is a classic marker for the presence of potential tumour suppressor loci. Southern blot analysis, using polymorphisms occurring within the human genome (RFLPs), identifies genetic alterations in the cancer cells. It involves homogenization of tissue samples to extract DNA, followed by cleavage of DNA with restriction endonucleases. Digested DNA is size-separated by gel electrophoresis and transferred to filters for hybridization to labelled probes to provide information on sequences of interest.

Limitations:

* Low sensitivity for detection of altered sequences.

* Large amounts of high-quality genomic DNA needed.

* Lengthy procedure.

Many of these have been overcome with the use of polymerase chain reaction (PCR) methodologies, but Southern blot analysis remains the standard in many situations.

Table 3.1 Landmarks in molecular oncology

1953	Watson & Crick, molecular structure of DNA.
1972	First recombinant DNA molecule made with ligase (Paul Berg).
1974	Doxorubicin, anti-cancer drug, receives FDA approval.
1975	DNA sequencing developed by Frederick Sanger.
1975	Southern blot technique developed to identify DNA fragments.
1976	SRC, the first human oncogene, discovered. (Now over 50 oncogenes are known.)
1976	Genentech, the first biotechnology firm, founded.
1978	Cisplatin and Tamoxifen, anti-cancer drugs, receive FDA approval.
1978	Restriction fragment length polymorphisms (RFLPs) discovered.
1979	p53 gene discovered.
1981	First recombinant vaccine for hepatitis B virus in liver cancer.
1982	Transgenic mouse overexpressing growth hormone.
1985	Polymerase chain reaction (PCR) invented.
1986	RB1 (retinoblastoma gene), the first of over 20 known tumour suppressor genes, cloned.
1990	Human Genome Project launched.
1991	Expressed sequence tags (ESTs) developed.
1991	First human gene therapy for cancer (melanoma).
1992	Paclitaxel, anti-cancer drug, receives FDA approval.
1993	hMSH2, the first of the hereditary non-polyposis colon cancer genes, cloned.
1994/1995	BRCA1/BRCA2, inherited breast cancer genes, cloned.
1996	First eukaryote genome sequenced, *Saccharomyces cerevisiae*.
1996	Topotecan, anti-cancer drugs, receives FDA approval.
2000	Completion date for sequence of the complete human genome.

PCR

A huge resource of micro-satellite markers distributed throughout the genome can be used to map and characterize genetic alterations. Primer pairs flanking regions of interest can be used to amplify the region; the size of product reveals information on the genetic change.

Table 3.2 Tools of the trade

Genetic analysis	Molecular Cytogenetics
	Fluorescence *in situ* hybridization
	Interphase cytogenetics
	Comparative genomic hybridization
	Southern blot analysis
	PCR
	DNA microchip technology
RNA analysis	*In situ* hybridization
	Northern blot analysis
	RT-PCR
	Gene expression microarrays
	Gene expression profiling
	Differential display RT-PCR
	Serial analysis of gene expression (SAGE)
	Suppression subtractive hybridization
Protein analysis	Immunohistochemistry
	Western blot analysis
	ELISA assay
	Enzyme assays
	Electrophoretic mobility shift assay
	DNA footprinting
Analysis of gene function	Gene transfer into tissue culture cell models
	Transgenic mice
	Knockout mice
DNA sequence analysis—bioinformatics	Database homology searching
	GeneBank database of DNA sequences
	BLAST sequence similarity analysis
	Gene identification
	Pattern identification e.g. transcription factors
	DNA structure and composition
	Sequence assembly and contig management

Major advantages:

- Speed of analysis.
- High-density coverage of the human genome with markers.
- Automation.
- Small amounts of sample required.

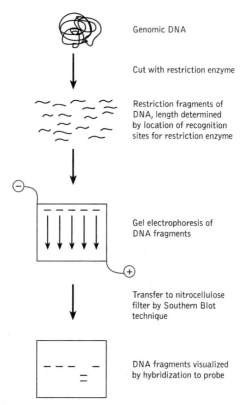

Genomic DNA

Cut with restriction enzyme

Restriction fragments of DNA, length determined by location of recognition sites for restriction enzyme

Gel electrophoresis of DNA fragments

Transfer to nitrocellulose filter by Southern Blot technique

DNA fragments visualized by hybridization to probe

Southern blot analysis.

Combined with micro-dissection of fixed tissue samples, PCR approaches can also study heterogeneity and separate normal and cancerous areas for independent analysis.

Fluorescence *in situ* hybridization (FISH)

Molecular cytogenetics is a rapidly evolving field; techniques like comparative genomic hybridization (CGH) and interphase cytogenetics are having major impact on tumour genetics. FISH is a sensitive method for analyzing genetic change in solid tumours, allowing visualization of the genetic make-up of individual cells within their histological context. FISH uses chromosome and region-specific probes to assess and rapidly copy the number and rearrangements of chromosomes and genes. Genetically abnormal cells are detected by an aberrant hybridization pattern in the interphase nuclei (interphase cytogenetics).

Major advantages

• Utility in routinely processed pathology specimens.

• Speed.

• Non-radioactive.

A disadvantage is the need for cloned probes. CGH resolves this by using tumour DNA as a complex probe. Thus CGH detects and maps genetic alterations in tumours without the bias of probe selection.

RNA analysis

Identification and quantitation of gene expression

Northern blot hybridization and reverse-transcription polymerase chain reaction (RT-PCR) are commonly used methodologies for detection and quantitation of gene expression.

Northern blot: standard method for determining transcript size and for comparison of messenger abundance between samples. For Northern blot analysis, RNA is extracted from tumour lysates and size-separated by gel electrophoresis. After transfer to filters, specific RNA species are detected by probe hybridization.

RT-PCR: RNA is first converted into cDNA and specific genes analysed using gene-specific primers in PCR reactions. RT-PCR is extremely sensitive but generally lacks the quantitation of Northern analysis. A complementary approach is RNA *in situ* hybridization, identifying cellular distribution of RNA sequences within a tumour section, allowing study of tumour heterogeneity and subclone development.

Gene expression profiling

Limitations of Northern blot and RT-PCR: analysis is restricted to only a few genes at a time, and sequence must be known in order to generate probes. Each cell may express 10 000–50 000 genes, so gene expression patterns may be tumour-specific. It has been difficult to monitor expression patterns of thousands of genes simultaneously until recently.

SAGE: Serial Analysis of Gene Expression (SAGE) can be applied in laboratories with PCR and sequencing capabilities. SAGE is based on generations of clones of short sequence tags derived from mRNA extracted from target tissue. Each individual tag represents a single mRNA, so sequencing of concatenates describes the pattern and abundance of mRNAs in target tissue. It is thus possible to screen several thousand tags in a few weeks. Sequences are screened against existing databases for known genes, and previously uncharacterized sequences are analysed in more detail. With SAGE, data are digitized and reusable, so once sequence information is obtained it can be reused and rescreened against any existing or developing genome database.

Bioinformatics: Bioinformatics is the use of computers to analyse biological information; a rapidly developing area of cancer research, given the vast amounts of sequence data produced by molecular biology projects. Nucleotide sequences can be used to interrogate public sequence databases for homology and identification over the internet. They can also be used to identify putative gene regulatory elements and gene features. The establishment of the Cancer Genome Anatomy Project (CGAP) means tumour-specific patterns of gene expression are now being held in databases.

Cell cycle and its regulation

Cell cycle phases

The somatic cell cycle consists of two alternative phases:

• S phase, where DNA is replicated.
• M phase where the cells divide.

Separating these are two phases where neither DNA replication nor cell division take place:

• G1 between M and S.
• G2 between S and M.

New findings

Cell cycle research has led to the identification of many molecules that drive and regulate the cell cycle. One important group are proteins called cyclins—so-named because concentrations rise and fall in a regular pattern during the cell cycle. This enables them to activate cyclin-dependent kinases (CDKs) whose activity is needed to propel cells through the cycle. Additional sub-units also regulate CDK activity, including cyclin-inhibitory proteins (CKIs).

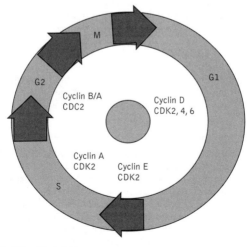

Basic cell cycle control.

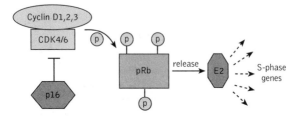

Rb-type proteins and the Rb pathway.

This complexity ensures cells have precise co-ordination of events that allow DNA duplication and subsequent cellular division. In addition, regulation guarantees maintenance of DNA fidelity and protects against a loss of genetic information. Basic cell cycle control is shown in the first figure.

Research has established many direct links between disruption of cell cycle control and cancer.

G1-S transition

Enzyme synthesis

Transition from G1 to S phase involves assembly and activation of transcription factors allowing the synthesis of enzymes required for DNA replication. At the heart of this process are Rb-type proteins and the 'Rb pathway' as seen in the second figure. The retinoblastoma protein, Rb, and the related p107 and p130 proteins, bind to a number of transcription factors. These activate genes required for progression through S-phase, such as DNA polymerases and nucleotide kinases.

Progression through G1 requires the phosphorylation of Rb-type proteins, allowing the release of transcription factors and subsequent S-phase entry. Phosphorylation of Rb-type proteins is controlled primarily by the cyclin-D-dependent kinases, CDK4 and CDK6. Kinase activity is regulated by fluctuating levels of D cyclins and CKIs from the p16^{INK4} and kip families, particularly p16 itself.

Timing of transition

Exactly when a cell embarks on a G1-S transition is tightly controlled to ensure survival, with factors such as cell size, metabolic state, growth factor availability, and DNA damage affecting whether a transition takes place. Not all signaling pathways involved have been unravelled. However, cyclin-D synthesis and subsequent activation of CDK4/6 has been linked to growth factor availability. It is suggested that cyclin D acts as a cellular sensor with cyclin synthesis allowing cells to cycle in the presence of appropriate mitogens.

Pathways

Superimposed over cyclin/CDK systems are pathways to detect problems such as DNA damage and cell growth inhibition. The most important is the p53 pathway, which plays a key role in G1 arrest, apoptosis, and genomic stability. Cells exposed to DNA-damaging agents often become arrested in G1 in a p53-dependent manner. p53 activation increases transcription and therefore protein levels of p21, a CKI that blocks cell cycle progression via its ability to inhibit Cdk enzymes. p53 upregulation does more than induce G1 arrest; in many cases programmed cell death or apoptosis is seen. G1-phase arrest and apoptosis are very divergent responses; the mechanisms involved in determining which of these dominates is still largely unknown. Variables such as the extent of DNA damage and levels of p53 may play a role.

p53 is the most commonly mutated gene in human cancer—not surprising since loss of control of genomic stability is central to cancer development and p53 is a critical factor in monitoring genomic integrity.

S phase

First steps: the first step in DNA duplication is the formation of initiation complexes and it appears that cyclin and CDK pairs, such as cyclin A and CDK2, are involved.

Regulation: maintenance of the replicative state may also be regulated by members of cyclin/CDK families. CDKs have been shown to phosphorylate several DNA replication factors involved in elongation including sub-units of the DNA-binding protein, RPA and DNA polymerase. Both are phosphorylated from the onset of S phase and remain so through G2 up to the end of M phase.

G2-M transition

The transition of cells from G2 to mitosis is dependent on the activity of the cylin/CDK complex, CDC2/cyclin B. Phosphorylation by CDC2 has been linked to several events required for mitosis entry, with targets including nuclear lamins and chromatin proteins. The activity of CDC2 is tightly regulated to ensure mitotic events do not begin until DNA replication is complete. Activation of CDC2 is a result of accumulation of cyclin B occurring as cells progress through S phase, peaking in late G2. Inactivation of CDC2 occurs by phosphorylation while dephosphorylation is associated with G2-M transition.

Delayed transition is commonly observed in G2-phase cells exposed to agents such as radiation and chemotherapy. The resulting G2 block is thought to allow time to repair DNA damage, while loss of this G2 checkpoint is often observed in cancerous cells.

Summary

Regulation of cell cycle is crucial for maintaining a normal cellular state. Conversely, perturbation of the cell cycle may occur in all tumour cells. The view of cancer as a disease of the cell cycle is rapidly becoming accepted; the design of novel drugs and gene therapy strategies to treat hyperproliferative cancers is now an integral part of medical research.

Growth of cancer

The basic mode of growth of tumours is exponential, though deviations do occur. One cubic centimetre of tumour tissue may contain over 10^8 neoplastic cells (in addition to many normal host cells) and their production from an initial transformed cell requires around 30 *generations* of cell multiplication. During this period of active tumour growth the tumour will be below 1 cm^3 and undetectable; five further doublings of cell number will give a volume of around 32 cm^3; and five more, a volume of over 1000 cm^3. Exponential growth from a single cell thus gives the impression of a long 'silent period' followed by apparently rapid growth.

Growth rate of tumours

Volume doubling time is the usual measure of tumour growth rate. Doubling times range from a few weeks to over a year, with an average of 3 months. Even a 1-month doubling time implies that the duration of the 'silent period' between initiation of a tumour and the appearance of symptoms could be a number of years.

Cellular basis of tumour growth

Three factors determine the growth rate of a tumour:

- **The average cell cycle times**. Values for human tumour cells usually range from 1–5 days.

- **The growth fraction** i.e. the proportion of tumour cells that are proliferating. Out-of-cycle cells are common in tumours, leading to growth fractions that are often less than 50%.

- **Cell loss.** The rate of loss of cells from tumours can be very high, often reaching 90% of cell production, and this is the principal reason why the volume doubling time is so much longer than the average cell cycle time. Cell loss occurs mainly by cell death, either as necrosis or apoptosis. Exfoliation and metastasis are other modes of cell loss.

Potential doubling time

Labelling of proliferating tumour cells with ^{3}H-thymidine or radiolabelled bromodeoxyuridine allows calculation of the expected tumour growth rate in the absence of cell loss. Such *potential doubling times* are often less than one week. When tumours recur following radiation therapy this is often due to rapid tumour cell re-population.

Therapy implications

The kinetics of tumour growth impinge on clinical management in various ways:

- Time to recurrence following treatment depends very much on the cellular re-population rate.

- The effectiveness of proliferation-dependent chemotherapeutic agents is limited by out-of-cycle cells, and therefore by a low growth fraction.

- Surviving tumour cells appear to accelerate after the start of radiation or cytotoxic drug treatment. To allow a gap in a course of therapy is therefore much more serious than delaying the start of therapy by the same period.

- Rapid tumour cell re-population provides a rationale for accelerated radiation therapy.

Oncogenes and tumour suppressor genes

Gene types

Most cancers are monoclonal, arising from a single cell that has accumulated key mutations leading to uncontrolled cell proliferation. Such mutations can cause gene function to be either enhanced (activated) or lost (inactivated).

Genes whose function becomes lost or inactivated in carcinogenesis are termed tumour suppressor genes. Both gene copies must be inactivated before the tumour suppressor function is completely lost (i.e. absence of normal protein) so they can be thought of as recessive.

Genes whose function becomes enhanced are termed proto-oncogenes and their mutated form is an oncogene. Proto-oncogenes play an essential role in controlling cell proliferation and encoding growth factors, growth factor receptors, signal transducers, cytoplasmic regulators, and transcription factors. Oncogenes generally behave in dominant fashion.

Cell mutations

DNA mutations occur with a high frequency in mammalian cells (due to radiation exposure, metabolic accidents, and exposure to environmental carcinogens). Exceptionally efficient DNA repair mechanisms normally ensure that less than 1:1000 accidental base changes in DNA causes a mutation. Mutations take a variety of forms:

- Point mutations (substitution of one base pair of a DNA sequence by another).
- Translocations (gene arrangement due to chromosomal breakage and rejoining).
- Gene amplification (multiple copies of a gene).
- Deletions (loss of genetic material—from a single base to a whole gene).

Oncogenes

A large number of oncogenes have been isolated from transformed cells, oncogenic viruses, and human and animal tumours. Mutations in *ras* genes occur in approximately 20% of human tumours—K-*ras* mutations are particularly prevalent in pancreatic cancer (75–90%).

Table 3.3 Human oncogenes

Gene	Normal function	Associated neoplasm	Class of mutation
H-ras	Signal transduction (membrane-associated G protein)	Melanoma; carcinoma of the colon, lung, and pancreas	Point mutations (codons 12, 13, 59–61).
K-ras	Signal transduction (membrane-associated G protein)	Melanoma; carcinoma of the thyroid; acute myelogenous and lymphoblastic leukaemia	Point mutations (codons 12, 13, 59–61).
N-ras	Signal transduction (membrane-associated G protein)	Melanoma; carcinoma of genitourinary tract and thyroid	Point mutations (codons 12, 13, 59–61).
myc	Transcription factor (operates as heterodimer with protein partner Max)	Burkitt's lymphoma; carcinoma of lung, breast and cervix	Translocation; (t(8:14) 75% of cases)
L-myc	Transcription factor (operates as heterodimer with protein partner Max)	Carcinoma of lung	Amplification
N-myc	Transcription factor (operates as heterodimer with protein partner Max)	Neuroblastoma; small cell lung carcinoma	Amplification
erb-B1	Growth factor receptor (EGF)	Astrocytoma; squamous cell carcinoma	Amplification
erb-B2(neu)	Growth factor receptor (BGF)	Adenocarcinoma of stomach, breast, and ovary	Amplification
Src	Signal transduction (non-receptor protein tyrosine kinase)	Carcinoma of colon	Point mutations; deletions (also altered protein phosphorylation)
Abl	Signal transduction (non-receptor protein tyrosine kinase)	Chronic myelogenous leukaemia	Rearrangement (t(9:22) — Philadelphia chromosome — bcr-abl fusion protein)

Table 3.4 Human tumour suppressor genes

Gene	Chromosomal function	Normal function	Associated neoplasm
p53	17p	Transcriptional regulator—promotes DNA repair, apoptosis, and differentiation (activates Bax, GADD45, p21, mdm2, Cyclin G; represses Bcl-2, myc, fos, PCNA)—is induced by DNA damage and hypoxia; G1/S checkpoint control gene	Carcinoma of the breast, lung, pancreas, colon; brain tumours; sarcomas; Li-Fraumeni syndrome
p73	1p	A p53 relative with similar functions but unlike p53 is not produced in response to DNA damage (only one functional copy—other is inactivated via imprinting)	Neuroblastoma
Rb	13q	Nuclear phosphoprotein (phosphorylation pattern regulates availability of E2F transcription factors—important regulators of cell cycle)	Retinoblastoma; osteosarcoma; small cell lung carcinoma
WT1	11p	Regulator of transcription and RNA splicing (represses IGF-2, PDGF A chain can activate EGR-1 under certain circumstances)	Wilm's tumour
MTS1 (p16)	9p	Cell cycle regulator (inhibitor of Cdk4/ cyclin—progression through G1)	Glioma; melanoma; mesothelioma; carcinomas of lung, bladder, and pancreas
BRCA1	17q	Transcription factor (p53 coactivator, transactivates expression of p21)	45% of familial breast cancers (80–90% of combined breast and ovarian cancers
BRCA2	13q	Transcription factor (interacts with the RAD51 protein i.e. participates in DNA repair; has intrinsic HAT activity i.e. histone acetylation)	Approx. 30% of familial breast cancers (14% of combined breast and ovarian cancers)
APC	5q	Forms complex with a- and b-catenin and tubulin	Colorectal carcinoma (familial and sporadic)

Table 3.4 (*continued*)

Gene	Chromosomal function	Normal function	Associated neoplasm
DCC	18q	Cell adhesion molecule (receptor for netrin-1 — axonal chemoattractant)	Colorectal carcinoma
DPC4	18q	Involved in TGFb-induced growth suppression	Carcinoma of the pancreas
nm23	17q	Nucleoside diphosphate kinase (involved with proliferation, differentiation, motility (microtubule assembly and disassembly), and development.	Loss of gene is associated with increased metastatic ability; breast and colorectal carcinoma

Tumour suppressor genes

Examination of familial cancer syndromes (e.g. retinoblastoma) and experimental evidence (particularly from somatic cell hybrid experiments) has demonstrated the existence of a different class of cancer gene—tumour suppressor genes. p53 is the most frequently-altered gene in human tumours. Approximately 37% of all cancers have a p53 mutation (incidence is much higher with cancers of the lung and colon). Certain specific tumour mutations are associated with particular carcinogens e.g. hepatocellular carcinoma is linked with hepatitis B and aflatoxins correlates with a high incidence of mutations in codon 249 of p53.

Products of tumour suppressor genes have a variety of functions within the cell. A large number of genes have now been isolated, as can be seen in the table.

Multi-step carcinogenesis

The development of cancer is a multi-step process characterized by repeated cellular insults resulting in the accumulation of mutations. The steps involved in the development of colorectal cancer have been particularly well characterized (see figure). Single mutations (e.g. APC) can lead to benign cellular proliferation (familial polyposis coli) that predisposes to the development of malignancy. Mutations in DNA repair genes (e.g. MMR—mis-match repair) speed up this process of mutation accumulation.

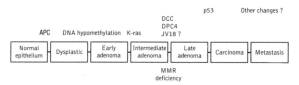

Genetic alterations associated with colorectal carcinogenesis. Mutation frequencies in MMR-deficient cells are two to three times higher than in normal cells—such MMR mutations are found in > 70% of hereditary non-polyposis colorectal cancer (HNPCC) cases and > 65% of sporadic colorectal cancers exhibiting micro-satellite instability. These cases account for 15–17% of total colorectal cancers. (Adapted from Kinzler and Vogelstein).

Cytogenetics and cancer

Cytogenetic analysis in cancer is used to confirm diagnosis, to aid differential diagnosis, and (possibly) to indicate prognosis.

Nowell and Hungerford first described a specific chromosome abnormality associated with chronic myeloid leukaemia in 1960. Since then, numbers of chromosomal abnormalities associated with cancer have grown exponentially. Abnormalities can be structural, numerical, or both; they may be restricted in distribution or found in many different tumour types. Some chromosomal alterations are useful in the diagnosis and prognosis of malignancies; the significance of others is unknown.

Nomenclature

Last revised in 1995, cytogenetic abnormalities are described by the ISCN (International System for Human Cytogenetic Nomenclature). Summary of the nomenclature used:

+ or –   Gain or loss of chromosome following the symbol.

p   Short arm of chromosome.

q   Long arm of chromosome.

del   Deletion. A deletion in the chromosome distal to breakpoint, or between two breakpoints if two are stated.

der   Derivative. A chromosome derived from a rearrangement. Rearrangement (if known) is described.

dic   Dicentric. Chromosome has two centromeres derived from the two named chromosomes.

dup   Duplication. A segment of chromosome defined by two breakpoints is duplicated.

i   Isochromosome. Chromosome is composed of two identical arms rather than a p and q arm.

ins   Insertion. Segment from one chromosome is inserted into another.

inv   Inversion. Segment of chromosome defined by two breakpoints is inverted compared to its normal orientation.

t   Translocation. Swapping of segments distal to the stated breakpoints in named chromosomes.

Chromosomal abnormalities

- structural
- numerical

Examples include:

- Chronic myeloid leukaemia
    —small chromosome 22 (Philadelphia chromosome)

- Acute myeloid leukaemia
  —many cytogenic abnormalities (80% of patients)
- Therapy-related AML
- Myelodysplastic syndromes
  —50% have chromosomal abnormalities
- Myeloproliferative disorders
- Acute lymphocytic leukaemia
  —80% have chromosomal abnormalities
- Chronic lymphoproliferative disorders
- Lymphoma
  —many structural and numerical chromosomal abnormalities
- Neuroblastoma
  —deletion of 1p and amplification of N-myc
- Wilms' tumour (nephroblastoma)
  —many chromosomal abnormalities reported

Invasion methodology

Tumour invasion and metastases is a complex, dynamic, multi-step process:

- Initial invasion of tumour through basement membrane.
- Movement into connective tissue surrounding tumour cells.
- Invasion of tumour cells into blood vessels.
- Circulating tumour cells are arrested in blood vessels of a distant organ or tissue; tumour cells invade organ from blood vessels.
- Tumour cells then grow within tissue to form a metastatic tumour that may become clinically evident.
- Process of tumour invasion and metastases results from alterations in cell-to-cell and cell-to-matrix adhesion and increased matrix degradation.

Extracellular matrix degradation

Several stages during the process of tumour invasion and metastases require increased degradation or breakdown of extracellular matrix or connective tissue surrounding tumour cells. The extracellular matrix is a complex mixture of proteins including different types of collagen, elastin, fibronectin, and laminin. Digestion of extracellular matrix is carried out by several groups of proteolytic enzymes. Major groups of enzymes implicated in tumour invasion and metastases are:

Matrix metalloproteinases (MMPs)

A family of zinc-containing enzymes involved in the degradation of the extracellular matrix; considerable evidence indicates that individual MMPs have an important role in tumour invasion and tumour spread while expression of individual MMPs in tumours may be associated with prognosis[2]. MMPs are broadly classified into collagenases, gelatinases, stromelysins, and the recently-identified membrane-type MMPs.

MMPs are secreted proteins, produced as pro-enzymes and activated by cleavage of a N-terminal propeptide. Gelatinases, particularly MMP-2, appear to be important in initial stages of tumour invasion as they degrade components of the basement membrane, while other MMPs contribute to later stages of tumour invasion. Membrane-type MMPs that are membrane-bound appear to be involved in activation of MMP-2, which is capable of activating other MMPs.

Activity of MMPs is regulated by interaction with naturally occurring inhibitors, tissue inhibitors of metalloproteinases. Clinical interest in MMPs is considerable since the use of synthetic, low-molecular-weight, broad-spectrum inhibitors of MMPs can prevent tumour spread in human tumour xenografts. Several MMP inhibitors are being developed for clinical use.

Plasmin system

Urokinase-type plasminogen activator (uPA) is a serine protease that catalyzes the activation of plasminogen to plasmin—a broad-spectrum protease that in turn can break down a variety of extracellular matrix components. Plasmin can also promote the activation of MMP-2, thus linking plasmin system and MMPs in tumour invasion.

Cathepsins

A group of lysosomal proteolytic enzymes that also degrade many components of the extracellular matrix. Widely expressed in tumour cells, stromal cells, and endothelial cells. Cathepsins can be activated by uPA.

Cell adhesion

Tumour invasion and metastasis is also characterized by alterations in both cell-to-cell and cell-to-matrix adhesion. Cellular adhesion both to adjacent cells and surrounding extracellular matrix is mediated by a variety of molecules including:

Cadherins

Transmembrane glycoproteins involved in cell adenomatous polyposis coli (APC) gene product. The most important cadherin in relation to tumour invasion is E-cadherin whose expression is downregulated in various types of malignant tumour; loss of E-cadherin frequently appears to correlate with tumour invasion and metastasis.

Integrins

Transmembrane proteins involved in cell to matrix adhesion. Individual integrins are receptors for a variety of matrix proteins including specific types of collagen, fibronectin, and vitronectin. Cell signalling pathways and expression of MMPs is also partially regulated by integrins. Altered regulation (often downregulation) and expression of integrins contributes to tumour cell invasion.

CD44

A cell surface glycoprotein that functions as an adhesion molecule. CD44 variants can be expressed on the surface of a variety of tumour cells. Specific splice variants of CD44 are associated with increased tumour invasion.

Angiogenesis

New blood vessel formation (angiogenesis) is an important factor for continued growth and development of both malignant tumours and metastases. Development of new blood vessels in tumours is stimulated by a wide variety of angiogenic factors produced by both tumour cells and stromal cells. In addition, several naturally occurring anti-angiogenic factors have been identified, most notably angiostatin and endostatin. New blood vessel formation in tumours is a complex and dynamic process requiring:

- Proliferation of endothelial cells from pre-existing capillaries or venules.
- Breakdown of extracellular matrix.
- Migration of endothelial cells.

Growth and development of blood vessels within tumours requires the same factors (i.e. increased matrix degradation and altered cell-to-cell and cell-to-matrix adhesion) that are crucial to tumour cell invasion.

New blood vessel formation is important in allowing tumour cells to enter the circulation and a high degree of tumour vascularity increases the likelihood of this. Newly formed blood vessels may be more permeable to tumour cells.

There is extensive interest in angiogenesis as a therapeutic target to prevent both tumour growth and metastases with both naturally occurring and synthetic anti-angiogenic compounds being intensively investigated for possible clinical use.

Formation of metastases in specific tissues

Some tissues and organs are more susceptible to the formation of metastases (e.g. liver, lung, and bone), whereas metastases are relatively uncommon in other tissues (e.g. kidney and heart). Several factors have been proposed to explain the formation of metastases in particular tissues including the expression of specific cell adhesion molecules in vascular endothelium of particular organs that are able to arrest circulating tumour cells. Another feature of metastases is the phenomenon of dormancy or latency of metastatic tumours such that many years can elapse between the diagnosis and the apparent curative treatment of the primary tumour and the clinical appearance of metastatic tumours. Dormancy appears to occur when growth of the metastatic tumour is balanced by an equivalent or even higher rate of tumour cell death by apoptosis.

---

1   Kinzler, K.W. and Vogelstein, B. (1996) The lessons from hereditary colorectal cancer. *Cell* 87, 159–70.

2   Murray, G.I., Duncan, M.E., O' Neil, P. *et al.* (1996) Matrix metalloproteinase-1 is associated with poor prognosis in colorectal cancer. *Nat Med* 4, 461–2.

Key website resources

New England Journal of Medicine: *http://www.nejm.org/collections/ molecularmedicine/TOC/1.htm*

National Center for Biotechnology Information: *http://www.ncbi.nlm.nih.gov/*

Chapter 4
Pathology of cancer

Cancer is a genetic disease at cellular level. The final result of synchronous or sequential lesions usually involving more than one gene is the capability acquired by the transformed cell(s) to undergo clonal, autonomous and purposeless growth into measurable masses. These masses comprise tightly packed cells with a varying amount of extracellular matrix of variable density incorporating disorderly distributed, newly formed blood and lymphatic vessels. Malignant cells' proliferation rate is influenced by numerous factors, but is finally characterized by aggressiveness that consists of invasion of adjacent normal tissues and distant metastatic spread by several routes.

Each germ cell and each somatic cell—some 200 cell types—can be a tumour's starting point. Several hundred tumours exist due to the large but not unlimited constellation of genetic alterations responsible for neoplastic proliferation at various body sites, each with its own natural history. About 12 are responsible for over 80% of cancer deaths (carcinoma of breast, lung, colon and rectum, prostate, stomach, pancreas, urinary tract, ovary, liver, kidney, melanoma, leukaemias and lymphomas).

Tumour types

Tumours can be related to four basic tissue types:
- Epithelial.
- Connective.
- Musculoskeletal.
- Nervous, or precursors of germ cells.

Benign tumours recapitulate normal cell morphology, lack invasiveness and metastatic potential, are slowly growing, but may cause severe damage and death because they are strategically placed (e.g. CNS, larynx). Benign tumours may transform into malignant (e.g. Schwannoma).

Tumour cells proliferate autonomously, escaping to an unpredictable extent the control of hormones and growth factors. They show varying degrees of atypical morphology, in terms of degree of maturation, and differentiation. The malignant appearance (phenotype) of cells include:
- Anaplasia (lack of differentiation).
- Cytoplasmic basophilia (increase of ribosomes).
- Nucleolar hypertrophy.
  and/or:
- Increase in number of the nucleoli.
- Increase of the mitotic index.
- Presence of bizarre mitotic figures.
- Variations in cell size and shape.
- Increase of nucleo-cytoplasmic ratio.

Disorderly structure and deviations from the normal tissue architecture, such as loss of polarity, are reflected in atypical growth.

Histological identification

Histological identification of the malignant nature is the critical issue; some lesions escape the criteria mentioned previously. Examples are:

- Small-sized renal cell carcinomas (erroneously called adenomas because of their size).
- Highly differentiated 'lipoma-like' liposarcomas.
- Controversial pigmented skin lesions ('dysplastic' naevi).
- Questionable soft tissue tumours—such as atypical fibro-histiocytoma, fibromatosis, haemangiopericytoma; myelodysplasia.

While lesion classification uncertainty has decreased in recent years, 'borderline' ovarian tumours are still controversial; for some time they were classified as (cyst)adenocarcinomas of low malignant potential, but now as (cyst)adenomas with uncertain malignant potential or atypical proliferating tumours.

Lesions preceding malignant tumours are as various as the natural histories of the subsequent cancers. At some sites (e.g. uterine cervix and prostate) pre-malignant lesions may persist for a long time, others are short-lived. Among the former, some lesions permit reproducible histological typing and even grading, whereas ductal carcinoma *in situ* of the breast can be sub-typed and graded according to cell differentiation. At other sites the current criteria allow only a reproducible overall diagnosis of carcinoma *in situ*. Examples include:

- Bronchi.
- Prostate.
- Uterine cervix.
- Most organs lined by squamous epithelium (skin, upper respiratory and alimentary tract).
- Transitional epithelium (lower urinary tract).

Melanoma *in situ* is recognized as a stage in melanoma tumour progression. 'Dysplasia', though vague, is nonetheless well established and employed to define pre-malignant changes of, for example, larynx, uterine cervix, and Barrett's oesophagus.

Malignant potential without well-defined or reproducible histopathological features is attributable to hypercellular leiomyomas of the uterus, hyperplasia of plasma cells in the bone marrow accompanied by monoclonal gammopathy, nodular hyperplasia of regenerating cirrhotic liver, dysplastic naevi with random atypia, large congenital cutaneous naevi, and lymphomatoid granulomatosis.

Although clonality is a basic feature of malignancy in early phases of proliferation before multiple subclones develop due to additional mutational events (genetic instability), it is not a synonym of malignancy as shown by the curable, occasionally self-limited, local lesions of Langerhans' cell histiocytosis (eosinophilic granuloma) whose monoclonality was recently proven.

Epithelial tumours comprise over 80% of neoplasms; adenoma being the most common epithelial benign growth and carcinoma the general term for the malignant counterpart. The latter may be additionally classified according to:

- Origin (adenocarcinoma, Merkel-cell ca.).
- Structure (papillary ca., tubular ca.).
- Extracellular matrix (desmoplastic ca.).
- Cellular content (glycogen-rich ca., lipid-rich ca.).
- Cell products (mucinous ca., keratinizing ca.).
- Cell-size (small or large cell ca.).
- Cell shape (spindle cell ca.).

The proliferating cell type is recalled in the names of tumours of soft parts and of myoid origin, both benign and malignant (e.g. fibroma vs. fibrosarcoma, leiomyoma vs. leiomyosarcoma). Most of the latter are subject to grading, and several systems have been proposed.

The central nervous system (CNS) displays an array of cell types from which several tumours may arise (astrocytes, ependymal cells, neuroblasts, etc.). A few CNS tumours are histologically benign (gangliocytoma, central neurocytoma); all others show a broad range of grades of malignancy. Progression from low to high-grade malignancy is a common event.

Mixed benign epithelial-stromal tumours are common in salivary glands (pleomorphic adenoma) and breast (fibroadenoma). Despite phenotypic multi-cellularity, clonality was recently proven for these tumours, supporting a totipotential stem-cell divergence hypothesis. Developmental errors are probably responsible for teratomas, which mostly arise along the midline of the body and in the gonads—these commonly display immature and malignant features in the testes and mature benign features in the ovaries.

Tumour-like conditions are non-neoplastic lesions that mimic neoplastic growth. Their importance lies in the differential diagnostic work-up. Chronic reactive inflammatory response may produce deceptively neoplastic-looking lesions such as nodular fasciitis of soft tissue. Other common lesions which simulate a neoplasm indicate:

- Aneurysmal bone cysts.
- Traumatic neuromas.
- Intravascular papillary endothelial hyperplasia.
- Central giant-cell granuloma of bone.
- Reactive hyperplastic nodules of mesothelium.

Tumour-like conditions also include hamartomas (e.g. pulmonary and hepatic bile duct)—local circumscribed developmental errors—and choristomas which are aggregates of ectopic tissue (e.g. nasal glial heterotopia, accessory spleen).

Tumour classification

Classification and typing of tumours still relies on histopathology and aspirated cell material. Tissue and cellular samples are submitted fresh or fixed (usually in formalin) with all relevant pieces of information (present and past clinical history, operative findings, and radiological data). Description of gross features of the organ or surgical specimen containing the tumour is essential. Size, shape, colour, consistency, appearance of the cut surface, and tumour-host interface (neoplastic pseudocapsule), presence/absence of ulceration, necrosis, and cystic spaces have to be recorded. Important histological features include:-

- Mitotic index.
- Lymphocytic infiltration (e.g. medullary carcinoma of breast, cutaneous melanoma).
- Extent and the type of necrosis (e.g. breast cancer and soft tissue tumours).
- Presence/absence of peritumoral vascular invasion (e.g. germ cell tumours of testes).
- Type of lesions adjacent to the tumour (e.g. atrophic gastritis, carcinoma *in situ*).

Grading

Grading of carcinomas is mandatory for adequate treatment (e.g. prostate, breast, endometrium, liver, kidneys) and several systems are available. Simplest consists of counting mitotic figures in defined microscopic areas. For some cancers micro-staging procedures are routinely applied (melanoma, carcinomas of organs with a cavity such as urinary bladder, gut, endometrium, uterine cervix, vulva) and consist of depth of invasion, tumour thickness, and type of margins (pushing, infiltrating).

For final diagnosis pathological reports should employ standardized nomenclature and coding using dedicated, computer-assisted reporting systems. Where appropriate, checkpoints for technical quality assurance should be incorporated. Due to rapidly expanding immunological, cytogenetic, and molecular techniques careful planning of supplementary methods is required; a tissue bank of snap-frozen samples of tumours and the corresponding normal tissues of the same patient is recommended.

Frozen section examination

Frozen section examination is still useful to establish/rule out malignancy and ascertain the status of surgical resection margins. On frozen section, tumour typing is often feasible. Enlarged non-metastatic lymph nodes and suspicious *in situ* or borderline lesions (breast nodules, polyps, ovarian cysts) are often unsuitable for frozen section procedures and require a definitive deferred diagnosis. Routine H and E staining of paraffin-embedded tissue section has to be supplemented by special stains, some of which are still used despite the advent of immunocytochemistry (ICC). Useful stains and methods are:

- Alcian blue cationic dye at pH 2.5 for intracytoplasmic epithelial acid mucin (e.g. mucin-producing carcinomas).
- Periodic acid-Schiff reaction (PAS) which visualizes glycoproteins and glycogen (e.g. Ewing's sarcoma, alveolar sarcoma, some carcinomas) and basement membranes.
- Romanowsky–Giemsa panoptical method for haematological proliferation.
- Reticulin fibre silver impregnation method.
- Stein's method for bile.
- Grimelius technique for argyrophilic substances.
- Several stains for micro-organisms.

Most enzymes are now identified by ICC, exploiting immunogenic properties of enzymatic proteins; the majority are hydrolases, oxidases, and dehydrogenases.

Transmission electron microscopy (TEM)

Diagnostically useful detectable structures include:

- Myofibrillary elements.
- Neurosecretory dense-core granules.
- Birbeck's granules of Langerhans' cells.
- Melanosomes.
- Cell junctions.
- Weibel-Palade bodies.
- Some virions (HPV).
- Bacteria.

Even more valuable are the results of a combination of immunological techniques with TEM.

Immunocytochemistry (ICC)

Use of ICC for detecting antigens in tissue sections for diagnostic purposes is now routine. Preservation of the antigen(s) and validation of antibodies are critical technical prerequisites, whereas interpretation of results supplemented by positive and negative controls are the histopathologist's responsibility. Many antibodies (most of them monoclonal) are now available, working on paraffin-embedded material with/without antigen retrieval. Targets are:

- Structural antigens (e.g. intermediate filaments).
- Matrix antigens.
- Functional antigens (secretory products).
- Lineage antigens (immunoglobulins).
- Membrane-bound antigens (receptors, glycoproteins).
- Miscellaneous cell constituents.

Rarely does a single antibody afford a specific diagnosis; mostly a small panel of antibodies yields more reliable information. Anaplastic tumours whose differential diagnoses include carcinomas, large-cell lymphomas, sarcomas, and melanoma, and small round-cell tumours in childhood which include neuroblastoma, the Ewing's sarcoma family (including PNET), lymphomas, and some rhabdomyosarcomas, are particular targets for immunocytochemical scrutiny.

A second level of investigation is represented by the array of malignant lymphomas, both of Hodgkin's and non-Hodgkin type. Their categorization on the basis of the recent REAL classification is facilitated by the antibodies that offer a cluster designation (CD).

An additional use of ICC is tumour staging consisting of a search of malignant cells by means of appropriate antibodies in lymph nodes, bone marrow, in lumina of peritumoral vessels, and at surgical resection margins.

Markers of proliferation, diagnostic cell products, and expressions of (onco)-gene protein products are also targets of the immunocytochemical diagnostic approach. Antibodies against chimeric fusion proteins are now available; the first example was an anti-p80 (chimeric NPM-ALK protein) antibody to detect t(2;5) (p23;q35) in anaplastic large-cell lymphoma.

Flow cytometry

Flow cytometry is used mainly to quantitate average cellular content of DNA (ploidy) and assess the cycle's DNA-synthetic phase. Another useful application is quantitative and qualitative evaluation of nuclear, cytoplasmic, or cell surface proteins stained with fluorescent dyes.

Classical cytogenetic analysis is useful in detecting consistent, non-random chromosomal lesions such as translocations and deletions. It is applied mainly to haematological and soft tissue tumours.

Chapter 5
Aetiology of cancer

Viral oncogenesis

Approximately 15% of tumours worldwide can be attributed to viruses; the majority of these are represented by hepatocellular and cervical carcinoma and are the sequelae of infection by two DNA viruses, the hepatitis B virus and the human papillomavirus respectively.

Other viruses directly linked to human tumours include:

• Epstein–Barr Virus (EBV).
• Human herpes virus 8 (HHV-8).
• Human T-cell leukaemia virus (HTLV-1).
• Human immunodeficiency virus (HIV).
• Herpes simplex virus (HSV).
• Cytomegalovirus (CMV).

Viruses indirectly linked include:

• HHV-3.
• HHV-6.

Although viral infection plays a significant role in the initial step towards carcinogenesis, acquisition of malignant phenotype requires additional genetic alterations.

Most tumour viruses are ubiquitous; prevalence of infection is much higher than the incidence of the respective form of tumour, and development of associated tumours requires many years of infection. This latent period may last decades. Other co-factors are necessary for development of virally-linked tumours, including genetic, immunological, hormonal, and environmental factors.

DNA and RNA viruses

Human papillomavirus (HPV)

HPV are small, double-standard DNA viruses that specifically infect squamous epithelial cells. HPV represents a heterogeneous group of viruses with over 70 different HPV genotypes identified. Only keratinocytes can be infected, and the virus has evolved a unique model of replication with absolute dependence upon the micro-environment of differentiating squamous epithelium for infection, replication, viral capsid synthesis, and particle assembly.

HPV virus and tumours

• Skin warts—types 1/2.
• Anogenital warts—types 6/11.
• Cervical cancer—types 16, 18, 31, 33, 35.
• Anal tumours.

- Vulval tumours.
- Penile tumours.

Convincing epidemiological studies have implicated an infectious agent in the aetiology of cervical cancer. Longitudinal studies have established high-grade cervical intra-epithelial neoplasia (CIN) as a pre-malignant precursor lesion to invasive cancer. Genital warts show an identical epidemiological pattern to cervical cancer and, in addition, HPV induces cellular changes previously interpreted as cervical dysplasia in cervical smears and tissue. Molecular confirmation of this association using PCR has demonstrated 'high-risk' HPV types in high-grade CIN lesions and other squamous intra-epithelial lesions such as PIN: penile intraepithelial neoplasia, AIN: anal intraepithelial neoplasia, and VIN: vulva intraepithelial neoplasia.

Studies of HPV-positive cervical cancer have shown integration of viral DNA; the E6 and E7 genes are regularly overexpressed. Proteins encoded by E6 and E7 in high-risk HPV types are oncoproteins, p53 being targeted for degradation by E6 protein, whilst E7 protein inactivates retinoblastoma (Rb) protein. Conversely, the E6 and E7 proteins encoded by 'low-risk' HPV types 6/11, show dramatically lower activity in these functions when compared to those encoded by 'high-risk' HPV types.

The role of HPV types in other tumour types such as oesophageal, laryngeal, and oropharyngeal cancer needs to be further defined. Epidemiological evidence suggests that HIV-infected patients have a higher incidence of HPV-associated anogenital tumours, namely cervical cancer in women and anal cancer in men.

Hepatitis B (HBV) and C (HBC) viruses

HBV is a small DNA virus of 3000 base pairs. Primary infection produces either acute hepatitis B or a subclinical infection. The majority of infections resolve with clearance of virus and lifelong immunity; 5% fail to clear the virus and go on to develop a lifelong persistent hepatic infection, resulting in a spectrum of hepatocellular injury and the development of chronic persistent hepatitis or chronic active hepatitis. Chronic HBV infection is associated with a 100-fold increase in hepatocellular carcinoma (HCC) risk.

Hepatocellular injury is thought to trigger a proliferative response in the liver. This response increases the chance for cellular mutations to occur over time and for cells to consequently escape normal cellular growth control. However, cases of HHC do arise in non-cirrhotic livers, so raising the possibility of another mechanism, such as the existence of a specific HBV oncogene. Unproven candidates include ORF X that encodes for a small regulatory protein that may bind to and inactivate p53. Alternative molecular mechanisms may involve viral genome integration. However, no one common integrated viral encoding site has been demonstrated.

Hepatitis C (HCV) is a single-stranded RNA virus and primary infection results in acute hepatitis C infection. HCV infection is linked to the development of HCC.

Herpes viruses

Epstein–Barr virus is an endemic lymphotrophic herpes virus. Primary infection of the oropharyngeal epithelium produces pharyngitis and subsequent B lymphocyte infiltration. Infection results in lifelong latent infection within lymphoid tissue and B-lymphocytes. A number of EBV encoded proteins have oncogenic potential (EBNA 1 and LMP 1). T-cell surveillance restricts the ability of these proteins to deregulate cell growth/apoptosis with consequent emergence of a lymphoproliferative disorder.

EBV is associated with a number of human tumours including:

- Endemic Burkitt's lymphoma (BL).
- Non-endemic/sporadic BL.
- Undifferentiated nasopharyngeal carcinoma (NPC).
- Hodgkin's disease.
- Lymphoproliferative disease and immunoblastic lymphomas, in immunocompromised host.

Endemic Burkitt's lymphoma (BL)

The majority of tumours in endemic form of BL contain EBV DNA sequences. In addition, malaria *P. falciparum* infection occurs coincidentally. Malaria infection is thought to depress cytotoxic T-cell function, thus rendering the patient relatively cytotoxic T-cell deficient and allowing the EBV infection to escape T-cell surveillance. The role of EBV in non-endemic and AIDS-related BL is complex and less definitive. EBV DNA is detectable in only 10–15% of patients with non-endemic BL and 50% of patients with AIDS-related BL. Immunoblastic lymphomas associated with chronic immunosuppression in allograft recipients or AIDS patients and undifferentiated NPC invariably contain EBV DNA sequences. In Hodgkin's disease, 50% of tumours contain EBV-infected cells and, in addition, the EBV genome has been demonstrated in the Reed–Sternberg cells of Hodgkin's disease.

Kaposi's sarcoma (KS)

Kaposi's sarcoma (KS) is commonly associated with AIDS, but was originally described in elderly men of Mediterranean, Middle Eastern, or Eastern European ethnic origin—so-called 'classic' KS. It has also been documented in chronically immunosuppressed organ transplant recipients. Within the HIV-infected population, variations in development of KS exists; the risk of KS is highest in HIV-infected homosexual/bisexual men, compared with only a minority of HIV-infected haemophiliacs, thus supporting the role of a sexually transmitted agent in the development of KS.

Using PCR, herpes-like DNA sequences have been demonstrated in AIDS-associated KS lesions. These sequences have been shown to be non-human and closely related to gamma herpes viruses, EBV, and the simian herpes virus (HVS). These herpes-like DNA sequences have been identified in all KS tissue and are thought to represent a new herpes virus, HHV 8 or KS-associated herpes virus (KSHV). This supports earlier epidemiological data suggesting an infective agent in the development of this tumour. Like EBV, HHV8 is lymphotrophic and has also been identified in peripheral blood mononuclear cells and two lymphoproliferative conditions, the rare body cavity lymphoma and in multicentric Castleman's disease.

Retroviruses

Sero-epidemiological and molecular data have established a causal role for HTLV-1 in adult T-cell leukaemia (ATL). ATL presents with either a leukaemic or non-Hodgkin's T-cell lymphoma type picture, characterized by malignant organ infiltration, immunodeficiency, lymphadenopathy, and hypercalcaemia. HTLV-1 is also associated with a chronic non-malignant disorder, tropical spastic paraparesis. HTLV-1 is trophic for CD4+ human T-cells, resulting in transformation of infected cells.

Human immunodeficiency virus

A number of specific tumours are associated with HIV infection and are AIDS-defining. However, this association is not due to a direct oncogenic effect of the HIV virus, but is the result of chronic immunosuppression. A long natural history of virus-associated tumours is accelerated in HIV-infected patients, again the result of failure of immune surveillance.

Chemical carcinogenesis

Chemical carcinogens are a principal cause of cancer and can be induced by certain lifestyles e.g. smoking tobacco, exposure to chemicals in the community or workplace, some drug taking. Chemical carcinogenesis is a multi-stage process.

Initiation and promotion

When cells are initially exposed to a carcinogenic agent, genetic carcinogens interact with DNA to form an adduct or to induce chemical alterations of DNA. DNA adducts may result in damage by inducing point mutations, deletions, or chromosomal translocations. When changes are induced in genes involved in cell growth regulation or differentiation (e.g. oncogenes and tumour suppressor genes), cell transformation can result.

The majority of chemical carcinogens are metabolically activated, leading to the formation of reactive species—the ultimate carcinogen. Metabolism is frequently mediated by cytochrome P450 but in tissues and organs with low levels of cytochrome P450, the peroxidase component of prostaglandin synthetase or lipozygenase can activate. Metabolism involves enzymes mainly in the body's entry routes—respiratory tract, gastrointestinal tract, and liver—though metabolism may occur elsewhere, leading to organ-specific tumours.

Cytochrome P450 exists as a number of isoforms, each having a different substrate selectivity. Activity and substrate specificity of both activating and detoxifying enzymes varies from organ to organ, individual to individual, and species to species, resulting in organ- and species-specific carcinogencity. If the affected cell neither dies nor reverts to a normal cell through error-free DNA repair, initiation becomes irreversible after the cell undergoes replication.

The initiated tumour cell, with altered genotype and phenotype, may remain dormant for a long time before becoming a tumour, in the presence of a promoter, which may be one of a wide variety of chemicals. Promotion is reversible, so for an initiated cell to continue to replicate, it must be exposed to a promoter more or less continuously. Carbon tetrachloride is a well-known example of a promoter resulting in liver cancer in animal studies. Hormones can also act as promoters e.g. thyroid hormone is a promoter of thyroid cancer. Like initiation, progression is an irreversible process.

Epigenetic carcinogens

Epigenetic carcinogens do not damage DNA, but act at a later stage through non-genotoxic mechanisms. They are frequently promoters.

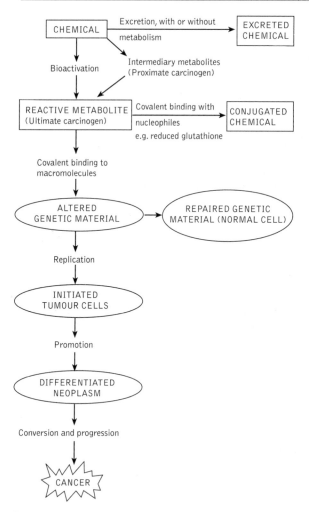

Genotoxic carcinogens and induction of cancer.

Their mode of action is based on induction of cell division. They may be mitogenic agents, cytotoxic agents, or immunosuppressive agents.

Peroxisome proliferators are an interesting class of epigenetic carcinogens, a chemically heterogeneous group of compounds, including the lipid-lowering fibrate drugs and plasticizers such as di-(2-ethylhexyl)phthalate and di-(2-ethylhexyl)adipate. They induce an increase in the number of peroxisomes in hepatocytes, and also increase liver DNA synthesis and cell proliferation in the rat, but the effect is not seen in man, possibly due to a lower expression of peroxisome proliferator-activated receptor (PPAR).

Exposure

Workers at risk from industrial chemical exposure include:

- Dye and textile workers (naphythylamines)—bladder tumours.
- Chemical, rubber workers (benzene)—marrow tumours.
- Plastics, pesticide workers.
- Asbestos workers—lung cancer, mesothelioma.

Cancers resulting from lifestyle factors account for at least two-thirds of chemical induction of cancer. Tobacco smoke contains a broad range of carcinogens. The risk of neoplasia increases dose dependent, in particular for lung, throat, oesophagus, and urinary bladder cancer. Cigarette smoking has an important synergistic effect on the development of neoplasms caused by other carcinogens, for example in asbestosis, or miners exposed to radioactive elements.

In food, pyrrolysis can result in the formation of polycyclic hydrocarbons and heterocyclic amines. 2-Amino-3,8-dimethyl-imidazol[4,5-f]auinoxaline (MeIQx) and 2-amino-1-methyl-6-phenylimidaxzo[4,5-b]pyridine (PhiP) are potent genotoxic chemicals formed at parts per billion levels when meat is cooked. Aflatoxin B_1 is a potent hepatocarcinogen in rodents; in areas of extensive contamination of foodstuffs with *A. Flavus* there is a high incidence of human liver cancer.

Therapeutic drug use

Chemical carcinogenesis can also result from the therapeutic use of drugs. An early example was the use of high dose of diethylstilbesterol, where a small percentage of female offspring of mothers treated during pregnancy developed clear cell carcinoma of the vagina. Alkylating agents used to treat a number of neoplasms are carcinogenic. The development of second neoplasms after chemotherapy is striking; N-acetyltransferase (NAT) is a conjugating enzyme involved in the deactivation of aromatic amines.

In a group of arylamine-exposed workers, slow acetylators were found to be at increased risk compared with rapid acetylators. NAT2 rapid acetylation and fried meat intake represent a combined risk factor for colorectal cancer.

The most widely expressed glutathione transferase gene, GSTM1, is polymorphic, with four common phenotypes. About 45% of most populations are homozygous for deleted GSTM1*0 allele and do not express

GST—this value differs between countries and ethnic groups. GSTM1*0 homozygotes are more susceptible to several malignancies; in the case of lung cancer susceptibility, this is seen only in light smokers, pointing to the interactions between genetic and environmental factors.

Chemoprevention

- Selenium.
- Anti-oxidative vitamins (e.g. vitamin E).
- Diet.
- Derivatives of indoles, flavores, structurally related compounds of the brassia family.
- Green tea.

Radiation carcinogenesis and radiosensitivity syndromes

Ionizing radiation damages cellular contents, specifically DNA, by interacting with molecular cellular components like water, iron, and oxygen to generate free radicals. These then react with DNA leading to double- and single-strand breaks, base loss, and base mutation. Consequences of non-repair of these lesions are:

+ Failure of transcription.
+ Production of mutant or truncated proteins.
+ Cell cycle arrest.
+ Cell death.

Effects to the organism as a whole include:

+ Ageing.
+ Carcinogenesis.
+ Organ dysfunction.

Repair of induced damage is essential for cellular integrity and function. Deficiencies in cellular response to DNA damage result in a series of characteristic syndromes called genomic instability disorders. They share common phenotypes like early predisposition to cancer, immunodeficiencies, and sensitivity to DNA-damaging agents such as ionizing radiation and alkylating agents.

Radiation carcinogenesis

Cancers after atomic bomb explosions include:

+ Leukaemia.
+ Breast.
+ Stomach.
+ Lung.
+ Thyroid.
+ Skin.

At a molecular level, the initiating factor is felt to be an induced mutation in a tumour suppressor or proto-oncogene, with consequent aberrant loss or gain of function. Certain genetic syndromes (e.g. hereditary retinoblastoma) are associated with increased risk of second malignancies within the radiation field.

Radiosensitivity syndromes

Ataxia-telangiectasia (AT)

AT is an autosomal recessive disorder characterized by:

* Development of telangiectasia (particularly on the bulbar conjunctiva).
* Progressive cerebellar ataxia.
* Premature ageing.
* Variable immunodeficiencies.

Patients develop cancer (usually lymphoma and leukaemia) at an early age and show a hypersensitive response to therapeutic treatment with ionising radiation.

The defective gene responsible, ATM (AT mutated), has been identified and cloned. It lies on chromosome 11q22.23, is approximately 150 kb in length and contains 66 exons. The gene encodes a 3056 amino acid protein with molecular weight of 350 kDa. The protein is thought to function in the detection of oxidative DNA damage and DNA damage signal transduction.

Nijmegen breakage syndrome (NBS)

NBS is a very rare disorder characterized phenotypically by:

* Presence of 'bird-like' facies.
* Immunodeficiency.
* Growth retardation.
* Early development of cancer.

The NBS gene has been cloned and lies on chromosome 8q21. It encodes an 85 kDa protein known as p95 or nibrin that has an essential role in homologous recombination, which is important in double-strand break repair.

Bloom's syndrome (BS)

BS is characterized by:

* Growth retardation.
* Immunodeficiency.
* Early development of cancer.

Cells from BS show cytogenetic abnormalities characterized by an increased number of sister chromatid exchanges and *in vitro* sensitivity to alkylating agents and ionizing radiation.

The BS gene has been cloned and lies at chromosome 15.q26.1. It encodes a 150 kDa protein that has structural motifs suggesting a function as a DNA helicase (protein essential for DNA replication, recombination, and repair).

Fanconi's anaemia (FA)

Although not strictly a syndrome of radiosensitivity, FA is important because cells show sensitivity to DNA cross-linking and alkylating agents. FA is diagnosed by the presence of chromosomal aberrations when cells are exposed to mitomycin-C. Phenotypically, a number of characteristics may be seen:

- Absent thumbs and radius.
- Growth retardation.
- Bone marrow failure.
- Early susceptibility to cancer.

Five different complementation groups of FA have been described; genes for two—groups FAA and FAC—have been cloned. Individually, both lie within cytoplasm but combine to form a complex of unknown function in nucleus.

Others

A number of other syndromes have been described in which sensitivity to some form of DNA-damaging agent is seen:

- Gorlin's syndrome.
- Tuberose sclerosis.
- Usher's syndrome.
- Gardner's syndrome.

The relevance of clinical observation of sensitivity to the underlying genetic defect is still unclear. Perhaps a more interesting group of individuals are those (around 2–3%) who show undue sensitivity to conventional doses of ionizing radiation without any obvious pre-treatment phenotype apart from the presence of cancer. It is probable that the same individuals are also sensitive to chemotherapy that induces DNA damage. Investigation of such individuals has shown a variety of differing defects in DNA repair, cell cycle, and DNA damage signal transduction. Given this heterogeneity, it is likely that pre-treatment predictive tests will be developed at cellular—not molecular—level.

Treatment

Clinically obvious cases of AT, FA, NBS, or BS who develop cancer should be treated, if possible, with agents that do not cause DNA damage. If necessary, it is possible to assess cellular radiosensitivity before treatment and adjust doses accordingly, as normal radiosensitivity is reflected to tumour sensitivity.

Hormones in the aetiology of cancer

Different hormones and their related growth factors play a variety of roles in carcinogenesis in a number of malignancies, including cancer of the:

+ Breast.
+ Endometrium.
+ Prostate.
+ Ovary.
+ Thyroid.
+ Bone.
+ Testis.

In these sites the cancer results from excessive hormonal stimulation of relevant target cells. These effects occur independently of other aetiological agents like chemical carcinogens or ionizing radiation.

In the 1960s, daughters of women treated with diethylstilbestrol (DES) during pregnancy were found to develop vaginal adenocarcinoma as they reached menarche, an indication that hormones could be both directly carcinogenic and involved in tumour promotion. Now it seems DES causes persistence of Mullerian duct remnants in the vagina, and these are activated with the hormonal changes of puberty. There is some evidence that exposure of the male foetus to high levels of oestrogens can also have carcinogenic effects later in life, with increased risk of maldescent and testicular cancer.

The role of hormones in promoting cancer is further shown by the fact that women whose ovaries never secrete steroid hormones do not develop breast cancer. Hormonal factors associated with an increased risk of breast cancer are:

+ Early menarche.
+ Late menopause.
+ Nulliparity.
+ Late age at first pregnancy.

As with breast cancer, an increased risk of ovarian cancer is associated with nulliparity. It is thought that promoters of ovarian cancer are growth factors that control normal repair after ovulation (the fewer numbers of ovulations, the less risk of ovarian cancer). In endometrial cancer the risk of disease is related to exposure of the endometrium to oestrogens, unopposed by the effects of progesterone (HRT, obesity, sequential oral contraceptives, late menopause).

In laboratory animals, prostate cancer can be produced by exposure to large doses of exogenous testosterone; in man, castration at an early age provides lifelong protection from this common tumour. However, circulating testosterone levels have not shown consistent differences between prostate cancer cases and controls, and studies of alteration in androgen receptors have so far been inconclusive.

Pimentel, E. (1987) Hormones, grown factors and oncogenes. Chapman and Hall, London.

Hodges, G.M., Rowlatt, C. (1993) Developmental biology and cancer. Chapman and Hall, London.

Chapter 6
Staging of cancer

Imaging in the oncology patient

The radiologist is involved at every stage from the initial diagnosis through staging, radiotherapy planning, patient management, and follow-up. He/she participates in:

* Recurrence detection
* Re-staging
* Assessing complications of the disease and its treatment
* Interventional procedures both curative and palliative
* Terminal care techniques including pain relief

Common tumours such as those of the lung, breast, and colon are often initially diagnosed by imaging (chest X-ray, mammography, and barium enema), to be confirmed by cytology or histology. Further imaging will depend on tumour type, methods of spread, and the ability of the diagnostic and interventional radiologist to help manage a particular patient.

The primary tumour

The radiological diagnosis of a primary tumour depends partly on the size and site of tumour and mode of clinical presentation. For example, a small pituitary gland tumour may be only just visible on high-resolution magnetic resonance (MR) imaging yet be clinically obvious, whereas an asymptomatic 10 cm pulmonary carcinoma may only be discovered accidentally on a chest X-ray performed prior to anaesthesia. The appearance of primary tumours on imaging may be characteristic but only cytology and histology give definitive proof of tumour type.

Tumours may produce their clinical effects by:

* Size
* Site
* Spread
* Paraneoplastic effects

Spread of tumour

Tumours may spread by:

* Local invasion
* Lymphatic and vascular channels
* Transcoelomic dissemination

Local spread may affect clinical presentation, staging, management, and prognosis. For example, a tumour in the apex of a lung (Pancoast tumour) may spread into the chest wall and into the brachial plexus, causing characteristic pain and neurological deficit. Where tumours abut tissue planes, imaging will often not indicate if the tumour has crossed such a plane. Pleural involvement by a peripheral lung carcinoma, for instance, will only be apparent at operation.

Transcoelomic spread is often seen in colorectal and ovarian carcinomas. Neither CT nor MR are good at showing peritoneal plaque disease, although both can readily demonstrate ascitic fluid and bulk of a tumour. While imaging may suggest that ascites is due to peritoneal disease, cytological proof will be necessary.

Tumours may show characteristic spread via lymphatics e.g. bronchial carcinoma to mediastinal nodes, melanoma to regional nodes, and testicular tumours to para-aortic nodes. Other tumours (e.g. lung and breast carcinomas) spread by haematogenous means to the liver, brain, bone, lung, and adrenal glands. The liver is a favourite site for spread from primary tumours in the gastrointestinal tract via the portal venous system. It acts as a venous filter with tumour emboli lodging and growing in the capillary bed.

Contrast-enhanced CT will detect 90% of metastases greater than 1 cm, although solitary lesions require biopsy to confirm their nature.

Monitoring treatment

The primary tumour and any metastatic spread may be monitored by serial examination using the most appropriate technique. Such examinations allow measurement of tumour response to radiotherapy, chemotherapy, or other intervention. Recurrence of primary tumour after surgery can also be assessed by serial monitoring, though there may be difficulty in differentiating post-operative haematoma, fibrosis, and tumour. Modern techniques, including Gadolinium-enhanced MR, are becoming more reliable and specific.

Interventional procedures

These include:-

+ Percutaneous fine-needle or core biopsy for cytology or histology under imaging control (U/S, CT)
+ Embolization of vascular tumours pre-operatively
+ Placement of intravenous and intra-arterial chemotherapy catheters
+ Insertion of stents into malignant strictures e.g. gut, bile duct
+ Laser surgery
+ Pain relief

Screening for cancer

Mammographic screening of women aged >50 years is widely accepted and improves the detection rate for early tumours and reduces breast cancer mortality. Such screening programmes necessitate high standards of quality assurance and quality control, in particular the use of skilled radiologists.

Radiotherapy planning

The basic principles include defining:

- Tumour volume, often by CT or MR
- Target volume, which is tumour volume plus a margin of healthy tissue
- Treatment volume to achieve desired effect while avoiding radio-sensitive areas such as the spinal cord

All aspects of such planning require imaging to ensure accurate and appropriate tumour irradiation

Radionuclide imaging

Technetium 99^m is an ideal diagnostic imaging radionuclide because of its photon energy, short half life of 6 hours, easy production, and ability to attach to a wide variety of radiopharmaceuticals. Some tumours have characteristic properties lending themselves to imaging with such agents. Neuroendocrine and carcinoid tumours concentrate MIBG (meta-iodo-benzyl-guanidine) and thus can be used both for diagnostic and therapeutic purposes. Medullary carcinoma of the thyroid has a high uptake of Technetium 99^m DMSA (dimecapto-succinic acid). Cyclotron-generated isotopes used dynamically in PET (positron emission tomography) scanning show potential in certain areas including pancreatic and lung tumours with lymph node spread.

Biochemical markers

Tumour markers are detectable substances present in a concentration suggestive of a tumour. A tumour marker is not tumour-specific, but may be secreted or shed into blood and other body fluids or expressed at the cell surface in larger quantities by malignant cells than by non-malignant cells. Tumour markers can be assayed either by measuring the concentration of marker in body fluids (usually by immunoassay) or by detecting the marker's presence on the cell surface in paraffin section or fresh biopsies (by immunohistochemistry).

The potential clinical uses of tumour marker estimation are:

- Screening
- Diagnosis
- Prognosis
- Monitoring response to therapy
- Early diagnosis of relapse

Gestational trophoblastic tumours

Diagnosis and screening

Elevated levels of human chorionic gonadotrophin (HCG) are always seen in choriocarcinoma, but can also be found in normal pregnancy, ectopic pregnancy, in some patients with germ cell tumours, and, occasionally, in patients with non-germ cell tumours. Following diagnosis and evacuation of a hydatidiform mole, patients are followed using serial HCG measurements in blood or urine. Screening allows patients with persistent trophoblastic disease to be detected on the basis of plateauing or rising tumour markers before clinical evidence of a tumour develops.

Prognosis/monitoring response to treatment

The level of HCG at presentation is a major factor in deciding if a patient falls into a good or poor prognostic group. Serial HCG estimation is used to monitor response to chemotherapy and to detect development of drug resistance. It has a serum half-life of 18–36 hours. Plateauing or rising of HCG values during a course of chemotherapy indicates the development of drug resistance and the need to change chemotherapy.

Detection of recurrence

Serial measurement of HCG will detect any recurrence of trophoblastic tumour with 100% sensitivity. Accurate measurement of HCG in urine increases the ease of monitoring and obviates the need for frequent hospital visits. A rise in HCG is not, however, diagnostic of recurrent disease and a new pregnancy must always be considered and ruled out by ultrasound examination.

Germ cell tumours

Alpha-feto protein (AFP) and HCG are elevated, either singly or in combination, in more than 80% of patients with disseminated non-seminomatous germ cell tumours (NSGCT) and in about 60% of patients with stage 1 disease prior to orchidectomy. Another marker useful in patients with germ cell tumours is lactate dehydrogenase (LDH). Placental alkaline phosphatase (PLAP), although elevated in about 50% of patients with seminomas, is also raised by cigarette smoking, and adds little to clinical management.

Diagnosis

All patients suspected of having a germ cell tumour should have a baseline tumour marker estimation before excision of the primary tumour. Patients whose clinical status could be compromised by biopsy should be considered for an NSGCT if disease distribution is compatible with such a tumour and there is gross elevation of either HCG or AFP. An elevated HCG can be found in patients with pure seminoma but a patient with an elevated AFP should never be considered to have a pure seminoma, regardless of histological findings.

Failure of tumour marker levels to fall to normal post-operatively indicates the presence of occult metastatic disease.

Prognosis and staging

Patients should be classified according to the risk factors shown in the table.

Monitoring response to treatment

Successful chemotherapy is invariably accompanied by a fall in serial HCG and AFP levels. The serum half-life of AFP is 5–7 days. An initial rise in tumour marker levels may occur soon after starting the first course of chemotherapy, due to tumour lysis. Occasionally, a plateau or even a rise in AFP levels may occur, despite evidence of response from all other investigations. This is due to AFP production by the liver in response to toxicity, most commonly after hepatotoxic drugs such as methotrexate and ifosfamide.

Early recurrence detection

All patients with germ cell tumours should continue to have serial tumour marker estimation after completion of chemotherapy to detect relapse early. Serial marker estimation is also invaluable as part of the surveillance programme of patients with stage 1 disease

Table 6.1 Assessment of prognosis by marker in germ cell tumours

	AFP ng/ml		HCG IU/L		LDH × upper limit normal
Good risk	>1000	*and*	<500	*and*	<1.5 × upper limit normal
Intermediate	1000–10 000	*or*	5000–50 000	*or*	1.5–10 × upper limit normal
Poor risk	>10 000	*or*	>50 000	*or*	>10 × upper limit normal

following orchidectomy. Because tumour markers can double rapidly, it is important that they are measured at least monthly, and more frequently if raised.

Gastrointestinal tumours

The most widely used serum marker for colorectal cancer is carcinoembryonic antigen (CEA). CA 19.9 has an epitope structurally identical to the sialylated Lewis A antigen and is elevated in 75–90% of patients with pancreatic carcinoma.

Diagnosis and screening

Serum CEA is elevated in about 65% of patients with distant metastases, in 44% of Dukes' stage C, about 25% of Dukes' stage B, and fewer than 5% of patients with Dukes' stage A colorectal cancer. CEA can also be elevated in:

• Severe benign liver disease
• Inflammatory lesions, especially of the gastrointestinal tract
• Trauma
• Infection
• Collagen disease
• Renal impairment
• Smoking

A low incidence of high serum CEA levels in early disease and its poor specificity explain its lack of value in screening normal populations for colorectal cancer. A low sensitivity precludes it being useful for screening patients even in high-risk groups such as ulcerative colitis or familial polyposis coli.

Monitoring treatment

Serum CEA levels should fall to normal within 4–6 weeks of complete resection of a colorectal carcinoma. Levels usually rise with disease and fall with response to chemotherapy or radiotherapy. Failure of CEA to fall during radiotherapy usually indicates the presence of a tumour outside the radiation field. Several studies have shown that survival is longer in patients with a fall in serum CEA level during chemotherapy than in those in whom there is no change or an increased level.

Follow-up and detection of relapse

In about 65% of patients with recurrent colorectal cancer, a rise in serial serum CEA values predicts recurrence, on average 11 months before it becomes clinically apparent.

Ovarian cancer

CA 125 is the most commonly used tumour marker for ovarian cancer and is found in derivatives of coelomic epithelium, including pleura, pericardium, and peritoneum, but not in normal ovarian tissue.

Diagnosis

CA 125 is elevated in >95% of patients with advanced (stage III or IV) ovarian cancer, but in <50% of patients with stage I disease. Levels >30 IU ml^{-1} are frequently seen during the first trimester of pregnancy in patients with endometriosis or cirrhosis, especially if ascites is present. It is elevated in >40% of patients with advanced non-ovarian intra-abdominal malignancies and in 1% of healthy controls.

Screening

Apart from women at high risk of familial ovarian cancer, screening for ovarian cancer should not be offered to women outside a clinical trial. CA 125 has no proven value in screening for ovarian cancer.

Prognosis and response to treatment

Very high CA 125 levels prior to surgery are associated with a worse prognosis. In women with stage I disease a pre-operative level >65 U/ml is a powerful adverse prognostic indicator, and such patients are candidates for chemotherapy rather than surveillance. Elevated CA 125 levels after one, two, or three courses of chemotherapy are important adverse prognostic factors for survival. Serial changes in CA 125 are recognized as one of the best methods for monitoring therapy.

A persistently elevated CA 125 after oophorectomy for suspected stage I disease is evidence of residual tumour.

A biological response based on CA 125 has been defined as either a 50% or a 75% reduction in CA 125 levels. To reduce the chance of falsely predicting a response, the 50% CA 125 response definition requires four CA 125 levels—two initial elevated samples, and the sample showing a 50% decrease requires confirmation by a fourth sample. The 75% CA 125 response definition requires only three CA 125 levels, with a serial decrease of at least 75%. In both 50% and 75% response definitions, the final sample has to be at least 28 days after the previous sample.

Detection of progression or relapse

A serial rise of CA 125 of >25% is the most accurate method of predicting progression of ovarian cancer during therapy. There is controversy however over the role of serial CA 125 measurements during follow-up. However, if relapse is suspected, a confirmed doubling from the upper limit of normal during follow-up predicts relapse with almost 100% specificity.

Prostate cancer

Prostate-specific antigen (PSA) has superseded prostatic acid phosphatase as a marker, as it is elevated in a higher proportion of men with prostate cancer.

Diagnosis, screening, and staging

Elevated levels of PSA (>4 ng ml^{-1}) occur in about 53% of men with intracapsular microscopic and 77% of men with intracapsular macroscopic prostatic cancer, but can also occur in 30–50% of men with benign prostatic hypertrophy (BPH). A combination of PSA and digital rectal examination, followed by prostatic ultrasound in patients with abnormal findings, is commonly used for screening in US but is not recommended in the UK. As yet, there is no definite evidence of survival benefit from screen detection of early prostate cancer. About 40% of patients with PSA levels of 4.0–9.9 ng ml^{-1} at screening will already have tumour spread outside the prostate.

The ratio of free to total PSA is being used to improve diagnostic specificity—more of the PSA is protein-bound in patients with prostate cancer compared with BPH. The ratio of free to total PSA is low (about 10%) in prostate cancer compared to $>16\%$ in BPH and prostatitis. Bone or lymph node metastases are usually, but not always, associated with an elevated PSA.

Prognosis/monitoring response/recurrence detection

A high pre-treatment PSA is associated with a poor prognosis. PSA levels fall rapidly to undetectable levels after complete removal of a tumour by radical prostatectomy. The rate of fall is slower and the nadir higher after successful radiotherapy or endocrine therapy. A serial rise in PSA frequently precedes other evidence of disease progression in the patient with a past history of prostate cancer. Development of bone pain in the presence of an elevated PSA level suggests the development of bone metastases.

Breast cancer

The most widely investigated mucin marker in breast cancer is CA 15-3.

Diagnosis and screening

Although elevated levels of CA 15-3 are found in 55–100% of patients with advanced breast cancer, serum CA 15-3 is raised in only 10–46% of patients with primary breast cancer and in about 10% of patients with early ($T_{1-2}NoMo$) operable disease, as well as 2–20% of patients with benign breast disease.

Prognosis/monitoring response to treatment

Elevated pre-operative levels of CA 15-3 are associated with a poorer prognosis. Although tumour marker levels can fall with reduction in tumour burden following system therapy, the variation between patients makes this tumour marker unreliable for assessing response.

Early detection of relapse

The observation that over 60% of patients who develop recurrent breast cancer have raised levels of CA 15-3 suggests potential value in early detection of recurrence.

Other cancers

- Serum AFP is elevated at presentation in 50–80% of UK patients with **hepatocellular carcinoma** and may be used in screening of high-risk populations.

- **Neuron-specific enolase (NSE)** is elevated in many patients with advanced small-cell lung cancers and in children with neuroblastoma.

- Paraprotein levels are very important in the management of patients with **myeloma**, where B_2-micro-globulin may be of prognostic value.

- **Carcinoid tumours** can be monitored by urine levels of 5-hydroxyindole acetic acid (5HIAA), and polypeptides such as gastrin or glucagon are useful in the management of rare gastrointestinal tumours.

- **Squamous cell carcinomas** are associated with elevated levels of squamous cell carcinoma antigen (SCC) as well as cytokeratin fragments. SCC and CA 125 give valuable prognostic information in patients with cervical carcinoma and may indicate relapse before scans.

- Calcitonin and calcitonin-related peptide are used in diagnosis and screening for **medullary thyroid carcinoma**.

- Serum S-100 and reverse transcriptase polymerase chain reaction to detect mRNA of tyrosinase on circulating melanoma cells are being studied for staging and follow-up of patients with **melanoma**.

TNM staging of cancer

Staging is the assessment of a patient's tumour burden. It rises from the observation that survival rates are higher for cases in which disease is localized rather than disseminated. It is performed prior to therapy and can be subdivided into clinical, radiological, and pathological.

Staging of cancer at presentation is essential for the patients, allowing accurate prediction of prognosis and planning of treatment modalities. It is also allows comparison of care to be made between different institutions and treatment approaches and for results between different chronological groupings to be compared.

A generic approach is the TNM system:

T—extent of the primary tumour.

N—absence or presence and extent of regional lymph node metastases.

M—absence or presence of distant metastases.

Adding numbers to these components indicates the extent of the disease and any progressive increase in the tumour burden.

Primary tumour (T)

Tx—primary tumour cannot be assessed.

T0—no evidence of primary tumour.

Tis—carcinoma in situ.

T1, T2, T3, T4—increasing size and/or local extent of primary tumour.

Regional lymph nodes (N)

Nx—regional lymph nodes cannot be assessed.

N0—no regional lymph node metastases.

N1, N2, N3—increasing involvement of regional lymph nodes.

Direct extension of primary tumour into lymph nodes is classified as lymph node metastases; involvement of nodes other than regional is classified as distant metastases.

Distant metastases (M)

Mx—presence of distant metastases cannot be assessed.

M0—no distant metastases.

M1—distant metastases.

The category M1 is often subdivided according to the following notation:

Pulmonary—PUL.

Osseous—OSS.

Hepatic—HEP.

Brain—BRA.

Skin—SKI.

Peritoneum—PER.

Marrow—MAR.

Pleura—PLE.

Using this methodology it is possible to assign a TNM class to any patient.

Specific rules for each subset of tumour type are published by the International Union Against Cancer (UICC) and the American Joint Committee on Cancer (AJCC).

Performance status

A patient's general condition profoundly affects treatment decisions, and his/her condition may be directly influenced by the underlying cancer or may reflect other concomitant illness, age, nutritional status, mental condition, etc. Patients with poor performance status tolerate therapy worse and response less often than those with good performance status.

Performance status does not necessarily parallel the stage of cancer. It does, however, provide additional prognostic information and should be recorded for all patients at presentation and throughout therapy and follow-up.

Two common systems are in frequent use:

Karnofsky scale (KPS)

- Normal; no complaints; no evidence of disease.
- Able to carry on normal activity; minor signs or symptoms of disease.
- Able to carry on normal activity with effort; some signs or symptoms of disease.
- Cares for self; unable to carry on normal activity or do active work.
- Requires occasional assistance but is able to care for most of own needs.
- Requires considerable assistance and frequent medical care.
- Disabled; requires special care and assistance.
- Severely disabled; hospitalization indicated although death not imminent.
- Very sick; hospitalization necessary; active supportive treatment necessary.
- Moribund; fatal processes progressing rapidly.
- Dead.

Eastern Co-operative Oncology Group (ECOG)

- Fully active; able to carry on all activities without restriction.
- Restricted in physically strenuous activity but ambulatory and able to carry out work of a light or sedentary nature.
- Ambulatory and capable of all self-care but unable to carry out any work activities; up and about more than 50% of waking hours.
- Capable of only limited self-care; confined to bed or chair 50% or more of waking hours.
- Completely disabled; cannot carry on any self-care; totally confined to bed or chair.

Part 2
Principles of treatment

Chapter 7
Surgical oncology

General considerations

Surgery is the mainstay of treatment—and principal hope of cure—for most patients with solid tumours. Surgery is most effective when cancer is localized, and substantial numbers of long-term survivors can be achieved with some tumour types that show metastatic disease at presentation.

Surgery has an advantage over radiotherapy as long-term morbidity of treating tissues without the primary tumour is significantly less; this must be balanced against disruption of normal anatomy inherent in radical resection of cancer, with potential loss of cosmesis and function.

Surgery has three main roles in the management of cancer patients:

- Diagnosis and staging
- Curative
- Palliative

Surgery is the longest-established treatment for cancer and remains the foremost curative treatment of choice for many localized cancers. It has a role to play in the treatment of both primary and secondary cancer as well as palliation.

Tumour behaviour

An understanding of tumour biology is essential to the planning of surgical treatment for cancer.

The behaviour of solid tumours is diverse and the implications for surgery are often paradoxical. The three principal methods of spread are:

- Direct infiltration
- Lymphatic
- Blood-borne

Most cancers disseminate by all three methods, although one method of spread may be predominant. Breast and colorectal cancer exhibit both blood and lymphatic spread whereas cancers arising in the upper gastrointestinal tract and the upper airways metastasize via the lymphatics. Even cancers arising from the same cell type behave differently—papillary and follicular tumours of the thyroid give rise to lymphatic and haematogenous metastases respectively. Different surgical approaches will be required depending on tumour type.

Surgical techniques

The *en-bloc* technique is most often used in cancers with a predominantly lymphatic spread and is best developed in surgery of head and neck cancer. It is increasingly being used for stomach and oesophageal cancers. No advantage has been reported for aggressive *en-bloc* resection of loco-regional lymphatics in surgery of large bowel cancer.

Surgery is often more successful in the treatment of cancers with haematogenous spread compared to those with more developed local and lymphatic metastases.

Growth rates of cancers vary enormously. Patients with breast cancer may relapse many years after primary treatment while those with upper gastrointestinal tumours usually die within two years of diagnosis. There are real differences in growth rate. Endocrine-related cancers often have very slow growth rates and metastases may appear years after initial resection. Repeated excision of metastatic disease may lead to long-term survival in such tumours but this approach would be futile for gastric or oesophageal cancer.

Diagnosis and staging

The development of cross-sectional radiology, ultrasound, CT, and MRI—together with the radiologist's ability to perform core biopsies or fine-needle aspiration cytology combined with use of endoscopy and biopsies or cytological brushing, allows pre-operative diagnosis to be made in most cases.

A significant advance in reducing unnecessary suffering for patients has been the use of these procedures to stage accurately cancers prior to surgery. This has been most important where surgical treatment carries significant morbidity and mortality, such as in major resection of the stomach or oesophagus.

The approach should be to establish a histological diagnosis by endoscopic biopsy with radiological staging, using a combination of endoscopic ultrasound, CT, or MRI. A useful adjunct to this is laparoscopy that will detect small peritoneal or liver metastases and is helpful in determining fixation. Using these methods, the numbers of 'open and close' laparotomies for unresectable cancer can be reduced to <5%, avoiding unnecessary surgery for patients at a disease's terminal stage.

Curative surgery

The long-term outcome after cancer surgery depends on tumour type and the stage of presentation. Survival rates for some cancers have improved due to earlier presentation following public awareness and screening programmes e.g. breast and cervical cancer. Improving techniques mean larger resections can be carried out with low risk, often with excellent functional results e.g. limb-preserving surgery for osteosarcoma. In the CNS, vital structures continue to inhibit the extent of resection.

For some cancers results are good—5-year survival rate in breast cancer is over 75% and for large bowel cancer it approaches 70%. Unfortunately, the cure rate for pancreatic and gastric cancer remains low with 5-year survival rates significantly less than 10% for patients treated in Europe.

Long-term tumour control can only be expected if all the cancer is removed at the operation. Such operations for rectal cancer result in very low recurrence rates in patients with localized disease. Conservation surgery for breast cancer has to be diligently performed to ensure complete removal of tumour. This requires close collaboration between the surgeon and pathologist.

With the development of high-quality radiological imaging and more accurate staging, more localized, low-morbidity operations can be performed e.g. perianal excision of early rectal cancer. Minimal access surgery is associated with less trauma for the patient, a shorter hospital stay, and a quicker return to normal function, but its role in cancer surgery is still unproven.

Palliative surgery

Surgical palliation falls into several different categories, requiring a broad range of expertise and knowledge. A patient's life expectancy may vary from weeks to years depending on their condition, and the surgeon must know when not to operate and to utilize palliative care teams and interventional radiology, as well as to decide when and what operation is required.

Bowel obstruction

Patients with colon or ovarian cancer make up the bulk of those developing small or large bowel obstruction. In a colon cancer patient, confirmation of incurability will usually be made at laparotomy, following a decision to treat a large bowel obstruction. Where possible, these patients should have the primary cancer excised and intestinal continuity restored by primary anastomosis. Management of the obstructed ovarian cancer patient is usually more difficult as the key decision is often whether or not the patient should have the operation.

Many patients will have multiple obstruction sites, with their small and large bowel studded with tumours on the serosal surface. Such patients are not suitable for surgical palliation. Others will have 1 or 2 site obstructions e.g. a segment of terminal ileum embedded in pelvic tumour. They can benefit from debulking, resection, and anastomosis or bypass surgery.

Differentiating these categories of patient can usually be done by a history of crampy abdominal pain, clinical examination revealing a distended tympanitic abdomen (as opposed to an abdomen with multiple sites of palpable tumour and ascites), plain X-rays revealing many loops of distended bowel with air fluid levels and CT evidence of pelvic or other single-site tumour deposit.

Laparoscopy will sometimes be helpful in the obstructed patient who has not had previous abdominal surgery.

Fistulas

Fistulas caused by pelvic tumours or post-radiotherapy include:-

- Rectovaginal
- Enterovaginal
- Colovesical
- Vesicovaginal
- Combination of above

Pre-operative assessment to determine the exact type is important. A proximal end sigmoid colostomy, which can usually be performed without a formal laparotomy, is the treatment of choice for most rectovaginal fistulas. Patients with combined rectovaginal and vesico-vaginal fistulas may need an end colostomy and ileal conduit. A covered stent, delivered endoscopically or at X-ray, should be considered for patients with a colovesical fistula. Patients with an entero-vesical fistula will require laparotomy resection of small bowel segment and anastomosis.

Jaundice

Obstructive jaundice can be palliated surgically by choledocho-enterostomy or cholecystenterostomy, although these procedures have been largely superseded by endoscopic and radiological placement of stents. Stents can become blocked, resulting in repeated cholangitis. A recent trial has demonstrated a shorter overall hospital stay and decreased morbidity for surgical palliation of jaundice compared to endoscopic stenting and should be considered in medically fit patients. Selected patients with inoperable hilar tumours will be best treated by segment III biliary enteric bypass.

Ascites

Peritoneal-venous (Leveen) shunts can be inserted to relieve ascites in selected cases. Careful pre-operative assessment should be undertaken to ensure that ascites is not loculated and that the tumour is not muci-nous, otherwise the shunt will become blocked. These are usually inserted using local anaesthetic and sedation, with >50% of patients achieving good, long-term palliation.

Pain

There are a number of options open to oncological surgeons to help patients with pain:

• Surgical debulking of large, slow-growing tumours (e.g. intra-abdominal, soft-tissue sarcomas in otherwise fit patients where expected morbidity of the procedure is low).

• Stabilization of pathological fractures and bone metastases involv-ing >50% of cortex.

• Neurosurgical approaches for pain control including cordotomy.

• Thoracoscopic splanchnectomy for intractable pain secondary to pancreatic cancer. (Results comparing this technique with percuta-neous chemical ablation of coeliac splanchnic nerves are awaited.)

Gastrointestinal bleeding

A wide array of endoscopic and radiological techniques are available to stop bleeding from benign and malignant causes in incurable can-cer patients, including injection sclerotherapy (benign ulceration), laser coagulation (neoplastic ulcers), and radiological embolization (should the other methods fail). Surgery should be reserved for those with a life expectancy of 3 months or more for whom these methods fail.

Palliative resection of the primary tumour

Up to 10% of patients with breast cancer will present with metastatic disease; patients with visceral metastases have a poor prognosis but patients with the more frequent bone metastases have a median survival of 2 years. Resection of the primary tumour to achieve loco-regional control may improve patients' quality of life, preventing fungation or uncontrolled axillary metastases.

Patients with colorectal cancer are increasingly staged prior to surgery to determine the most appropriate therapy. In those in whom unresectable liver metastases are identified, primary tumour resection should still be considered to minimize the risk of bleeding, perforation, or obstruction, which may subsequently occur.

Surgery for metastatic disease

Lymphatic clearance

* May be curative
* May avoid need for adjuvant chemotherapy or radiotherapy
* Useful in
  —breast cancer
  —colorectal cancer
  —gastric cancer (controversial)
* No role for prophylactic block nodal surgery in melanoma
* May be role for sentinel node dissection in breast (trials awaited) and melanoma

Liver metastases

* Most secondaries are unsuitable for resection
* Benefit to selected patients with colorectal secondaries
  —33%, 5-year survival
  —2%, operative mortality
  —20%, post-operative morbidity
* Better survival if one lobe (compared to two)
  —if size of secondary <5 cm
  —if margin >1 cm
  —if metachronous resection as opposed to synchronous
* A further later liver resection is possible

Treatment options

* Cryotherapy
* Laser (may have a role but unproven currently)
* Radio-frequency ablation
* Injection of alcohol

Lung metastases

* 10–60% 5-year survival after resection of solitary lung secondary
* Long-term survival in patients with primary tumours of
  —oropharynx
  —kidney
  —testis
  —colon
  —sarcoma
* Occasionally repeated resection is beneficial

Bone metastases

- Internal fixation is useful if
  —weight-bearing bone, especially if lesion is >2.5 cms or involves circumference
  —painful secondary after radiotherapy
  —will improve mobilization and nursing care
  —patient is fit
  —Bone quality will support fixation
- Considerations in spinal secondary
  —stability of spine
  —spinal cord compression

Treatment options

- Radiotherapy
- Hormone manipulation
- Surgery—stabilization

Brain metastases

- Good palliation
- Underused
- Occasionally curative
- Post-operative radiotherapy helps
- Anatomical site important

Further reading

Gilbert, J.M., Jaffrey, I., Evens, M. *et al.* (1984) Sites of recurrent tumour after curative colorectal surgery: implications for adjuvant therapy. *British Journal of Surgery* 71, 203–5.

Rao, A.R., Kagan, A.R., Chan, P.M. *et al,* (1981) Pattern of recurrence following curative resection alone for adenocarcinoma of the rectum and sigmoid colon. *Cancer* 48, 1492–5.

Veronesi, U. (1987) Rationale and indications for limited surgery in breast cancer: current data. *World Journal of Surgery* 11, 493–8.

Kaibara, N., Sumi, K., Yonakawa, M. *et al.* (1990) Does extensive dissection of lymph nodes improve the result of surgical treatment of gastric cancer? *American Journal of Surgery* 159, 218–21.

Chapter 8
Principles of radiation oncology

Radiobiology of normal tissues

Effects of radiation on tissues are generally mediated by one of two mechanisms:

• Loss of mature functional cells by apoptosis (active form of cell death, usually within 24 hours of irradiation).

• Loss of reproductive capacity.

Different cell types show large differences in radiosensitivity to either of these processes and only a limited number of cell types predominantly respond by apoptosis. These include some cells of haemopoietic lineage and salivary glands. As most tissues or organs have redundant functional cells, they may lose a significant fraction of this cell population by apoptosis without clinical impairment of tissue function. Usually lost cells are replaced by proliferation of surviving stem cells or progenitor cells. These may be cells surviving in irradiated tissue or cells migrating from unirradiated margins.

When cell loss occurs predominantly through loss of proliferative capacity, the rate of cell renewal (proliferation) of a particular organ determines the time of appearance of tissue damage, varying from days to even years after irradiation. This has led to the arbitrary distinction of acute and late effects of radiation, with acute effects being restricted to changes developing during a fractionated course of radiotherapy of 6–8 weeks.

Acute and late effects of radiation

Acute effects of radiation comprise the dose-limiting normal tissue reactions during a course of radiotherapy and involve mainly the mucosa and the haemopoietic system. Although initial cell loss may be partly through apoptosis, the predominant effect is loss of reproductive capacity, interfering with the replacement of lost cells. Thus, tissues with fast normal cellular turnover (epithelia of skin and gut, bone marrow) display effects of irradiation earliest.

Timing of radiation effects also depends on rate of dose administration. After a single dose of 10 Gy, the mucosal lining of the intestinal tract is depleted in a few days, while it may take several weeks during a fractionated course of radiotherapy with daily doses of 2 Gy.

The speed of recovery of acute reaction depends on the level of stem cell depletion, and varies from a few days to several months. If the number of surviving stem cells is too low, severe epithelial damage may persist as a chronic ulcer.

Late effects occur predominantly in slowly proliferating tissues (such as the lung, kidney, heart, liver, and the central nervous system) but are not necessarily restricted to these slowly renewing cell systems (e.g. in the skin, in addition to the acute epidermal reactions, late changes such as fibrosis, atrophy, or telangiectasia can develop up to several years later).

The distinction between acute and late effects has important clinical implications. Since acute reactions are usually observed during the course of a conventionally fractionated radiotherapy schedule (1.8–2 Gy per fraction, five times a week), it is possible to adjust the dose in the event of unexpectedly severe reactions, allowing a sufficient number of stem cells to survive. Surviving stem cells will repopulate and restore the integrity of the rapidly proliferating tissue. When overall treatment time is reduced, the acute reactions may not reach maximal intensity until after completion of treatment. This precludes adjustment of the dose regimen to the severity of reactions. If intensive fractionation schedules reduce the number of surviving stem cells to below the level needed for effective tissue restoration, acute reactions may persist as chronic injury, called **consequential late complications**.

By definition, late radiation reactions are not apparent until a considerable time after irradiation and these are by no means always predicted by the severity of the acute reaction. Although the total dose of radiation is most important, another major determinant of late radiation effect is the dose of radiation per fraction of treatment.

The time elapsing between radiation and the clinical appearance of a radiation-induced lesion has basically no relationship with the radiosensitivity or tolerance of the relevant normal tissue. Some acutely responding tissues such as the skin and mucosa are relatively resistant, in contrast to the highly radiosensitive haemopoietic tissues and germ cells. Conversely, typically late responding tissues like the lung and kidney are among the most sensitive, while the brain is in the more resistant part of the spectrum.

Radiation effects in specific tissues

Skin

+ Erythema—week 2–3
+ Desquamation—later
+ Ulceration—later
+ Shorter course increases severity of acute skin reaction
+ Dose per fraction is less important in acute reaction
+ Tolerance for late effects decreases with increasing dose per fraction

Late effects include:
+ Atrophy
+ Contraction
+ Radiation fibrosis
+ Telangiectasia

Oral mucosa

+ Severe mucositis after a dose of 70 Gy in 6 weeks
+ Severity relates to treatment time and volume irradiated

Gastrointestinal tract

+ Acute mucositis causes diarrhoea and gastritis; if occurs, cease treatment for a few days
+ Late effects—mucosal ulceration, atrophy, fibrosis, necrosis

Nervous system

+ Dose of 50 Gy—low risk of injury
+ Dose of 60 Gy—5% risk of major complications
+ Early reaction (6 months)—demyelination; brain (somnolence); spinal cord (Lhermitte's syndrome)
+ Later reaction (1–2 years)—radiation necrosis, initially in white matter; then telangiectasia, focal haemorrhage
+ Peripheral nerves may be more radioresistant

Lung

+ Responds late
+ Radiation pneumonitis—2–6 months after treatment
+ Dose tolerance—10 Gy in single treatment; 25 Gy in 2 Gy fractions
+ Lung fibrosis—6 months to years

Kidney

+ Responds later
+ Large reserve capacity, therefore effects occur up to 10 years later
+ Radiation nephropathy—proteinuria, hypertension

Heart

+ Pericarditis (6 months–2 years); settles spontaneously
+ Cardiomyopathy—decreased ventricular ejection; conduction blocks (10–20 years)

New developments

High-precision or conformal radiotherapy

A combination of new imaging technologies (MR, CT, portal imaging), new treatment planning approaches, and high-precision accelerators permit higher radiation doses to more precisely delineated target volumes. By these high-precision techniques, smaller volumes of normal tissue are irradiated, but to a higher dose.

Normal tissue tolerance to re-treatment

Recent studies have shown some tissues and organs have a substantial ability to recover from subclinical radiation injury, allowing the re-treatment of previously irradiated sites. The large capacity of long-term regeneration of the CNS allows the possibility to re-treat parts of the brain or the spinal cord and offers new clinical possibilities for tumours recurring in or near these critical structures.

Endovascular irradiation

Although not strictly belonging to the field of oncology, prevention of restenosis by endovascular irradiation with small beta- or gamma-emitting radioactive sources is a rapidly expanding application of radiation in the cardiology clinic. Radiation has been shown to prevent or delay the formation of new plaques by inhibition of proliferation of the vascular endothelium or smooth muscle cells. This immediate benefit needs to be counterbalanced by the risk of late complications.

Radiotherapy fractionation

Objective

To choose the most appropriate combination of the number of treatments (fractions), overall time, and total dose to achieve the required level of effect on the tumour with the minimal effect to surrounding normal tissues.

Basis of practice

Mathematical models based on clinical and laboratory studies have been developed and the *linear quadratic* has now replaced Ellis as the preferred formula for relating dose and fractionation.

At clinically relevant doses, tumours and early reacting tissues respond to ionizing radiation with a linear relationship between dose and effect—*the linear or α component*. In the late reacting tissues, in the clinically relevant dose range, a large part of the effect is related to the square of the individual dose given—*the β or quadratic element*.

The important implication of the linear quadratic model is that by giving radiotherapy in many small doses, changes in the late reacting tissues should be spared, with little or no alteration in the response of the early reacting normal tissues and of the tumour.

Number of treatments

Advantages of few fractions:

+ Fewer attendances
+ Sparing of resources
+ Quicker response.

Advantages of many fractions:

+ Less severe acute and a lower incidence of late reactions
+ Higher tumour doses can be achieved, so giving the greatest chance of cure.

Expression of radiation dose

The important elements of a course of radiotherapy—fractionation, overall time, and total dose—must always be considered together in order to assess the likely effect of a regime. The dose in the tumour target volume is normally prescribed at the centre of the tumour where the beams employed usually intersect (the intersection dose), but the maximum and minimum levels also need consideration.

Radiosensitivity of tumours

Some tumours, such as lymphoma and seminoma, may be controlled by doses approximately half that required for many carcinomas and sarcomas; others including gliomas and sarcomas, tend to be resistant.

Radiosensitivity of normal tissues

Some tissues are particularly radiosensitive and doses to them must be limited in order to minimize the risk of late damage. If 2 Gy doses are given, then total doses should not exceed 10 Gy to the lens of the eye; the whole kidney, 20 Gy; whole lung, 20 Gy; the spinal cord, 50 Gy; the brain, 60 Gy; and the brachial plexus, 60 Gy. The risk of severe damage rises above 1% at these levels.

The regime chosen must balance risk against likely benefit.

The interfraction interval

After a radiation treatment, some of the damage induced is complete but some can be repaired. With a single daily exposure, all or nearly all of the repairable damage is complete before the next treatment is given. If more than one treatment is given during a day, the duration of time between the fractions must be chosen with care to allow for as much repair as possible in the normal tissues. If this is not followed, then there will be an increase in effect, most importantly, in the late reaction of normal tissues.

Hyperfractionation

By giving many small treatments, usually in a twice-a-day schedule, a higher total radiation dose may be achieved without an increase in the incidence of late morbidity. Such a regime was shown to be superior to conventional radiotherapy in a randomized controlled trial in oropharyngeal carcinoma. This is now being[†] tested more widely in head and neck tumours in a further EORTC trial in which cytotoxic chemotherapy is being incorporated.

Overall time and accelerated radiotherapy

There is now evidence that squamous cell carcinoma in the head and neck and in the lung has the capacity to rapidly proliferate and, in some cases, the tumour cell numbers may double in a few days. This can occur during a course of treatment and be the cause of radiation failure. By shortening the overall duration, the opportunity for this to occur is reduced.

....

† EORTC   European Organization for Research and Treatment of Cancer

In a randomized controlled trial, the CHART† regime, in which treatment is given 3 times on each of 12 consecutive days, proved superior to conventional radiotherapy in non-small cell lung cancer (NSCLC). A split course regime of accelerated radiotherapy was shown to be superior to conventional radiotherapy in head and neck cancer but there was some increase in normal tissue morbidity.

There is now evidence from randomized controlled clinical trials that a reduction of one week in the duration of radiotherapy in head and neck cancer gives major improvement without significant increase in late morbidity.

The optimum regimen

The clinical circumstances dominate the choice of regimen. In palliation, the fewer the attendances, the shorter the course, the sooner a response is achieved, the greater is the benefit for the patient. Regimens used for palliation generally carry a low risk of morbidity and long-term effects are usually irrelevant. Where the highest doses must be given to achieve tumour cure, as when radiotherapy alone is employed with the intention of cure, a low dose per fraction—not exceeding 2 Gy—should be employed in order to minimize the risk of late radiation damage.

A clinical oncologist should employ a wide range of schedules to best deal with all the situations where radiotherapy may benefit the cancer patient.

† CHART   Continuous Hyperfractionated Accelerated Radiotherapy Trial

External beam radiotherapy

Basic principles

Treatment with beams of ionizing radiation produced from a source external to the patient is known as external beam radiotherapy. Superficial tumours are often treated with X-rays of low energy, in the range 80–300 kV. Electrons, emitted from a heated cathode, are accelerated across an X-ray tube, strike a tungsten anode, and undergo bremsstrahlung interactions. The beam size is selected by using metal cone-shaped applicators of different sizes.

The main limitations of such beams are:

- Inherent delivery of high dose to the skin
- Relatively rapid 'fall off' of dose with depth
- Higher absorbed dose in bone compared with soft tissue

Deeper-seated tumours are mostly treated using megavoltage photons. One option is to use a source of Co-60, emitting gamma rays of average energy 1.25 MeV. Source strengths of about 350 TBq are required to achieve a sufficiently high dose rate.

It is more common to use megavoltage X-rays produced by linear accelerators, in which electrons are accelerated to near the speed of light in a waveguide, before striking a thin transmission target. The resultant X-rays can have energies in the range 4–20 MV. Such beams offer advantages of higher penetration, higher dose rate, and better collimation than beams of Co-60.

Megavoltage photons

- Maximum dose below skin surface
- Skin sparing
- Absorbed dose falls off exponentially with depth
- Sharp 'fall off' of dose at beam edge (penumbra)
- Whole-body radiation can be used
- Beam shape modified by metal shields or multi-leaf collimators
- Metal filters can be used to gradient dose
- Treatment from any direction can be used
- Crossfire technique with 2–4 beams gives higher target dose

Some linear accelerators are also configured to produce beams of electrons of various energies, usually in the range 4–20 MeV. Such beams can uniformly treat from skin surface down to a certain depth (related to the energy), with a fairly rapid fall-off in dose beyond that. For

(a)

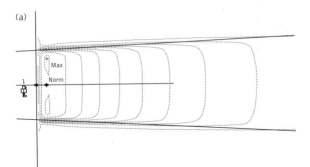

Isodose curves for open beams of 6 MV X-rays.

(b)

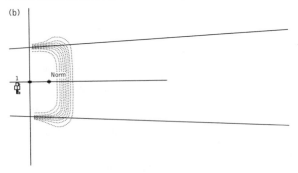

Isodose curves for 12 MeV electrons.

example, 6 MeV electrons will treat to about 1.5 cm deep and 20 MeV to about 5.5 cm. Electrons offer a good alternative to kilovoltage X-rays for treating superficial tumours.

The planning process

There are six major steps in designing and delivering external beam radiotherapy treatment:

1. Beam dosimetry

The pattern of dose distribution from each linear accelerator has to be measured prior to clinical use. Due to absorption properties at such high energies, these measurements can be made using a small ionization chamber dosimeter in a tank of water. The dosimeter tracks across the beam at preset depths and dose profiles are recorded for a range of beam sizes, with and without wedges. It is also essential to measure calibration factors (known as output factors) which define irradiation time required for a specified absorbed dose.

2. Planning Computer

Simple planning can be carried out using tables or plots of measured beam data. Mostly, planning is performed using powerful computers with specialized application software. Calculations are based on measured beam data but also depend on algorithms that allow for varying attenuation and scatter of X-rays in tissues of different densities. This density information is based on CT scans performed with the patient in the treatment position.

3. Target drawing

The most important step in planning radiotherapy is defining the target i.e. volume of tissue to be irradiated. This includes the gross tumour (e.g. as visualized clinically or by imaging) together with surrounding tissues that might have microscopic invasion of tumour cells or which are known to be at risk of spread of disease. A further margin has to be allowed for uncertainties in treatment set-up; these include variations in patient positioning, internal organ movement, and tolerances of machine calibration. It is also essential to define the position of critical organs i.e. those with a lower tolerance to radiation such as the spinal cord, eyes, and kidneys. All can be drawn directly into the planning computer on a set of CT images covering the full extent of the involved area. For less sophisticated treatments, the target and critical organs are defined using anterior and lateral radiographs.

4. Dose planning

The objective of dose planning is to design a treatment plan such that the target is uniformly irradiated to a high dose whilst ensuring that critical organs do not exceed tolerance doses. Parameters that can be varied include:

- Beam size
- Beam direction
- Number of beams
- Relative dose per beam (beam weight)
- Wedging
- Use of compensators

5. Treatment verification

It is essential that beams are correctly positioned and critical organs not over-irradiated. Beams are usually verified by taking radiographs on a radiotherapy simulator prior to treatment; this can also be done during treatment with radiographs or Electronic Portal Imaging Devices (EPID).

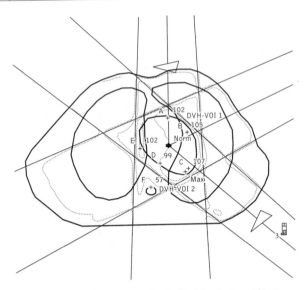

Three radiotherapy beams converging on CT defined volume of lung cancer.

6. Treatment prescription and delivery

The clinical oncologist prescribes the appropriate dose and fractionation schedule. Together with beam configuration information, these form a data set completely describing the intended treatment. They are entered into a computer verification system on the linear accelerator and control set-up and delivery of each treatment.

Areas of development

3D planning

Perhaps the most significant change in radiotherapy practice in the past 15 years has been the direct use of CT scanning for planning. The advantages of CT planning are significant:

- Tumour and critical structures are more readily defined
- Dose calculation is more accurate
- The planning process is truly 3D, offering more options for optimizing the treatment plan

In certain circumstances, adequate coverage of the target whilst avoiding critical organs can only be achieved using beams that are non-coplanar; these calculations can only be performed in 3D utilizing the CT information.

Conformal treatment/multi-leaf collimators

It has always been the aim of radiotherapy to conform high dose volume to the target. Normal practice was to use rectangular beams with limited use of blocking. Inevitably, some normal tissue was unnecessarily irradiated to high doses. Improved levels of conformation can be achieved by positioning shaped alloy blocks in the beam and, automatically, with a feature on the accelerator known as multi-leaf collimators (MLC). Here, the beam can be shaped under computer control by sliding a series of 1 cm-wide leaves into the beam.

By minimizing the amount of normal tissue irradiated to high dose, it may be possible to deliver higher doses to the target, thereby improving tumour control without increasing morbidity.

Target drawing/image fusion

The push toward conformal radiotherapy has highlighted the need to improve tolerances of target drawing. Imaging modalities other than CT (MRI, nuclear medicine, and PET scanning) may improve target definition and there are benefits in overlaying or 'fusing' various image sets.

Dynamic radiotherapy/intensity modulated radiotherapy

With standard techniques it can be difficult to treat an irregularly shaped target in close proximity to a critical organ. This may be improved by using dynamic therapy, where the machine rotates around the patient, continuously emitting X-rays, and with the beam shape constantly changing. Alternatively, the intensity of radiation across stationary beams may be modulated.

Biological planning

Radiotherapy prescription is based on absorbed dose even though different tumours and normal tissues are known to react differently to a given radiation dose. Using mathematical models to compute a 'biological' dose it would then be possible to predict the tumour control probability (TCP) and the normal tissue complication probability (NTCP) associated with various proposed treatment plans, thus forming a better basis for selecting the optimal plan.

Electron beam therapy

Electron beams have been used in treating malignant disease for over three decades. Although electron radiation is radiobiologically equivalent to photon radiation, the physical characteristics of electron beams are preferred over photon beams in the treatment of certain anatomical sites. Unlike photons, electrons possess charge and so interact frequently as they penetrate tissue; the resulting nearly continuous energy loss leads to a well-defined range in tissue (radiation dose deposited beyond a certain depth in tissue in negligible). This treats the target volumes lying within a few centimetres of the skin's surface while sparing any underlying critical structures.

The frequent interactions between the penetrating electrons and the tissues have several deleterious effects. Specifically:

- Large-beam penumbra
- 'Hot' and 'cold' spots beneath surface discontinuities
- Significant changes in dose near inhomogeneities

Production of electron beams

Production of electron beams necessitates the use of electron accelerators such as betatrons, microtrons, or linear accelerators. All these accelerators are capable of producing clinically useful beams of X-rays or electrons. With an X-ray beam, a narrow electron beam emerging from an accelerator strikes a thick, high-atomic-number target to produce bremsstrahlung photons. An appropriately shaped flattening filter converts the forward-directed bremsstrahlung beam into a clinically useful beam of uniform intensity. In an electron beam, the X-ray target is removed and the emerging electrons are scanned magnetically or scattered in foils to produce a uniform broad beam. Most radiation therapy facilities have high-energy accelerators capable of producing both X-ray and electron beams. Thus, radiotherapists have both treatment modalities at their disposal in the design of an optimal treatment.

Since electrons scatter significantly in air, beam-defining cones or 'trimmer' bars are fitted to the head of the treatment machine in order to collimate the beam near the skin's surface. The beam may be shaped further either by fitting a lead or 'cerrobend' aperture at the end of the cone (often called an electron cut-out), or by using lead sheet laid directly on skin.

Dosimetric characteristics of electron beams

The various dosimetric aspects of electron beams in *homogeneous* tissue are as follows:

Depth dose characteristics

Dose builds up slowly to a maximum value and then falls off rapidly, reaching nearly zero dose at a depth equal to the practical electron range. Beyond the practical range, any radiation dose is due entirely to contamination photons produced in the head of the linear accelerator and tissues themselves. The magnitude of the contamination dose varies but is usually 1–5% of maximum dose depending on the energy of the beam and design of accelerator.

Effect of field size

The shape of a depth dose curve is independent of field size when all field dimensions are larger than the practical range. For smaller fields, depth of dose maximum shifts towards shallower depths while dose fall-off becomes less steep.

Effect of incident energy

The depth of penetration of an electron beam is determined by its incident energy. Practical range (in centimetres) of an electron beam in water is given approximately by:

$$R_p \approx \frac{E_0}{2}$$

where E_0 is incident beam energy expressed in mega electron volts (MeV).

Similarly, the clinically useful range—the depth at which the dose falls to 80% of its maximum value—is given by:

$$d_{80} \approx \frac{E_0}{3}$$

The surface dose (commonly defined as dose at 0.5 mm depth) is significantly higher for an electron beam than for a megavoltage photon beam and ranges from about 85% of dose maximum at low energies (less than 10 MeV) to about 95% at higher energies. The rate at which dose falls off beyond the depth of dose maximum is also energy-dependent, with the rate of dose fall-off decreasing as the beam energy increases.

Accelerators that offer an electron beam mode generally allow selection of one of several available electron beam energies. Beam energies may range from as low as 4 MeV up to 50 MeV in some cases. However, energies most commonly used clinically tend to be in the range 6–15 MeV.

Beam profile and penumbra

Beam penumbra tend to be larger for electron beams than for photon beams. For electron beams, dose falls to 90% of central axis value approximately 1 cm inside the geometric field edge for depths near the dose maximum; a 10×10 cm^2 beam, for instance, produces an 'effective' field size of only 8×8 cm^2. The corresponding distance for a photon beam is only about 0.5 cm. Thus, a larger electron beam is required to cover a given target to a clinically useful dose. This property of electron beams makes abutting of photon and electron beams problematical since a uniform dose across a field junction cannot be achieved at all depths.

Near-surface irregularities and tissue inhomogeneities

Variations in the surface contour and composition of tissue (i.e. tissue inhomogeneities) strongly influence the shape of the electron beam dose distribution. Depending on the anatomical site, these effects may be clinically significant and an estimate of their magnitude may be required.

Methods of dose calculation

Dose calculations for electron beams are not as accurate as those for photon beams. As a result, the use of electron beams may be prevented where the accuracy of the delivered dose distribution is critical. However, accuracy of predicted dose distributions will improve as better methods of dose calculation evolve.

Ray-line method

This is the earliest (and simplest) form of dose calculation. Electrons are assumed to travel along ray-lines originating from a single 'virtual' source. An appropriate shift of the percentage depth dose curve along these ray-lines accounts for the effect of tissue inhomogeneities. Dose distribution calculated in this manner does not reflect the lateral scattering of electrons near the edge of inhomogeneities or near-surface irregularities. Since these effects can lead to considerable dose perturbations, the ray-line method has been largely supplanted by the pencil beam method.

Pencil beam method

This method of dose calculation decomposes a broad electron beam into a set of narrow 'pencil beams'. The dose at any given point in irradiated tissue is the summation of the contributions from each of these pencil beams. Individual pencils can be altered appropriately to allow for the effects of inhomogeneities. Thus, some account is taken of lateral scattering of the electrons as well as changes along the ray-lines. However, the methods used for altering the pencils beams are, by necessity, approximate.

'Monte Carlo'

A direct computer simulation of individual penetrating electrons is now emerging as a clinically viable tool for dose calculation. This calculational technique simulates individual electron trajectories using random numbers to sample theoretical electron-scattering cross-sections; its reliance on random numbers has earned the technique the name 'Monte Carlo'.

Clinical applications

Breast cancer

- Treatment of breast or chest wall after surgery
- Photon beams delivered tangentially or perpendicularly
- Possible side-effect on underlying lung but rare due to rapid dose fall-off

Skin

- Useful for skin lesions
- Wire meshes used to increase skin dose
- Safe over cartilage and bone e.g. ear
- Lip and eyelid shields used to protect eye and mouth
- Total skin irradiation possible e.g. mycosis fungoides

Head/neck

- Useful for positive neck nodes in head/neck cancer
- Photon beams used to irradiate entire region including spinal cord
- Electron beams used additionally, except for spinal cord

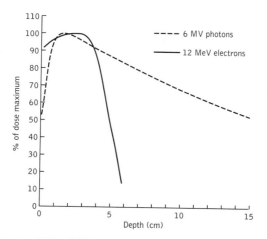

Tissue penetration of different types of radiotherapy beams.

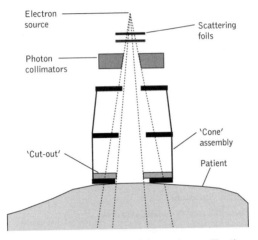

A schematic representation of a typical electron beam collimation system (some components are not shown).

Intra-operative electron therapy

Intra-operative radiotherapy using electron beams has also been used clinically. This technique involves exposing the target surgically, thus allowing a specialized applicator (i.e. collimator) to be used to irradiate the target. In this way, any normal tissue overlying the target is spared. The labour and resource intensive nature of this technique limit its widespread use.

Treatment planning

The radiation oncologist decides optimum radiation dose distribution for a patient prior to commencing treatment planning. The aim of treatment planning is to model that dose distribution as closely as possible using a number of radiation beams of appropriate modality and energy. The direction and size of each beam has to be determined, together with radiation dose to be given and any modification that may be required to the inherent dose distribution of the beam. To achieve this aim, it is necessary to know the precise dose distribution that will result from any treatment beam. This is obtained from prior radiation measurements in unit-density tissue-equivalent material, made available as a set of charts or tables (known as the *depth dose distribution*). These data specify the dose at any point in the beam relative to a reference point (usually the point of maximum dose on the central axis of the beam). The depth of the reference point increases with increasing beam energy and is in the range 1–3 cm for commonly available megavoltage (MV) treatment beams.

Dose distributions are required for a whole range of clinical settings available on a treatment machine. The relative dose distribution for the patient is obtained by summing the individual distributions for all beams and is displayed as a map showing lines of constant dose, known as *isodose lines*. The radiation oncologist prescribes an absolute dose to an isodose line and to achieve this dose each individual beam must be calibrated in terms of the number of machine units required to give a specified dose to its reference point.

The machine units control the quantity of radiation given in an individual exposure. This absolute calibration is again carried out by prior radiation measurements, provided in tabular form as a set of output factors. These also vary with the possible clinical machine settings and must be measured over the complete range to be used.

Types of radiotherapy

There are two types of radiotherapy:
* *Palliative*, where the aim is the relief of symptoms.
* *Radical*, where the aim is to achieve a cure.

Palliative radiotherapy

Treatment planning for palliative radiotherapy is a simple procedure as treatment usually consists of a single or parallel opposed treatment beams, where the patient is considered to be unit-density tissue-equivalent material of uniform thickness.

For single beams the dose is usually prescribed to the reference point, which is the point of maximum absorbed dose in the central axis of the beam (or occasionally to a point at depth). Parallel, opposed pairs of beams are normally prescribed to mid-separation of the patient, again in the central axis of the beam.

In all cases, treatment planning can be performed manually from the set of depth dose and output tables for the treatment beams as already described. Prescribed doses for palliative irradiation are usually low, so doses to vulnerable organs close to or within the treated volume are not a problem.

Radical radiotherapy

Treatment planning for radical radiotherapy provides a more complicated problem and is carried out with computerized treatment planning systems. The main aim is to provide a high and uniform dose to the target volume while ensuring that the dose to any vulnerable organs is kept as low as possible and within specified constraints. It is important to determine carefully the anatomy of the patient in the region to be treated and the location of the target volume within this region, so that the dose distribution can be calculated accurately. Methods used depend on whether the dose calculations are to be performed on a single two-dimensional plane through the patient or over the full three-dimensional treatment volume.

The simplest method is to determine the external contour by a mechanical or optical device and the target position from AP and lateral radiographs. Use of a treatment simulator can also provide the information required for two-dimensional planning especially if it is equipped with a computerized tomography (CT) option.

Full CT scanning is essential for three-dimensional planning and is by far the best technique, as it provides all the necessary information as well as a density map of the patient that can be used for dose calculation.

Magnetic resonance (MR) scanning can provide better diagnostic information than CT but produces geometrical distortions in the image that must be corrected. MR scanning is therefore only used in conjunction with CT planning.

In all cases it is essential during the treatment planning process that patients consistently remain in the treatment position; immobilization devices can assist in this.

The correct determination of the planning target volume (PTV) is obviously essential to the success of radiotherapy. The gross tumour volume (GTV) is that which is palpable or radiologically demonstrable, but must be surrounded by a margin to allow for microscopic spread, giving a clinical target volume (CTV).

A further margin must be applied to the CTV to allow for geometrical inaccuracies in the treatment set-up and patient/organ movement during treatment, and this defines the planning target volume. Progression from the GTV to the PTV is straightforward in two-dimensional planning. However, enlarging the CTV to the PTV, slice by slice on CT may not give correct margins in three dimensions when there is a significant difference in the size of the CTV on adjoining slices. Further problems exist in defining margins at the superior and inferior limits of the CTV due to the width of the CT slice. Problems can be overcome by the use of three-dimensional volume-growing algorithms that are available on computerized planning systems.

Beam arrangements

Optimum beam arrangements required to treat a particular site have been widely investigated and adopted into protocols in each radio-therapy centre, with little variation from one centre to another. However, some sites in the head and neck and the chest may require individualized beam arrangements.

In general, co-planar beam arrangements are used, but the avail-ability of fully three-dimensional treatment planning systems allows the placement of non-coplanar fields. The number of beams required is less with a high-beam energy and a small depth to the centre of the target. In the pelvis, three or four beams are used at the highest avail-able energy, preferably 12–16 MV. Three beams are sufficient in the chest, using an energy of 6–8 MV, as at higher energies the range of the secondary electrons in lung tissue makes the calculation of the dose distribution uncertain. In the head and neck region, two fields are generally sufficient, using an energy 4–6 MV, as it may be necessary to provide a high dose close to the entrance surface while minimizing the exit skin dose.

The central axis of the beams pass through one point (known as the isocentre) which is placed at the centre of the PTV, with the directions of the treatment beams chosen to avoid the irradiation of sensitive structures. Placing the beams uniformly around the patient is advan-tageous in obtaining a uniform dose distribution over the target, and the selection of beam directions where the depth of the target is kept small reduces the overall dose to the patient.

Beam size

Beam sizes should be chosen so that the resulting high-dose volume encompasses the PTV with a minimum dose not <95% of the iso-centre dose. To achieve this, field dimensions must be larger than the PTV due to the fall off in dose towards the edge of the beam. The margins required are typically in the region of 6–10 mm and depend on how many beams contribute to the fall off in dose.

A development arising from three-dimensional treatment planning that assists greatly in the determination of beam size is the beam's eye view (BEV) approach. Here the observer is placed at the radiation source and the projection of any structure that has been outlined on a CT image set is displayed on a plane normal to the central axis of the beam. A projection of the beam portal is superimposed and its size can be determined according to the projection of the PTV. The approach also assists in the selection of the optimal beam directions with respect to the separation of the target and vulnerable organs.

The technique of conformal radiotherapy is increasingly used in which the beam shape is matched more closely to the PTV. This is achieved by the use of customized blocks or multi-leaf collimators (MLC) on individual beams, and in both cases the use of BEV is essential.

Beam weight

The relative contribution of a beam to the treatment plan is known as the beam weight. The definition varies between centres and is defined either as the relative contribution of the dose to the isocentre or to the reference point. The adjustment of beam weights is a method of achieving uniformity of dose over the PTV and giving approximately the same dose to the isocentre from each beam will give good uniformity. Care should be taken to ensure that the entrance dose under the beam portals is not excessive.

The inherent dose distribution of a beam can be altered by the insertion of a wedge-shaped filter that produces a dose gradient in one dimension across the beam. Wedges can be used to compensate for obliquity at the skin surface or to assist in obtaining dose uniformity in the PTV when the beams are not uniformly spaced around the patient. Wedges are characterized by the angle through which the isodose lines are tilted and normally a selection are available (or can otherwise be achieved), producing tilts of up to 60°.

Selection of the optimum beam weights and wedges is assessed by the closeness of the resulting dose distribution to that required by the radiation oncologist. Modification of the inherent dose distribution over the beam in two dimensions is possible by the use of physical compensators or, more recently, by the dynamic movement of the leaves of an MLC.

The use of the treatment simulator depends on the patient data used for planning. In three-dimensional CT planning, the radiation oncologist usually outlines the CTV on the relevant CT slices together with the outline of any vulnerable organs. The CT data represent the patient with computer graphics used to simulate the treatment beams. This can be thought of as virtual simulation and the patient only visits the treatment simulator at the end of the treatment planning process to have the treatment verified.

Treatment sheet

The final action of the treatment planning process is to produce a treatment sheet that provides a set of instructions to allow the treatment radiographer to set up the patient as planned and to deliver the correct dose distribution, including the number of monitor units to be applied to each beam. Accuracy has to be assured by a set of checks at all stages of the planning process, and these should form part of a quality assurance system, such as ISO 9002, with fully documented procedures and work instructions.

Total body irradiation (TBI)

Treatment intensification with high doses of chemotherapy and/or radiotherapy is used to try to improve cure rates for sensitive tumours. In some benign diseases such as aplastic anaemia and thalassaemia, myelo-ablative therapy, usually with chemotherapy alone, precedes engraftment of normal donor marrow to overcome the underlying host problem.

Aims

- To eliminate any residual malignant disease.
- To ablate residual marrow to permit engraftment of peripheral stem cells or bone marrow.
- To produce immune suppression (especially for non-haplotype identical grafts).

Indications for high-dose therapy

Acute lymphatic leukaemia

- Patients at very high risk of relapse (such as those presenting with a white cell count of >100 000 or with specific chromosome abnormalities) may be treated in first remission.
- Second or subsequent remission—any patients who are not excluded by age or probability of complications.

Acute myeloid leukaemia

High-dose consolidation therapy with chemotherapy, TBI, and bone marrow transplantation or stem cell rescue should be considered for all patients aged 2–50 years with a compatible donor.

Lymphoma

Consider treatment for patients with high-grade non-Hodgkin's lymphoma after a first relapse; and for Hodgkin's disease patients with primary chemoresistant disease or widespread disease after remission induction or after relapse.

Myeloma

Best tolerated in patients <50 years with good performance status and response to initial chemotherapy.

Other malignancies

These include advanced germ cell tumours, neuroblastoma.

Types of haemopoetic reconstitution

- **Autologous** Transplant may be peripheral stem cells or cryo-preserved marrow obtained before high-dose therapy.
- **Allogeneic** Matched or mismatched (1 haplotype identical) bone marrow is usually used, and may be obtained from a family member or from a donor panel.

Pre-treatment screening

- The patient's disease should be in remission.
- There should be adequate renal, cardiac, hepatic, and pulmonary function to cope with the toxicity of chemotherapy and TBI.
- Exposure to medication with the same side-effects as TBI, or likely to potentiate its side-effects, should be assessed. Common interactions: neurotoxicity with asparaginase, renal with platinum or ifosfamide, pulmonary with methotrexate or bleomycin, cardiac with cyclosphosphamide or anthracyclines.
- The need for additional therapy to sites such as the central nervous system, testes, mediastinum i.e. areas of sanctuary or bulk disease.
- Informed consent must be obtained.

Preparation

TBI is usually preceded by high-dose cyclophosphamide given 48–72 hours before treatment. Experimental results suggest the possible benefit of giving cyclophosphamide after TBI as used in the Memorial Sloan Kettering protocol. Other combinations of chemotherapy may also be used before TBI.

Anti-emetics, including a 5HT antagonist, are given with dexamethasone, intravenously, 1 hour before treatment starts. If additional sedation is required phenobarbitone or diazepam may be used. For very young children, anaesthesia with ketamine may be necessary.

Technique

- Linear accelerator or cobalt unit—optimum energy around 6 MV.
- Fractionated TBI is preferred for reasons of convenience.
- Patient lies on couch behind a perspex sheet (to provide full skin bolus) either on their side or back and side alternately.
- Treatment is given by opposed fields for half each treatment time.
- The couch is placed at an extended distance from the machine to obtain the field size required to cover the whole body.
- The dose distribution will be inhomogenous because of variation in AP/PA separation along the body and because of density differences (especially the lung). This can be compensated for by using

bolus or lung shielding but is unnecessary using schedules described here, where doses do not exceed tolerance for any normal tissues.

• The maximum risk of damage is to the lung.

Calculation of dose

Paired lithium fluoride dose meters or diodes are used to measure dose distribution throughout the body. These are placed on the skin at defined sites in the upper and lower lung, mediastinum, abdomen, and pelvis. Midline doses are taken as the average of AP and PA dose meter readings or CT scanning of the whole body can be used with a planning computer to calculate doses throughout the body.

Dose schedules

Adults

The optimum fractionated doses are determined as 13.2 Gy–14.4 Gy depending on the point of dose prescription. The maximum lung dose is preferred, as this is the dose limiting toxicity, and should not exceed l4.4 Gy.

Children

May tolerate slightly higher doses than adults. In the MRC protocol, treatment is given in 8 fractions of 1.8 Gy over 4 days. Many other dose schedules are in common use and have been found by experience to be satisfactory.

Toxicity of treatment

Acute effects

• Nausea and vomiting commonly starts about 6 hours after the first fraction.
• Parotid swelling—occurs in the first 24 hours and then resolves spontaneously, although often leaving dry mouth.
• Hypotension.
• Fever—abolished by steroids.
• Diarrhoea—occurs at day 5 as a result of gastrointestinal mucositis.

Delayed toxicity

• Pneumonitis presenting with dyspnoea and characteristic X-ray appearances.
• Somnolence due to transient demyelination occurs at 6–8 weeks and is characterized by sleepiness, anorexia, and in some cases nausea which settles spontaneously within 7–10 days.

Late toxicity

- Cataracts occur in <20% of patients, incidence increases at 2–6 years, but then appears to plateau.

- Hormonal changes—azoospermia and amenorrhoea with consequent sterility are the norm; very occasionally fertility has been maintained leading to normal pregnancies with no increased incidence of abnormalities in the offspring

- Hypothyroidism may result from damage to the thyroid alone or in combination with pituitary damage.

- In children, there may be impaired production of growth hormone which, added to the effect of early epiphyseal fusion from TBI, results in stunting of growth.

- Induction of second malignancy—there is a 5-fold increase in the risk of second malignancies. Brain tumours may be attributed to the TBI and oral and rectal carcinomas have been reported.

- Malignancy of the lymphoid system may result from the prolonged immune suppression.

Clinical outcome

Clinical trials have shown better survival after high-dose therapy with appropriate rescue than after conventional chemotherapy for selected patients with acute myeloid and acute lymphatic leukaemia. Some benefit has been shown for patients with high-risk node-positive breast cancer, stage IV neuroblastoma, and high-grade lymphoma, but the role of high-dose therapy in these settings needs further clarification.

Comparisons of chemotherapy with and without TBI for conditioning are not conclusive. TBI is preferred where more immune suppression is needed (e.g. mismatched grafts). Chemotherapy is preferred for benign disease because of the increased risk of second tumour induction with TBI. Otherwise, choices are based on the differing patterns of toxicity of the modalities of conditioning.

TBI may be considered for more frequent use in adults where growth and developmental problems are less important.

Brachytherapy

A form of radiation treatment where the radiation sources are placed within or close to the target volume i.e. the sources are placed at the heart of the tumour.

Indications

- The extent of the neoplasm must be known precisely, as treatment is often given to a relatively small volume and 'geographic miss' of tumour is a significant risk.

- The site should be accessible for both inserting and removing sources and allowing satisfactory geometric positioning of those sources.

Advantages

- The probability of local tumour control increases with increasing radiation dose, but so does the probability of normal tissue damage. Brachytherapy allows the delivery of a localized high radiation dose to a small tumour volume, increasing the chance of local control. There is a sharp fall-off of radiation dose in the surrounding normal tissue, therefore the risks of complication are reduced.

- The overall duration of brachytherapy is short, generally between 2–7 days. The constant low-dose irradiation takes advantage of the different rates of repair and re-population of normal and malignant tissue to produce differential cell killing, enhancing the therapeutic ratio.

- Hypoxic cells are relatively resistant to radiation treatment. Re-oxygenation may occur during low-dose-rate radiotherapy, with initially resistant hypoxic cells becoming well aerated and sensitive.

- The dose distribution within the tumour volume is often not homogeneous. Treatment is often prescribed to the minimum dose received around the periphery of the treated volume. Areas close to the radiation sources in the centre of the tumour volume often receive up to twice this dose. Hypoxic cells are situated in avascular, sometimes necrotic areas in the centre of tumours and the higher doses received in the centre help to compensate for the relative radio-resistance of these hypoxic cells.

- Irregular-shaped tumours can be treated by judicious positioning of radiation sources and critical surrounding normal tissues can be avoided.

Disadvantages

• Many sources emit gamma rays and nursing and medical staff may be exposed to low but significant doses of radiation from the patient. Staff exposure can be minimized by after-loading techniques or the use of low-energy radionuclides.

• Large tumours are usually unsuitable, although brachytherapy may be employed as a boost treatment following reduction in size by external beam radiotherapy and/or chemotherapy.

• Radiation dose falls off rapidly from the sources according to the inverse square law. In order to treat the required tissue volume adequately, accurate geometric positioning is critical. The spatial arrangement of sources used varies, depending on the type of source applicator, the anatomical position of the tumour, and the surrounding dose-limiting normal tissue. Accurate positioning of sources or applicators requires special skill and training and this is not universally available.

• Surrounding structures such as lymph nodes that may contain overt or microscopic cancer will not be irradiated by the implant or intracavity treatment.

Types

• Intracavity—radioactive material into body cavities
  - *Uses*—gynae cancers
    - —bronchial cancers
    - —oesophageal cancers
    - —bile duct cancer
• Interstitial—radioactive material in tissues
  - *Uses*—breast cancer
    - —tongue cancer
    - —floor of mouth cancer
    - —anal cancer
• Surface of tumour
    - —skin
    - —eye

Implants can be classified as manually inserted, after-loading, or remote after-loading. Manual insertion of radiation sources should be avoided if possible owing to the radiation hazards to operating staff and nurses. After-loading is when radioactive material is loaded into hollow needles, catheters, or applicators that have been inserted into the tumour area previously. Manipulation of these 'cold' applicators carries no radiation hazard to medical and nursing staff, so that time can safely be taken to ensure optimal source geometry.

After-loading with radioactive material can be manual or remote (using machines such as the Selectron, commonly used to treat gynaecological cancer). For remote after-loading stainless steel pellets containing, for example, caesium in glass, are moved pneumatically from a computer-controlled lead-lined safe into intrauterine and vaginal applicators. This completely eliminates irradiation of theatre and nursing staff.

Some remote after-loading devices work at a very high dose rate e.g. the Microselectron (high-intensity iridium sources) or the Cathetron (high-intensity cobalt sources) and treatment is over in a matter of minutes.

Most implants are of the removable type—the radiation sources are removed after the delivery of the prescribed treatment dose. However, permanent implantations can be performed using relatively short half-life isotopes such as ^{125}I or ^{198}Au, which are implanted into the tumours in the form of seeds which remain after the radiation has decayed virtually completely.

Radionuclides

Gamma emitters

Radium was used for many years as the major source of gamma rays for brachytherapy. This is now obsolete. The major source of gamma rays is the gaseous daughter product, radon. Radium tubes and needles must be gas-tight and frequently checked for leaks. The gamma rays used are very penetrating and very thick lead shields are required to provide adequate radiation protection. Caesium-137 has no gaseous daughter products, a very useful half-life of 30 years, and a somewhat less penetrating 660 KeV gamma ray—it has largely replaced radium, especially for gynaecological work.

Iridium-192 is manufactured in the form of flexible wire and has many advantages over traditional radium or caesium needles for interstitial brachytherapy. Thin wires (0.3 mm in diameter) can be inserted into flexible nylon tubes or after-loading needles previously implanted into the tumour. Thicker wires (0.6 mm diameter), in the form of hairpins, can be inserted directly into a tumour through suitable introducers. In the USA, iridium is also available in the form of seeds sealed in thin plastic coating. Iridium produces a gamma ray of 330 KeV and lead shields 2 cm in thickness provide good protection. The only major disadvantage of iridium is the relatively short half-life (74 days), so that fresh material should be used for each implant.

Iodine-125 has a half-life of 59.6 days and is used for permanent implants of the prostate. As well as having a relatively short half-life, the gamma rays produced by this radionuclide (27–35 KeV) are of very low energy and very little radiation is emitted from a patient following the implant, allowing early discharge from hospital.

Beta emitters

The major use of plaques emitting beta-ray radiation is in the treatment of eye tumours. Plaques can be made of Strontium-90 or Ruthenium-106/Rhodium-106.

Neutron emitters

Californium-252 has been used in the past to treat gynaecological tumours. The advantage of neutron-emitting sources is that they are more effective against hypoxic tumours. The radiation hazards involved have restricted the use of such sources.

Dosimetry

Radioactive material is implanted into tissues according to distribution rules that vary according to the system used. In Europe the classical Parker–Paterson and Quimby systems have largely been superseded by the Paris system which is particularly suitable for iridium wire implants. Wire of the same linear intensity is used and sources are arranged in parallel, straight, equidistant lines, 8–20 mm apart. To compensate for 'uncrossed' ends, the wires are 20–30% longer than the length required to treat the tumour. In a volume implant, sources in cross-section should be arranged in either equilateral triangles or squares.

The dose to the tumour can be calculated manually, using graphs such as Oxford cross line curves, or by computer. The basal dose rate (the mean of minimum values between sources) is first calculated. The treatment dose (e.g. 65 Gy in 7 days) is prescribed to the reference dose line (85% of the basal dose).

The prescription point for surface applicators such as moulds and some intracavity treatment is usually 0.5–1 cm from the applicator. A special case is intracavitary gynaecological treatment. The most frequently used prescribing point is the Manchester A point, defined as a point 2 cm lateral to the uterine canal and 2 cm above the cervical os. The dose calculated at this point is a good predictor of late radiation damage to the ureter, bladder, rectum, and other pelvic organs. The International Commission of Radiation Units (ICRU) Report 38[1] has proposed that the volume (defined in height, thickness, and width enclosed by a 60 Gy isodose line) should be used for reporting absorbed dose following gynaecological treatments.

Future developments

There is increasing use of sophisticated three-dimensional planning techniques incorporating CT or MRI scans to determine the dosage to the whole tumour and to critical normal tissues. As well as defining the dose in purely physical terms, the biological effects in different tissues may be expressed as biological effective doses.

Radiation exposure to staff has been reduced by the increased use of high-dose-rate remote after-loading machines. The complication rate following fractionated high-dose gynaecological insertions is less than that following manually inserted low-dose sources. Continuous low-dose-rate implants may be replaced by high-dose 'pulsed' insertions with optimization of the dose distribution and more homogeneous irradiation of the target volume.

Intra-operative radiotherapy

A fundamental problem with radiotherapy is targeting diseased tissues while avoiding unaffected normal structures. Various approaches are possible including:

• Increasing sophisticated planning and treatment delivery for external beam radiotherapy (EBRT)
• Brachytherapy
• Radio-immunotherapy
• Boron neutron capture therapy (BNCT)
• Intra-operative radiotherapy (IORT)

There is some overlap between these techniques e.g. implantation of brachytherapy sources will be done under general anaesthetic for a variety of diseases, including prostate cancer, and can thus be termed 'intra-operative'.

The attraction of IORT is that affected tissues can be surgically exposed and selectively treated with reduced morbidity to non-affected tissues The principal drawback is the need for specialist additional equipment in the operating theatre. Also, there is a consequent increased need for radiation protection for staff in the presence of therapeutic (as opposed to diagnostic) radiation exposure. The need for the radiation oncologist to be present throughout imposes a further constraint on IORT compared to EBRT where patients can be treated without this requirement.

Surveys

Long-term follow-up data are limited but animal studies suggest that IORT exposures up to 30 Gy carry little risk of long-term sequelae as long as sensitive structures such as major nerves, blood vessels, the spinal cord, or the small bowel are kept out of the irradiation field. The threshold for nerve damage is 20–25 Gy with a latent period of 6–9 months with little damage seen below 10–15 Gy in large animal models.

A further factor to be considered is late malignancy—a number of studies in dogs have reported a high incidence of sarcomas induced by IORT compared to other treatment modalities. Issues such as treatment planning are clearly complex, as only limited advanced data can be available.[2]

Specific tumours

Rectal cancer

• May be helpful in both primary and recurrent tumours
• Complex treatment

* High cost
* Little hard data

Stomach and oesophagus

* Dose of up to 20 Gy—safe
* Higher doses—significant complications
* No randomized data

Bile duct

* Limited benefit in unresectable bile duct tumours
* Complex treatment
* May be role in minimal residual disease

Pancreas

* Technique feasible
* Toxicity acceptable
* Little (no) benefit

Head and neck cancer

* Safe, tolerated
* Encouraging results from limited number of centres
* Little hard data
* May be helpful if minimal residual disease or recurrent disease

Brain

* Poor results
* Tumours spread along white tracts
* Boron neutron capture therapy (BNCT) Boron compounds exposed to a low-energy neutron beam undergo neutron capture, releasing lithium 7 nuclei and alpha particles—range less than 1 cell diameter. Early useful results; 15% long-term survival in Japan.

Other tumours

* May be of value in paediatric and soft-tissue sarcomas
* No randomized trials

Conclusions

IORT is a promising technique but limited by the technical and logistic problems already outlined. The continued development of conformal planning and delivery techniques for EBRT will reduce the therapeutic gain that can be obtained from intra-operative treatment. In addition, conformal radiotherapy (CRT) is more reproducible in set-up and dosimetry and poses no special radiobiological problems as in most cases fractionation is not changed significantly.

The lack of phase III data is likely to limit the development of IORT and restrict its use to specialist centres with a research base for evaluation of long-term results. At present, IORT cannot be regarded as part of mainstream radiation oncology practice.

The role of unsealed radionuclides

Nuclear medicine in oncology is used to localize the primary tumour, to determine tumour size, and to detect metastases. Radioactive tracers may also be used to monitor the response to therapy and detect recurrences.

Radio-labelled tracers

A radiopharmaceutical consists of a pharmaceutical attached to a radionuclide that emits gamma rays. The kinetics or distribution of the radiopharmaceutical may vary from the normal because of a pathological process e.g. a malignant tumour. Biochemical changes in tumours cannot be detected by morphology. In this respect scintigraphy, reflecting regional biochemistry, is unique compared with other imaging modalities. Anatomical and functional information are often complementary.

Several radiopharmaceuticals are used for both diagnosis and treatment; well-known examples are iodine[123] and ^{131}I which localize avidly in functioning thyroid tissue. Other simple radiopharmaceuticals are thallium-201 (^{201}T1) and gallium-67 (^{67}Ga). The ideal radionuclide for scintigraphic imaging does not exist, but technetiuin-99m (^{99m}Tc) has many favourable characteristics.

Scintigraphic methods

Traditionally, gamma cameras are used for scintigraphic imaging. Planar images and whole-body images are acquired during a period of several minutes by a stationary gamma camera. With single photon emission tomography (SPET), cross-sectional images can be obtained using computer techniques similar to those in CT. The main advantages of SPET are greater sensitivity and accurate three-dimensional localization of lesions.

Positron emission tomography (PET)

PET employs radionuclides that emit positrons and provides quantitative tomographic images. Glucose utilization is measured with ^{18}F-labelled fluorodeoxyglucose and cerebral blood flow has been studied with ^{15}O-labelled water. PET scanning may be useful to identify primary tumours and metastases, and to study tumour vitality, cell turnover rates, and metabolic response to therapy.

Applications in diagnosis and follow-up

Bone scintigraphy

Bone scintigraphy is normally performed 2–4 hours after the injection of 550 MBq of ^{99m}Tc-labelled methylene disphosphonate (^{99m}Tc-medronate, MDP) or hydroxymethylene disphosphonate (^{99m}Tc-oxidronate, HDP). Multiple planar images or a whole-body survey of the skeleton are obtained. Skeletal scintigraphy has high sensitivity for the detection of primary and metastatic bone lesions. In the absence of reactive osteoblastic activity, the lesion itself may appear on the bone scan as a 'cold' defect.

High sensitivity (80–100%) has been reported in patients with breast carcinoma, prostatic carcinoma, bronchogenic carcinoma, gastric carcinoma, osteogenic sarcoma, cervix carcinoma, Ewing's sarcoma, head and neck carcinomas, neuroblastoma, and ovarian carcinoma. Lower sensitivity, around 75%, has been found in melanoma, small-cell lung tumours, Hodgkin's disease, renal-cell carcinoma, rhabdomyosarcoma, multiple myeloma, and bladder carcinoma.

Liver scintigraphy

The conventional liver scintigram is performed after IV administration of 50–100 MBq of ^{99m}Tc-labelled colloidal particles varying in size from 0.3–1.0 mm. The radioactive agent accumulates in the cells of the reticulo-endothelial system by phagocytosis. The reticulo-endothelial system cells are homogeneously distributed in the liver and spleen, and to a lesser extent in bone, marrow, and lungs.

The most common indication for liver scintigraphy used to be the detection of space-occupying lesions. Nowadays, ultrasonography and CT are generally considered to be more effective modalities than scintigraphy.

The solitary non-cystic lesion may pose a clinical problem. Non-invasive differentiation between haemangioma and metastasis or between hepatoma, hepatocellular carcinoma, follicular nodular hyperplasia, and metastasis is important for the clinical management of the patient. Scintigraphic studies with ^{99m}Tc-labelled erythrocytes, iminodiacetic acids (IDA), or with ^{67}Ga can be used as non-invasive methods for a more specific characterization of the tumour in addition to colloid scintigraphy.

Thyroid scintigraphy

^{131}I as radioiodine, ^{123}I as sodium iodide, and ^{99m}Tc as sodium pertechnetate are the radionuclides used for scintigraphic visualization of the thyroid gland. Although ^{131}I is cheap and readily available, its major disadvantages are its long physical half-life and α-emissions, resulting in a considerable radiation dose to the thyroid and the gastrointestinal tract. ^{123}I has excellent physical properties for imaging and a physical half-life of 13 hours, but its use is limited due to its cost. ^{99m}Tc is trapped in the thyroid, but is not organified and washes out from the gland over time.

The indications for thyroid scintigraphy in oncology are:

• Evaluation of a solitary or dominant nodule.

• Follow-up after surgery for differentiated thyroid cancer.

Thyroid scintigraphy with ^{99m}Tc and ^{123}I can be used to assign probability of malignant disease on the basis of the functional status of the nodule. Hyperfunctioning nodules are almost always benign, but malignancy can be found in 4% of the hot nodules. The majority of non-functioning nodules represent benign cysts and adenomas; 16–20% of solitary non-functioning nodules contain thyroid cancer.

Scintigraphy of medullary thyroid cancer is possible with ^{201}Tl, ^{99m}Tc-DMSA-V, ^{131}I- or ^{123}I-labelled m-iodobenzylguanidine (MIBG), and ^{111}In- or ^{123}I-labelled somatostatin analogues. The sensitivity of these methods in detecting the primary tumour or its metastases is generally low. For the new tracer, ^{111}In-octreotide, the sensitivity for the detection of medullary thyroid cancer is 66%, compared with 35% for ^{131}I-MIBG. The value of ^{131}I-MIBG scintigraphy is to determine whether a patient may benefit from therapy with this radiopharmaceutical.

Imaging of neuroendocrine tumours

Phaeochromocytoma and other neural crest tumours can successfully be detected with ^{123}I or ^{131}I-MIBG. The molecular structure of MIBG has some similarity to noradrenaline. The scintigraphic study is done at intervals of 24, 48, and occasionally 72 hours after intravenous injections of 370 MBq of ^{123}I-MIBG or 37 MBq of ^{131}I-MIBG. With a sensitivity of 92% and specificity of nearly 100% in neuroblastoma, MIBG scintigraphy is a useful technique for the detection, staging, and follow-up of this disease. Additionally, it serves as an indicator for potential therapy using ^{131}I-MIBG.

Somatostatin is a polypeptide hormone with a short biological half-life. Receptors for this hormone are present on many cells of neuroendocrine origin. A long-acting analogue, octreotide, was synthesized for therapy. ^{111}In-octreotide was developed for imaging, performed 24 and 48 hours after injection of 111 MBq. The potential clinical value of somatostatin receptor scintigraphy is in the detection of occult primary tumours, screening of metastases for staging, follow-up of therapy, and selection of patients who might benefit from palliative treatment with unlabelled octreotide.

The cumulative sensitivity of ^{111}In-octreotide scintigraphy for the detection of endocrine pancreatic tumours is around 75%, and for carcinoid tumours, around 85%. These tumours are often small and not easily recognized on CT or MRI.

Monoclonal antibodies

The development of monoclonal antibodies that recognize human tumour-associated antigens has implications for nuclear medicine. Antibodies and fragments (Fab) can be labelled with ^{131}I, ^{123}I, ^{111}In, and ^{99m}Tc for scintigraphy. In colorectal cancer, scintigraphy with monoclonal antibodies is potentially valuable in detecting occult disease, localizing recurrent disease when serum markers are elevated, and differentiating between viable tumour and post-surgical fibrosis. The potential roles for radio-immunoscintigraphy in ovarian cancer are in the evaluation of chemotherapy, of pelvic masses after therapy for the presence of viable tumour, and of raised serum markers.

Imaging of tumour tissue

Nuclear medicine techniques have a limited role in the characterization of tumours. Modalities such as plain X-ray radiography, ultrasound, CT, and MRI offer superior anatomical detail. The value of tumour-seeking radiopharmaceuticals lies in the capability of distinguishing viable tumour tissue from a specific residual mass after therapy and in convenient screening for additional lesions using whole-body imaging.

Gallium scintigraphy is usually done 48–72 hours after the IV administration of 180 MBq ^{67}Ga-citrate. It is of limited value in the initial staging of Hodgkin's and non-Hodgkin's lymphoma, because of the difficulty of detecting lesions in the abdomen. In patients with Hodgkin's disease and other lymphomas, ^{67}Ga scintigraphy, including SPET is an indicator of residual viable tumour tissue with a better predictive value than CT.

Thallium-201 is widely used for myocardial perfusion imaging. Over the past few years there has been growing interest in the use of ^{201}Tl in oncology. It may be useful in the differentiation between low- and high-grade glial tumours and between tumour recurrence and scar tissue. Thallium-201 scintigraphy can assess residual tumour viability after chemotherapy in bone and soft-tissue sarcomas.

Assessment of organ and tissue damage related to cancer therapy

Ventilation/perfusion lung scintigraphy

Patients will lose a substantial part of their pulmonary capacity after surgery (pneumonectomy or lobectomy). With ventilation/perfusion scintigraphy, quantitative information on regional perfusion and ventilation can be obtained. Ventilation/perfusion scintigraphy is also useful in the assessment of pulmonary damage after radiation therapy. Typically, a reduction of perfusion is seen in the irradiated parts.

Left ventricular function in cardiac injury

Doxorubicin and other anthracycline derivatives are effective chemotherapeutic agents, but one of the major limiting side-effects is cardiotoxicity. An essential aspect in the treatment strategy is serial monitoring of left ventricular ejection fraction (LVEF) at rest. Radionuclide ventriculography can be performed under standardized conditions, ensuring a good reproducibility that is essential in serial measurements. A decline in LVEF is a relatively late symptom of cardiotoxicity. Recently, methods to detect directly the myocyte damage by ^{111}In-labelled antimyosin scintigraphy have been developed.

Lymphoscintigraphy

In patients with breast cancer, the evaluation of acquired lymphoedema caused by radiation therapy or lymph node resection is important in the assessment of competency of lymphatic drainage and/or to select the location for possible anastomotic surgery.

Therapy with open radioactive sources

Targeted radiotherapy using tumour-seeking radiopharmaceuticals has been employed for almost half a century. The radiopharmaceutical should have specific affinity for tumour tissue with a high target-to-background ratio and long retention time; the radiation emitted by the radioisotope should be sufficiently energetic for a therapeutic effect, but be absorbed over a short distance to irradiate the tumour target only. Some of the clinically useful radiopharmaceuticals for therapy are ^{131}I, ^{89}Sr, ^{32}P, [186]Re, [153]Sm, and [90]Y.

Iodine-131 therapy in differentiated thyroid cancer

[131]I has been used extensively in the treatment of benign thyroid disease and in differentiated thyroid carcinoma after surgery. [131]I is used for ablation of the remaining thyroid tissue following total thyroidectomy and for treatment of recurrent and metastatic disease.

[131]I-m-iodobenzylguanidine therapy in neural crest tumours

^{131}I-MIBG has been used successfully for radionuclide therapy of neural crest tumours. Post-therapy scintigrams, one week after administration, can be obtained for further documentation. In patients with malignant phaeochromocytoma, response is achieved in >50% of patients; with neuroblastoma the response rate is 35%. Some success is reported with ^{131}I-MIBG therapy for paraganglioma and medullary thyroid carcinoma.

Bone-seeking radiopharmaceuticals for intractable bone pain

Bone metastases occur in up to 85% of patients who have breast, lung, or prostate cancer. Bone-seeking radiopharmaceuticals have pharmacokinetic properties similar to either calcium or phosphate. Strontium-89 (^{89}Sr) is a calcium analogue. ^{32}P, ^{86}Re, HEDP, and ^{153}Sm are all phosphate analogues.

Application of ^{32}P-orthophosphate for the treatment of bone pain was effective, but bone marrow toxicity limited its widespread use. ^{89}Sr was the first radioisotope employed as a systemic treatment for bone metastases in prostate cancer. After IV administration of l50 MBq of ^{89}Sr the radiopharmaceutical is avidly accumulated in areas of high bone turnover, such as reactive bone surrounding a metastasis. A transient leucopaenia can be expected after 6 weeks. After a single administration of ^{89}Sr, in 75–80% of patients pain is promptly relieved and progression of further bone disease is delayed, with the response lasting 1–6 months.

Rhenium-186HEDP is a new radiopharmaceutical with similar chemistry and biodistribution to ^{99m}Tc-labelled diphosphonates. There is a tendency for palliative response to decrease approximately 7 weeks following injection in some patients. Haematopoietic toxicity is minimal. Samarium-153-EDTMP preferentially localizes in bone metastases and is rapidly cleared from the blood by the kidneys.

Intracavitary therapy

Injection of radiopharmaceuticals directly into the pleural cavity, pericardium, peritoneum, urinary bladder, cerebrospinal fluid, or into cystic tumours offers the potential advantage of direct access of radiopharmaceuticals to tumour tissue without a systemic burden. Colloids and monoclonal antibodies labelled with ^{32}P, ^{90}Y, or ^{131}I can be used for this purpose.

Monoclonal antibodies

Monoclonal antibodies were considered the ultimate 'magic bullets' for cancer therapy when introduced 20 years ago. The goal has been to develop antibodies that target active tumour cells specifically and act as carriers of radiation to treat the disease. At present radioimmunotherapy has met with more problems than successes and its future is uncertain.

---

1 ICRU Report 38 (1985) *Doses and volume specification for reporting intra-cavity therapy in gynaecology*. International Commission on Radiation Units and Measurement. Bethesda Md, USA.

2 ICRU Report 58 (1997) *Dose and volume specification for reporting interstitial therapy*. International Commission on Radiation Units. Bethesda Md, USA.

Further reading

1 Nag, S. (ed.) (1997) *Principles and Practice of Brachytherapy* Futura, New York.

2 Dische, S. and Saunders, M.I. (2000) Modified fractionation schemes. In *Oxford Textbook of Oncology* (2nd edn). Oxford University Press.

Chapter 9
Principles of chemotherapy

Rationale for combination therapy

Cytotoxic chemotherapy destroys cancer cells. Currently available drugs target:

- Chemistry of nucleic acids.
- DNA or RNA production.
- Mechanics of cell division (e.g. spindle poisons).

The discovery and development of cytotoxics has paralleled the understanding of the chemical processes involved. The lack of selectivity inherent in this approach has limited the ability to kill cancer cells while leaving normal dividing cells unscathed. There are only rare examples where single-agent therapy is sufficiently active to eradicate the clinically apparent cancer totally and lead to a durable remission or cure.

Cytotoxic agents can be classified by:

- Chemical properties or mechanisms of action (alkylators)
- Source (natural products).
- Propensity to be cell cycle or phase specific.

The following underlie the design of a potential combination therapy:

- Each drug should have single-agent activity in that tumour type.
- Each drug should have a different mechanism of activity.
- Drugs with non-overlapping toxicity patterns are preferable.
- Drugs that work in different parts of the cell cycle should be selected.
- Drugs should not all share the same resistance mechanisms.

Combination therapy aims to increase 'fractional cell kill' leading to improved overall response of the tumour. Higher doses of cytotoxic drugs tend to produce increased cell kill (at least within certain limits) thus it is important not to compromise on the dose of each agent (hence the need to select drugs with non-overlapping toxicity).

Tumour growth also needs to be considered. Tumour mass is usually composed of cells that are asynchronously dividing—thus combinations of drugs that act at different points in the cell cycle will theoretically kill more cells.

'Multi-drug resistance' is displayed by some tumour types, resulting from expression of an efflux pump on the cell surface that pumps the drug out of the cell. This resistance is then apparent to a set of agents known collectively as natural products. The combination should, therefore, not include two such agents.

There are other considerations in developing a combination regimen, including:

* Schedule of administration.
* Frequency of administration.
* Possible synergistic or antagonistic interactions.
* Possible pharmacokinetic or pharmacodynamic interactions.

Novel agents in development target other aspects of malignant behaviour, including:

* Angiogenesis.
* Autocrine and paracrine growth regulators.
* Cell matrix interactions.

The future challenge is to incorporate such drugs into new and existing combinations to improve patient outcomes

Alkylating agents

The oldest anti-cancer cytotoxic-alkylating agents—are anti-neoplastic drugs because they bind covalently via alkyl groups to DNA. They are divided into two groups:

- Unifunctional—with one reactive group.
- Bifunctional—with two reactive groups (more efficient at forming DNA cross-links).

Covalent binding to DNA occurs through the formation of a reactive aziridinium group.

The most common sites of alkylation are the N^7 and O^6 positions of guanine. Following cross-linking there is thought to be an arrest in G1-S transition followed either by DNA repair or apoptosis.

Clinical use

The following have been observed:

- As well as toxicity to mucus membranes, sulphur mustard and mustard gas caused lymphoid aplasia.
- Mustard gas exposure resulted in myelosuppression.
- Nitrogen mustard could be used to treat leukaemia and lymphoma.

More recently, the alkylating agents have become widely used in cancer chemotherapy.

Resistance

Resistance to alkylating agents is multifactorial and may differ between classes of alkylating agents e.g. resistance to nitrosoureas is probably mediated by increased expression of the enzyme O^6-alkyl transferase. In addition to DNA repair, resistant cells may exhibit an increased ability to detoxify alkylating agents. Such mechanisms include increased:

- Glutathione.
- Metallothionein.
- Glutathione-S-transferase.

Major groups of alkylating agents

Nitrogen mustards

The original mustard, mechlorethamine, was highly reactive with a half-life of minutes in biological fluids. Other members—melphalan and chlorambucil—are less chemically reactive and can be administered orally. Melphalan is a derivative of nitrogen mustard and the amino acid phenylalanine. The rationale behind this was that dividing cells might take up amino acids more rapidly (and hence melphalan), thus providing some tumour selectivity.

Chlorambucil is the phenylbutyric-acid derivative of nitrogen mustard, a well-absorbed alkylating agent with activity in both solid and haematological malignancies.

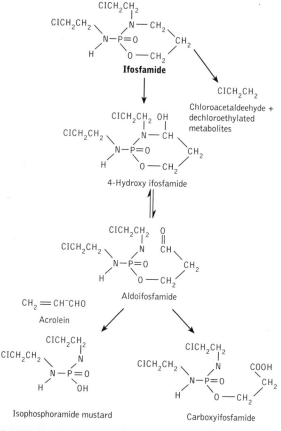

Metabolism of ifosfamide.

Oxazaphosphorines

The observation that tumours overexpressed phosphoramidases led to attempts to create an oxazaphosphorine that could be selectively cleaved by phosphoramidases within tumour cells, leading to the synthesis of cyclophosphamide. Subsequently, two other oxazaphosphorines were synthesized—ifosfamide and trophosphamide. By the 1960s it became apparent these drugs were not activated within tumours but within the liver.

It appears that the oxazaphosphorines are hydroxylated by Cytochrome P450 to the 4-hydroxy compound that is probably the transport form of the drug. 4-hydroxy compounds undergo a series of complex intracellular degradation to form the active mustard.

Cyclophosphamide is extensively used in cytotoxic chemotherapy. It is well absorbed and has nearly 100% bioavailability. Its major toxicities are:

• Myelosuppression.

• Hair loss.

• Emesis.

As a result of its relative lack of non-haematological toxicities, it is used in high-dose chemotherapy regimens.

Ifosfamide is an isomer of cyclophosphamide. In addition to the usual pathway of 4 hydroxylation, a significant proportion of the ifosfamide dosage can be N-dealkylated, liberating chloroacetaldehyde, that is thought to be responsible for some of the toxicity profile.

Ifosfamide nearly always causes alopecia and haemorrhagic cystitis, but this can be circumvented by co-administration of thiol mesna which is thought to chemically combine with acrolein, the metabolite thought to be responsible for this toxicity. Ifosfamide can also cause encephalopathy; this is more common with oral administration.

Alkylalkane sulphonates

Busulphan is the only member of the alkylalkane sulphonates group now used in clinical practice—a bifunctional alkylating agent with a special role in treating chronic myeloid leukaemia. It is well absorbed from the gastrointestinal tract. The dose-limiting toxicities are myelosuppression and hepatic veno-occlusive disease. It can also cause hyperpigmentation and, rarely, pulmonary interstitial fibrosis.

The nitrosoureas

The discovery in the 1950s of the anti-cancer properties of N'-nitroso-N-nitrosoguanidine led to synthesis of many chloroethyl nitrosoureas. They tend to form C-G DNA intrastrand cross-links.

Not all group members form cross-links e.g. methylnitrosourea and streptozocin modify DNA by covalent bonding of a methyl group at the O^6 position of guanine. BCNU is a small lipophilic molecule and is used to treat CNS tumours and as a conditioning agent in high-dose therapy. Toxicities include:

* Myelosuppression.
* Veno-occlusive disease.
* Pulmonary fibrosis.

CCNU[†] is very similar to BCNU[†], administered orally, but can also cause nephrotoxicity.

Aziridines

Thiotepa undergoes complex metabolism. The major, perhaps active, metabolite is TEPA. The principal toxicity is haematological and it is therefore used in high-dose chemotherapy.

Tetrazines

A group of molecules that undergo enzymatic or chemical conversion to liberate the highly reactive diazonium ion, which alkylates DNA at the O^6 position of guanine; as such they are monofunctional alkylating agents. Dacarbazine is a tetrazine that requires metabolic activation and is active in melanoma. Temozolomide is a tetrazine that undergoes non-enzymatic activation and appears to be active in glioma.

The future of alkylating agents

A number of compounds bind by hydrogen bonding to the minor groove of DNA and then form cross-links. They exhibit sequence selectivity as to which nucleotide sequences they bind. They may, thus, be useful in targeting certain tumours selectively. Other approaches to selective tumour kill involve the use of:

* ADEPT (Antibody-Directed Enzyme Pro-drug Targeting)—a tumour-specific antibody linked to an enzyme that is not normally expressed in human cells is given to the patient, followed by a pro-drug that is activated by this enzyme to a cytotoxic agent.
* GDEPT (Gene-Directed Enzyme Pro-drug Targeting)—similar to ADEPT but tumour is made to express the enzyme by gene therapy techniques.

Many of the pro-drugs currently being used are alkylating agents.

....

[†] CCNU: 1-(2-chloroethyl-3-cyclo-hexyl-1)- nitrosourea = lomustine
[†] BCNU: 1,3-bis(2-chloroethyl)-1-nitrosourea = carmustine.

Anti-tumour antibiotics

Some of most important anti-cancer drugs are products of microbial fermentation. Anthracycline antibiotics, doxorubicin and daunorubicin, are widely used in treating solid tumours and haematological malignancies respectively. Recently, liposomal formulations have entered clinical practice. Epirubicin was developed as a less cardiotoxic analogue of doxorubicin. Idarubicin is an analogue of daunorubicin with increased activity in AML and the only anthracycline that can be given orally. Mitoxantrone is the most important of anthracenediones, a group of compounds structurally related to the anthracyclines. Two other structurally distinct anti-tumour antibiotics are in use:

• Actinomycin D, active in childhood tumours.
• Mitomycin C, used both as a cytotoxic and a radiosensitizer.

Anthracyclines

Anthracyclines (doxorubicin, daunorubicin, epirubicin and idarubicin) are closely structurally related and have similar mechanisms of action and resistance, but have different patterns of clinical activity and toxicity.

Pharmacology

The anthracyclines have several effects, and their specific mode of action is unclear.

There are direct effects at the cell surface and also on signal transduction, specifically activation of protein kinase C-mediated cell signalling pathways. The role of these actions in mediating anthracycline cytotoxicity is undefined.

Their ability to undergo reduction to highly reactive compounds and generate free radicals has clinically important implications. Characteristic cardiotoxicity of anthracyclines appears due to the generation of free radicals in the heart where defence systems are less active.

The major target of anthracyclines is the enzyme topoisomerase II. During cell division topoisomerase II binds to DNA forming a 'cleavable complex' that makes transient 'nicks' in DNA, allowing torsional strain in DNA to be released, after which strands rejoin. Anthracyclines bind to the cleavable complex, disrupting this process, leading to DNA strand breaks and cell death.

Drug resistance

Some tumours are inherently resistant to anthracyclines whereas others initially respond but later become resistant.

The *MDR*1 gene codes for a P-170 glycoprotein (Pgp) that is a naturally occurring cell-surface pump. Its physiological function appears to be a protective mechanism, expelling toxic substances from the cell. Cell lines resistant to anthracyclines often have increased expression of Pgp and sensitivity can be restored by the addition of Pgp inhibitors such as verapamil or cyclosporin A. The importance of Pgp in the clinic is less clear. Though expression is increased in some human cancers before treatment or at relapse, attempts to manipulate Pgp have had limited success. It can be difficult to achieve potentially effective plasma levels of Pgp modulators without causing side-effects. Cyclosporin A and other modulators can also influence anthracycline pharmacokinetics, directly increasing exposure to the cytotoxic. To date, modulation of Pgp has shown most promise for patients with haematological malignancies. There remains a need for specific, well-tolerated inhibitors of Pgp.

A second efflux pump associated with expression of multi-drug resistance-associated protein (*MRP*) gene has been implicated in anthracycline resistance in the lab.

Reduced activity of the target enzyme topoisomerase II has also been associated with *in vitro* anthracycline resistance.

Pharmacokinetics and metabolism

After IV administration, anthracycline levels fall rapidly as it is distributed and binds to tissue DNA. Subsequent metabolism and elimination leads to a slow fall in plasma concentrations over several days.

The principal route of metabolism is by reduction and subsequent hepatic elimination. The significance of liver dysfunction in altering anthracycline kinetics has been controversial. Dose reductions are, however, recommended for patients with abnormal liver biochemistry tests as they are at risk of increased toxicity. Dose reductions are not usually required for patients with impaired renal function.

Structural differences affect the pharmacology and clinical use of anthracycline analogues. Epirubicin differs from doxorubicin only by the orientation of a single -OH group, but this enables glucuronidation in the liver and more rapid elimination.

Idarubicin has a different side-chain from daunorubicin making it more lipid-soluble and allowing oral in addition to IV administration. It is also distinctive in that the metabolite idarubicinol retains greater cytotoxic activity than metabolites of other anthracyclines.

Clinical use

The anthracyclines are among the most active cytotoxic agents.

- Doxorubicin and epirubicin are effective against:
  —breast cancer.
  —small-cell lung cancer.
  —sarcoma.

—haematological cancers.

—paediatric malignancies.

Usually used as combination agent; IV bolus or IV infusion every 3 weeks.

* Daunorubicin and idarubicin:

—main role in treatment of acute leukaemia.

—IV administration (idarubicin can be given orally).

Toxicity

The dose-limiting acute toxicities are:

* Myelosuppression and mucositis, both occuring 5–10 days after treatment.

* Alopecia occurs but is reversible.

* Extravasation injury can be severe and there is no proven, effective treatment.

Cumulative cardiotoxicity is specific to anthracyclines and appears to be caused by accumulation of free radicals in the heart. It is characterized by dilatation of sarcoplasmic reticulum and loss of myofibrils. Children appear more sensitive to these effects.

Cardiotoxicity typically presents with heart failure, the risk of which is dose-related. At doxorubicin doses below 450 mg/m^2, the risk is less than 5%, but increases substantially at higher doses. In most cases this threshold allows a full course of anthracycline to be given without risk. Irradiation of the heart, which may occur with radiotherapy to the left breast or chest, increases risk of cardiotoxicity, as does pre-existing cardiac disease.

Cardiotoxicity appears to be related to peak drug levels as doxorubicin is less cardiotoxic when given as a 96-hour infusion than by bolus administration. Liposomal encapsulation of doxorubicin also reduces cardiotoxicity.

Epirubicin is less cardiotoxic than doxorubicin, the 'threshold' dose being 900 mg/m^2. This two-fold difference in cardiotoxicity compares with 1.2-fold difference in therapeutic activity. In terms of cardiotoxocity, epirubicin has a 1.6-fold higher therapeutic index than doxorubicin, so more prolonged treatment may be possible with epirubicin before there is an unacceptable risk of cardiotoxicity. Daunorubicin and idarubicin also have less effect on the myocardium than doxorubicin.

Serial estimation of cardiac ejection fraction by gated isotope scanning or echocardiography detects changes in cardiac function before becoming clinically significant. Where patients do develop cardiac failure it often responds to standard treatment. Iron appears to generate free radicals that are associated with anthracycline treatment. The iron chelator ICRF 187 may protect against cardiotoxicity.

Mitoxantrone

One of the anthracenediones, synthesized as analogue of the anthracyclines. In common with the anthracyclines, mitoxantrone binds to DNA and interacts with topoisomerase II but appears less potent in generating free radicals. Mitoxantrone is also a substrate for Pgp.

Like doxorubicin, mitoxantrone is rapidly and highly tissue-bound. The main clinical use of mitoxantrone has been as an alternative to doxorubicin in advanced breast cancer, as it is substantially less cardiotoxic, less vesicant, and causes less alopecia. However, mitoxantrone is less effective than doxorubicin. It has some activity against other solid tumours, including non-Hodgkin's lymphoma and non-lymphocytic leukaemia.

Actinomycin D

Structurally distinct from the anthracyclines, Actinomycin D binds strongly to DNA by intercalation and inhibits synthesis of RNA and proteins. In pre-clinical models, reduced cellular uptake is associated with resistance to Actinomycin D; it also appears to be a substrate for the Pgp pump.

Actinomycin D is especially active against childhood tumours and is used in combination therapy for:

- Wilms' tumour
- Rhabdomyosarcoma
- Neuroblastoma
- Ewing's sarcoma

The dose-limiting toxicity is myelosuppression, maximal around 10 days after treatment. Actinomycin D can also cause:

- Nausea and vomiting
- Mucositis
- Diarrhoea
- Alopecia

Mitomycin C (MMC)

MMC is active against a range of solid tumours but is also used as a radio-sensitizer in chemo-irradiation.

MMC is inactive in its natural form and requires reduction before binding to DNA by alkylation to form adducts. This bioreductive activation may occur preferentially under the anaerobic conditions that are known to exist within some solid tumours.

Causes of resistance have not been well defined, but as a naturally occuring compound it appears to be a substrate for Pgp.

MMC is used in combination with other cytotoxics to treat breast cancer, non-small-cell lung cancer, and GI cancer. It is used as a radio-sensitizer in the treatment of anal cancer. MMC is effective in reducing recurrence of superficial bladder cancer where it is given intravesically, effectively eliminating systemic exposure to the drug.

The most important toxicity of MMC is myelosuppression, especially thrombocytopaenia, which is delayed and can be cumulative. Accordingly, MMC is given systemically every 6 weeks in contrast to the 3-weekly schedules usually used for other anti-tumour antibiotics.

Haemolytic-uraemic syndrome, pulmonary fibrosis and, cardiac complications are all uncommon, especially at low cumulative doses, but are potentially fatal. Other toxicities such as nausea and vomiting, alopecia, and stomatitis are usually mild, but extravasation can be serious.

Anti-metabolites

Anti-metabolites interfere with normal cellular metabolism of nucleic acids; they act with cell-cycle S-phase specificity. An early compound induced the first remissions in childhood ALL, and they now include some of the most widely prescribed cytotoxic agents, whose indications are not confined to treating malignancies.

Anti-folates

Understanding anti-metabolite action necessitates knowledge of folate biochemistry. The enzyme thymidylate synthase (TS) acts as rate-limiting step in the synthesis of thymidylate, converting dUMP into dTTP by transferring a methyl group from CH_2-FH_4. The supply of reduced folate is maintained by the enzyme dihydrofolate reductase (DHFR).

Methotrexate (MTX)

Widely used, MTX is effective in:

* Breast cancer
* Osteogenic sarcoma

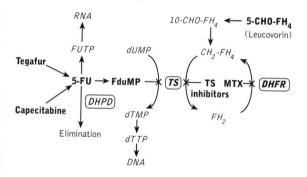

MTX   Cytotoxics (MTX—methotrexate; 5-FU —5-fluorouracil; TS inhibitors include ralitrexed)

dTTP   Normal metabolites

—X   Indicates enzyme inhibition

(DHPD)   Enzyme (TS—thymidylate synthase; DHPD—dihydropyrimidine dehydrogenase; DHFR—dihydrofolate reductase)

Main sites of action of anti-metabolites.

- Bladder carcinoma
- Gastric cancer
- Choriocarcinoma
- Head and neck cancers
- Leukaemia
- Lymphoma

Also used for psoriasis and rheumatoid arthritis, MTX is actively transported into cells where it is polyglutamated, binds tightly to and inhibits DHFR. It also:

- Inhibits other enzymes e.g. TS
- Impairs DNA repair
- Causes accumulation of dihydrofolate polyglutamates (that in turn inhibit folate-dependent enzymes)

Pharmacology

MTX is well absorbed orally below 25 mg/m^2, but is usually administered IV, except in maintenance regimens and treatment of benign connective tissue diseases. It is eliminated in three phases, the second and third phases each taking 10–24 hours; elimination is considerably lengthened by renal dysfunction. There is some hepatic metabolism to the active drug 7-OH-MTX and approximately 10% of the drug is cleared by biliary excretion. Dose adjustments are not usually necessary with hepatic dysfunction. Significant third-space effects occur in the presence of fluid collections (e.g. ascites, pleural effusions) and can increase toxicity through reduced clearance. MTX excretion can also be inhibited by:

- Probenicid
- Penicillins (and cephalosporins)
- Non-steroidal anti-inflammatory agents

Evidence shows synergy with 5-fluorouracil (5-FU), which is maximal if given 24 hours before the 5-FU. Resistance occurs through:

- Impaired uptake
- Gene amplification of DHFR
- Decreased polyglutamation

Toxicities include:

- Mucositis
- Myelosuppression
- Nephrotoxicity
- Acute and chronic hepatotoxicity
- Self-limiting pneumonitis
- Arachnoiditis and chronic demyelination (when given intrathecally)

High-dose MTX has been used in sarcomas, has the advantage of some CSF penetration, and may overcome resistance. Folinic acid can be used to 'rescue' normal cells from undue toxicity, usually given 24 hours after MTX.

Methotrexate analogues

Aminopterin has been surpassed by MTX, though no trial comparing them has been done. Edatrexate is an analogue, with better uptake characteristics and is active in breast, non-small-cell lung, and head and neck cancer. Trimetrexate is lipophilic, does not require poly-glutamation or the folate uptake pathway, and is currently under evaluation in clinical trials.

Thymidylate synthase (TS) inhibitors

New agents have been developed that directly inhibit TS (in contrast to indirect inhibitors e.g. 5-FU and MTX) and interact with the folate-binding site of TS. Glutamated members utilize the folate-carrier system for entry into cells and are polyglutamated, enhancing their efficacy and intracellular retention. Non-glutamated compounds are lipophilic and may have different effects.

Raltitrexed (Tomudex) is a glutamated compound that causes pro-longed inhibition of TS. It has triphasic elimination, with a rapid initial fall in concentration but very prolonged final phase. 50% of the drug is renally excreted unchanged. It is active in breast and colorectal cancer with toxicities including:

* Myelosuppression
* Diarrhoea
* Transaminitis

It is usually administered IV once every 3 weeks.

Fluropyrimidines

These pro-drugs are intracellularly activated and their products inhibit pyrimidine synthesis.

5-flurouracil (5-FU)

This widely prescribed example is active in:

* Breast cancer
* Most gastrointestinal cancers
* Head and neck tumours
* Ovarian cancer

It is metabolized to FdUMP that forms, in the presence of CH_2-FH_4, a stable complex inhibiting TS. It also inhibits RNA synthesis and pre-ribosomal RNA processing.

Pharmacology

Oral absorption is erratic so 5-FU is given IV both as a bolus and a prolonged infusion. It has a short initial half-life, with significant hepatic, renal, and lung clearance. Active metabolites (e.g. 5dUMP and FUTP) have variable pharmacokinetics.

Toxicities of 5-FU include myelosuppression and, particularly with 5-day schedules, stomatitis and diarrhoea. Prolonged infusion overcomes the initial rapid clearance, resulting in differing toxicities with minimal bone marrow effects. Instead, cutaneous toxicity known as hand–foot syndrome occurs. Neurotoxicity and cardiotoxicity may also occur.

Resistance to 5-FU therapy can be due to:

- Altered transport
- Folate depletion
- Changes in TS expression (due to gene amplification or post-transcriptional factors)

5-FU pro-drugs

Ftorafur (tegafur)

Orally active, usually given in combination with uracil in a molar ratio of 1:4. Ftorafur has preferential uptake in tumours and can be given for up to 28 days at a time. It is active in many tumours including:

- Breast
- Gastric
- Colon
- Lung

Capecitabine

Orally active, it is preferentially activated in tumour and liver tissue and has the potential to replace prolonged or continuous infusion 5-FU. Optimum schedule is thought to be twice daily for 2 weeks out of every 3. Active in breast and GI tumours. Its side-effects include:

- Mucositis
- Diarrhoea
- Hand–foot syndrome

2-fluoro-2′-deoxyuridine (floxuridine)

Given IV, this agent can be metabolized both into 5-FU and also directly into FdUMP, theoretically giving increased efficacy. Its clinical use has largely been confined to hepatic artery infusion, where trials show it to be superior to single-agent 5-FU for treating colon cancer.

Modulation of 5-FU

A number of agents have been combined with 5-FU in order to increase either its efficacy or therapeutic index.

Folinic acid   5-FU and folinic acid combinations are the mainstay of treatment of colon cancer. Folinic acid is given by infusion, before or concomitant with 5-FU. By increasing supply of CH_2-FH_4, folinic acid potentiates interaction between 5-FU and TS. Although more toxic, has higher response rate in advanced colorectal cancer with combined treatment than single-agent 5-FU.

Levamisole   the anti-helminth agent, levamisole, has some activity as an immune modulator and has been used in the treatment of colon cancer. It has been combined with 5-FU in the adjuvant setting and the combination is superior to no treatment, but not to intravenous 5-FU (with or without folinic acid). The mechanism of action is uncertain.

Interferon   Interferon may enhance TS inhibition. In combination with 5-FU (with or without folinic acid), it has not been shown to be superior to single-agent 5-Fu.

PALA   PALA (N-phosphonacetyl-L-aspartate) inhibits *de novo* pyrimidine synthesis, and thus increases 5-FU anabolism and incorporation into RNA.

DPD inhibitors   Inhibit the main catabolic pathway of 5-FU and may result in increased efficacy. Early clinical trials are in progress.

Anti-purines

Purine analogues are widely used to treat leukaemias and as immuno-suppressives (azathioprine) and anti-virals (acyclovir, gancyclovir).

6-Mercaptopurine (6-MP) and 6-Thioguanine (6-TG) both inhibit *de novo* purine synthesis and their nucleotide products are incorporated into DNA. HGPRT produces monophosphates, which inhibit early stages of purine synthesis, and then convert into tri-phosphates which are incorporated into DNA, causing strand breaks. There are synergistic effects with MTX, due to PRPP build-up, facilitating phosphorylation by HGPRT. Resistance develops due to HGPRT deficiency and reduced substrate affinity. Variable oral bioavailability may contribute to some treatment failures in childhood ALL.

Both drugs have a short half-life and are primarily metabolized—the important difference is that 6-MP is a substrate for xanthine oxidase, and dose alterations are necessary when co-administered with allopurinol. There is poor CSF penetration, but otherwise these agents are widely distributed.

Main toxicity is myelosuppression, but 6-MP can also cause hepatotoxicity. Nausea, vomiting, and mucositis can also occur, more commonly with 6-MP. The commonest indication is haematological malignancy: 6-MP is used for maintenance therapy of ALL, and 6-TG is used for both remission induction and maintenance in AML.

Cytosine analogues

Two main analogues are metabolized along similar pathways. Initially phosphorylated by deoxycytidine kinase, the active metabolite is triphosphate, incorporated into DNA. Agents are deaminated by cytidine deaminase, which is abundant in liver and GI tract tissues, and products are inactive.

Cystosine arabinoside (Ara-C)

Ara-C is actively transported, and its metabolite ara-CTP is incorporated into DNA, inhibiting DNA polymerases and possibly phospholipid synthesis. Unlike gemcitabine, no further normal nucleotides are added, so that damaged DNA is susceptible to DNA repair.

Ara-C is active in NHL and AML, but not in solid tumours. There is renal excretion of deanimated compound and because of rapid clearance better activity is observed when Ara-C is given by continuous infusion. CSF levels are about half-plasma concentration, Side-effects are:

* Nausea
* Vomiting
* Alopecia
* Myelosuppression

It can also cause 'ara-C syndrome' with fevers, myalgias, rash, keratoconjunctivitis, and arthralgias. Rarely, lung and pancreatic damage occurs. There are significant interactions with many cytotoxics, including:

* Hydroxyurea
* Cisplatin
* Cyclophosphamide
* BCNU

2,2-difluorodeoxycytidine (gemcitabine)

This fluorinated analogue has better membrane permeation and affinity for deoxycytidine kinase than Ara-C. Intracellular retention is prolonged, partly due to a unique self-potentiation in which the bi- and tri-phosphates facilitate the phosphorylation of the parent compound, as well as inhibiting its catabolism.

Active metabolite dF-CTP is incorporated into DNA, followed only by one more normal nucleotide, resulting in protection of the DNA from repair enzymes ('masked termination'). It is probably the saturable formation of dF-CTP that contributes to the clinical schedule dependency of gemcitabine, usually given IV, weekly for 3 weeks out of 4.

Toxicities include:

* Flu-like symptoms
* Transaminitis
* Peripheral oedema

- Myelosuppression
- Possible nephrotoxicity

There is some evidence for synergy with cisplatin, the extent of which appears to be schedule-dependent. It is active in pancreatic cancer (where there is improved symptom control in comparison with single-agent 5-FU) as well as in lung, breast, and bladder cancer.

Adenosine analogues

Three adenosine analogues have come into clinical practice, active in low-grade NHL, Waldenström's macroglobulinaemia, and CLL. All have similar effects and interact with enzyme adenosine deaminase (ADA), a deficiency of which causes severe combined immuno-deficiency. Toxicity includes myelosuppression with particular effects on lymphocytes, including depression of CD_3 and CD_4 levels, and reduced NK activity. Infective complications are more likely to be opportunistic than with most cytotoxics. Neurotoxicity can occur, usually, but not exclusively, associated with higher doses.

Fludarabine

Resistant to ADA, it is particularly useful in treating CLL. It is actively transported into the cells and its mode of action is a consequence of phosphorylation following which it is incorporated into DNA and, probably RNA, and may even cause topoisomerase II inhibition. Can cause haemolytic anaemia.

2′-deoxycoformycin (pentostatin)

Has a very high affinity for ADA, and the resultant complex is stable for over 24 hours, resulting in enzyme inhibition. Its major indication is treatment of hairy-cell leukaemia. Actively transported into cells, it is phosphorylated and incorporated into DNA and also produces inhibitory dATP. It inhibits both DNA synthesis and DNA repair.

2-Chlorodeoxyadensine

Resistant to ADA, phosphorylated and incorporated into DNA; and is used for hairy-cell leukaemia.

Hydroxyurea

This oral agent inhibits ribonucleotide reductase, which reduces availability of all deoxynucleotides. It crosses the blood–brain barrier, and is used in myeloproliferative disorders. Toxicities are:

- Myelosuppression
- Gastrointestinal toxicities
- Sometimes hyperpigmentation

Cisplatin and derivatives

Cisplatin is one of the most active anti-cancer drugs in clinical use since the early 1970s, with a very wide spectrum of anti-tumour activity. In view of its considerable toxicity profile, many attempts have been made to develop analogues with less toxicity, increased efficacy, or both.

Carboplatin

A large number of analogues have been subject to clinical trials but only carboplatin has emerged as a viable clinical candidate. All platinum compounds possess 'leaving groups' that are substituents on the platinum atom that are lost when DNA-platinum cross-links are formed. Physical properties for analogues suggests a correlation between reactivity of leaving groups and nephrotoxicity.

There is still a degree of controversy regarding the clinical equivalence of cisplatin and carboplatin; there are limited situations such as germ cell tumours where cisplatin still appears to be the agent of choice. However, carboplatin in most other circumstances has supplanted the use of cisplatin.

Side-effects of carboplatin

Significant

- Thrombocytopenia, worse at day 14
- Leucopenia, worse at day 14

Less significant toxicities

- Renal
- Neurological
- Otological
- Nausea and vomiting—occasionally
- Alopecia—absent/mild
- Visual disturbances—rarely
- Allergy—in 2%

Dosage of carboplatin

Initially, a dosage of carboplatin based on body-surface area resulted in a variable degree of thrombocytopenia with a number of patients requiring platelet transfusion. Pharmacokinetically-based dosing is now the adopted standard.

With simple pharmacokinetics, about 65% of an administered dose of carboplatin is excreted in the urine within 24 hours and renal clearance is virtually the same as the glomerular filtration rate (GFR). The remaining drug remains covalently bound to tissues for long periods (months to years) and is biologically inert.

Antiproliferative toxicities of carboplatin are related to drug concentration and time, which is given by the area under the plasma concentration time curve (AUC). The simple pharmacokinetics of carboplatin allow a dosing formula to be derived from which the dose required to achieve a specific AUC can be calculated for an individual patient. The most widely used formula is:

$$\text{Dose} = H(\text{GFR} + 25)$$

Where:

Dose is the total dose in mg to be given to the patient.

H is the desired AUC in mg/ml.mm. Typical AUCs are between 4 and 7, depending on frequency of administration, previous treatment, and the drugs being used in combination.

GFR is glomerular filtration rate of patient (ml/min), unadjusted for surface area (should ideally be measured by an isotope method such as ^{51}CrEDTA clearance, but a carefully performed 24-hour urinary creatinine clearance is also acceptable).

AUC-based dosing results in a predictable toxicity and the administration of a larger average dose. AUC has largely superseded surface area-based dosing. When high-dose carboplatin is used with stem-cell rescue regimens there appears to be a relationship between AUC and non-haematological toxicities.

Activity of carboplatin

Carboplatin can be regarded as a less toxic substitute for cisplatin and is used for similar indications. Patients resistant to cisplatin will also be resistant to carboplatin and vice versa. However, the increased thrombocytopenia seen with carboplatin may be a disadvantage in some combinations, while reduced non-haematological toxicities may be an advantage in others. Further, a low level of non-haematological toxicity makes carboplatin suitable for inclusion in high-dose regimens with bone marrow or stem cell rescue.

Indications for carboplatin

- Ovarian cancer
  —equal efficacy for carboplatin and CAP (cyclophosphamide, doxorubicin, and cisplatin)
  —less toxicity for carboplatin compared to CAP
  —addition of paclitaxel lessens risk of thrombocytopenia
- Germ cell tumours
  —testicular teratoma: lower relapse rate for cisplatin compared to carboplatin:

   —paediatric germ cell tumours: equal efficacy for cisplatin and
   carboplatin
   —seminoma: carboplatin, highly efficacious
* Paediatric cancers
   —cisplatin has role in many cancers
   —carboplatin less toxic
* Small-cell lung cancer
   —carboplatin, high response rate
* Non-small-cell lung cancer, bladder cancer, cervical cancer
   —carboplatin, slightly better response than cisplatin
   —carboplatin combined with paclitaxel, high response rate in
   non-small-cell lung cancer
* Head and neck cancer
   —carboplatin used as alternative to cisplatin
* Breast cancer
   —not used as first-line treatment
   —used in high-dose regimes
* Colon cancer
   —little activity
* Prostate cancer
   —little data
* Upper GI tumours
   —little data
* Brain tumours
   —response in medulloblastoma

Pharmacokinetic interactions with carboplatin

Unlike cisplatin, carboplatin does not affect hepatic cytochrome P450
enzyme and pharmacokinetic interactions with other drugs seem to be
rare.

Summary

Carboplatin has major advantages in terms of ease of administration
and non-haematological toxicities than cisplatin, although the higher
incidence of thrombocytopenia may be a problem in some circumstances. In the main, it can be regarded as an alternative to cisplatin,
but current data suggest cisplatin should still be used for treating
testicular teratoma. Unlike cisplatin, carboplatin can be used in high-
dose regimens. Carboplatin should generally be dosed on a pharmacokinetic basis. In the future, a major role for carboplatin is likely to be
in combination with paclitaxel for a variety of tumours.

Cisplatin mechanism of action

Cisplatin binds directly to DNA, inhibiting synthesis by altering the
DNA template via formation of intra-strand and inter-strand cross-

links. These cross-links are generated by an aquated complex that acts as a bifunctional alkylating agent. Cytotoxic effects of cisplatin are cell-cycle independent, and synergy between cisplatin and anti-metabolites has been demonstrated both *in vitro* and in clinical trials. The mechanism behind this synergy has not been fully explained; the most commonly held hypothesis is that this is due to a malfunction in DNA repair processing.

Side-effects of cisplatin

• Dose-dependant nephrotoxicity
  —prehydrate
  —may need diuretics
• Nausea, vomiting
  —all require anti-emetics
• Peripheral neuropathy
  —sensory loss
  —segmental demyelination
• Central nervous toxicity
  —less common
• Leucopenia
  —recovers in 21 days
• Thrombocytopenia
  —recovers in 21 days
• Anaemia
  —common

Dosage of cisplatin

Cisplatin is used in a variety of dosage schedules. The standard dose limit for high-dose therapy is 100 mg/m^2 as a single daily dose; higher doses have been explored in clinical trials, particularly in conjunction with neuroprotective agents. Alternate schedules such as five daily injections of 20 mg/m^2 are favoured in the treatment of teratoma.

The initial clearance of cisplatin is rapid, followed by a much slower decline due to binding to plasma proteins. Clearance is prolonged in patients with renal insufficiency. Unlike carboplatin, there is no clear evidence of a pharmacodynamic/pharmacokinetic relationship with cisplatin; therefore dosage is usually based on empirical body-surface calculations.

Clinical indications for cisplatin

Cisplatin was a major step forward in the treatment of testicular cancer. In patients with metastatic disease, cisplatin-based combination therapy results in a complete clinical response in over 80% of patients, with the majority of these achieving long-term cure. Cisplatin is also a major component of treatment of:

+ Ovarian cancer
+ Bladder cancer
+ Penile cancer
+ Cervical carcinoma
+ Other squamous carcinomas, particularly those in the head and neck and non-small-cell bronchogenic carcinoma

Combinations of cisplatin with other cytotoxic agents are common and are used in a variety of human solid cancers and paediatric tumours.

Oxaliplatin

Oxaliplatin is a platinum analogue that differs from carboplatin and cisplatin, in both chemical behaviour and possibly its mechanism of action. Availability is limited. *In vitro* oxaliplatin has a broad spectrum of activity with marked differences from the spectrum seen with cisplatin or carboplatin e.g. oxaliplatin appears to be active in those cell lines that are resistant to cisplatin, and a high level of activity is seen in colorectal cell lines. This has led to multiple Phase I, II, and III studies of the agent, evaluating its activity in colorectal cancer.

Dosage of oxaliplatin

Two commonly used regimens exist:

+ **First:** 85 mg/m^2 every two weeks as a 2–6 hour infusion.
+ **Second:** 130 mg/m^2 over a similar length of time repeated every three weeks.

However, a multitude of studies exist using a variety of different dosing regimens, including chronomodulated infusion together with 5-fluorouracil. When used as a single agent in colorectal cancer, an overall response rate of around 10% is achieved in patients who are resistant to 5-fluorouracil and around 20% in those not previously exposed to 5-fluorouracil. Of clinical importance, the highest response rates are seen when oxaliplatin is added to regimens with 5-FU and folinic acid. There is synergy between these agents. A study in first-line colorectal cancer has shown a marked increase in response rates in those patients given oxaliplatin; however there is no clear survival advantage.

Topoisomerase inhibitors

Topoisomerase enzymes are a family of nuclear proteins with essential functions in regulating the topology of the DNA helix. Topoisomerase proteins appear to constantly monitor DNA structure, looking for points of increased tension. The protein then alters DNA tertiary structure, by creating transient strand breakage in DNA backbone. Eukaryotics has two forms of topoisomerase enzyme:

- **Topoisomerase I** (topoI) binds to double-stranded DNA and cleaves and religates one strand of duplex DNA. Relaxation of supercoiled DNA is then used during processes of replication, transcription, and recombination.

- **Topoisomerase II** (topoII) creates transient double-stranded breakage of DNA, allowing subsequent passage of a second intact DNA duplex through the break.

Biochemical analysis has identified camptothecin (CPT) and its analogues as inhibitors of topoI, while epipodophyllotoxins, etoposide and teniposide, are inhibitors of topoII.

Topoisomerase I inhibitors

CPT has been identified as the active constituent of an extract isolated from the Chinese Tree *Camptotheca acuminata*. Mechanism of action studies demonstrated that CPT stabilized co-valent adducts between genomic DNA and topoI. Early clinical studies with CPT observed anti-tumour activity in a variety of common solid tumours. However, a high rate of severe and unpredictable toxicities, including haemorrhagic cystitis and gastrointestinal effects, were seen. This led to discontinuation of CPT's development.

The novelty of topoI as a cellular target for chemotherapy has resulted in the development of several analogues, such as irinotecan (CPT-11) and topotecan. Both CPT-11 and topotecan have greater aqueous solubility than CPT. Analogues of CPT with an amino group at the 9-position have enhanced activity, but are less soluble than topotecan or CPT-11. CPT and all CPT derivatives have a basic 5-ring structure. Reversible, pH-dependent non-enzymatic hydrolysis of the lactone ring of all CPT derivatives results in an open-ring carboxylate moiety. The two are in equilibrium in aqueous buffers, but the carboxylate form is a less potent inhibitor of topoI and a much less potent anti-tumour agent.

To date, two CPT analogues have received regulatory approval for use in patients with solid tumours:

- **Topotecan** (hycamtin) in Europe and the US for treatment of advanced ovarian and non-small-cell lung cancers.
- **CPT-11** (camptosar) in patients with advanced colorectal cancer.

Both agents are currently administered as a 30–90 minute infusion daily for five days every three weeks (topotecan) or weekly for four weeks, every six weeks (CPT-11). Alternate intravenous, intra-peritoneal, and oral schedules are under evaluation and demonstrate anti-tumour activity.

Side-effects

- Neutropenia—common
- Diarrhoea—common (early or late)
- Thrombocytopenia
- Anaemia
- Alopecia
- Nausea, vomiting

Clinical pharmacology

Clinical pharmacology of CPT-11 and topotecan is now relatively well developed. Both can be absorbed orally, with topotecan bioavailability of 30–50%; both are widely distributed throughout the body, with cerebrospinal fluid topotecan concentrations 30-50% of simultaneous plasma concentrations.

Topotecan undergoes negligible metabolism. CPT-11 is in itself relatively inactive and must be converted by carboxylesterases to SN-38 that has potent topoI inhibitory activity. SN-38 undergoes glucuronidation to inactive metabolite by uridine-diphosphosphate glucuronosylatransferase lAl and genetic polymorphism in the forma-tion of SN-38 glucuronide has been proposed.

Topotecan is primarily eliminated by the kidneys, with evidence for renal tubular secretion. A linear relationship between creatinine clear-ance and clearance of both total topotecan and lactone form has been demonstrated. Approximately 20% of the total dose of CPT-11 is excreted unchanged in urine, whereas less than 1% is excreted as SN-38. Glucuronidation and biliary excretion appear to be principal mechanisms of elimination for SN-38.

Several mechanisms of resistance to topoI inhibitors have been described in *in vitro* systems. These include:

- Factors that affect the stabilization of the topoI–DNA complex
- Alterations in drug accumulation
- Decreased activation of CPT-11
- Decreased cellular content/activity of topoI
- Mutations of the topo I enzyme

Little is know about mechanisms of resistance to CPT or its analogues in human tumours.

Topoisomerase II inhibitors

In the 1960s, podophylin derivatives—etoposide and teniposide— were found to have a unique mechanism of action, subsequently identified as inhibition of topoII. Etoposide and teniposide exert their action on topoII by:

* Inhibiting the ability of the enzyme to relegate the cleaved DNA complex

* Generating high levels of DNA with potentially toxic double-stranded breaks

* Promoting mutation

* Permanent double-stranded breaks

* Illegitimate recombination

* Apoptosis

Chemically, teniposide only differs from etoposide in the substitution of a thenylidene ring in place of a methyl group. However, teniposide is approximately 10% more potent then etoposide, in terms of both *in vitro* cytotoxicity and DNA strand breakage, but the difference is less apparent *in vivo* where teniposide is only 1.5–3 times more potent.

Etoposide and teniposide are poorly water-soluble and are formulated with a number of excipients including polysorbate (etoposide) or cremophor EL (teniposide). Etoposide can be administered by either oral or intravenous routes, teniposide only by intravenous injection. Recently, etoposide phosphate was introduced, a more soluble yet bioequivalent form of etoposide designed to decrease infusion-related toxicity.

Teniposide and etoposide are widely used in treatment of adult and paediatric malignancies. Etoposide has been more broadly used in front-line therapy for:

* Small-cell lung cancer
* Germ-cell tumours
* Kaposi's sarcoma
* As part of preoperative regimens for bone marrow transplantation

Both agents are used in front-line therapy for childhood cancer, including:

* Acute lymphoblastic leukaemia
* Neuroblastoma
* Rhabdomyosarcoma

The pattern of toxicity is very similar between both agents and includes:

- Neutropenia
- Alopecia
- Mucositis
- Infusion-related blood pressure changes
- Hypersensitivity reactions

Clinical pharmacology

Oral etoposide capsules have bioavailability of 60% with extensive variation. Etoposide absorption appears to be non-linear with decreased bioavailability at doses above 200 mg. Etoposide phosphate has a similar degree of bioavailability and suggestions of non-linear absorption.

Both etoposide and teniposide are heavily protein-bound; use in patients with low albumin concentrations will result in greater than expected systemic toxicity due to the larger free (unbound) drug concentrations. Although both etoposide and teniposide are distributed into the CSF, they achieve concentrations of 0.1–4% of that measured simultaneously in plasma.

Both etoposide and teniposide are extensively metabolized. Production of a catechol metabolite is mediated through P450 3A4 and may have intrinsic cytotoxic activity. Etoposide glucuronide has been found to account for up to 30% of the administered dose.

Etoposide is more rapidly eliminated than teniposide with:

- Faster systemic clearance
- Greater renal clearance
- Shorter elimination half-life

Linear relationships between etoposide systemic clearance and creatinine clearance have been described for both adult and paediatric patients. Both etoposide and teniposide have demonstrated pharmacodynamic relationships, where measures of systemic exposure (AUC, Css, trough concentrations, etc.) are correlated with haematological toxicity.

Anti-microtubule agents

Tubulin-interactive agents, commonly known as 'spindle poisons' have a long history of use in cancer treatment. They act by binding to specific sites on tubulin, a protein that polymerizes to form cellular microtubules. Microtubules are important structural units involved in a number of cellular activities, including formation of the mitotic spindle.

Agents that bind to tubulin can be categorized according to their main tubulin binding site:

- Vinca alkaloid binding site
- Colchicine binding site
- Rhizoxin/maytansine binding site
- Tubulin sulfhydryl groups
- A separate class of as yet uncharacterized binding sites

The table focusses on important anti-microtubule agents in pre-clinical and clinical development, grouped into families to summarize:

- Mechanism of action
- Major indications
- Administration
- Pharmacokinetic data for clinical practice
- Selected important information for the clinic

Tubulin is an important target for anti-cancer drug development; several anti-tubulin agents have significant anti-cancer activity in the clinic. Taxanes were the most encouraging development in anti-cancer chemotherapy of the 1990s; paclitaxel, when incorporated in a first-line chemotherapy regimen for advanced ovarian cancer leads to significant prolongation of survival, while docetaxel can make a small but significant impact on survival of metastatic breast cancer patients, even when given in a second- or third-line setting to heavily pre-treated patients.

Recent progress observed with taxanes has led to renewed interest in anti-microtubule analogues or drugs interacting with different sites on tubulin. In particular, agents with an improved pharmacological profile and/or activity in vinca/taxane-resistant cell lines are of interest. Several new anti-tubulin agents are in pre-clinical development.

Most of the basic research into drug resistance has involved using pairs of sensitive and resistant tumour cells derived from the same parental cell line, usually by serial passage in increasing concentrations of the drug under investigation. This is an artificial situation

Table 9.1 Anti-microtubule agents

Class of spindle poison (mechanism of action)	Useful indications	Drug administration (IV doses in mg/m²)	Main toxicities	Pharmacokinetics and metabolism	Comments of clinical interest
Vincristine (VCR) (destabilization of polymerised tubulin (β-tubulin))	Leukaemias, lymphomas, paediatric tumours, small-cell lung cancer, multiple myeloma	0.5–1.4 q 1–4 w (total individual dose: 2 mg)	Neuropathy	Metabolized in the liver	VCR induces multi-drug resistance (MDR) by P-glycoprotein (PgP). Mutations in α and β tubulin proteins enhance stability against depolymerization.
Vinblastine (VBL) (same as VCR)	Lymphomas, germ cell tumours, Kaposi's sarcoma, breast cancer	6–10 q 2–4 w	Neutropenia, neuropathy	Metabolized in the liver	Neuropathy occurs less frequently than with VCR
Vindesine (VDS) same as VCR, prostate,	Non-small-cell lung cancer (NSCLC), breast cancer, lymphomas	2–4 q 1–3 w	Neutropenia, neuropathy	Metabolized in the liver	Randomized trials (breast, NSCLC, sarcomas, and melanoma) with VDS showed no advantage over treatments without VDS.
Vinorelbine (NVB) (same as VCR)	NSCLC, breast cancer	25–30 / w combinations: cisplatin (NSCLC) and doxorubicin or 5FU (breast). Oral form in clinical development	Neutropenia, constipation, neuropathy	Metabolized in the liver	Selective binding to the Tau family of microtubule–associated proteins → tubulin aggregation into spirals and paracrystals.

Table 9.1 (*continued*)

Class of spindle poison (mechanism of action)	Useful indications	Drug administration (IV doses in mg/m²)	Main toxicities	Pharmacokinetics and metabolism	Comments of clinical interest
					NVB not active and associated with severe neurotoxicity in paclitaxed pre-treated breast cancer patients.
Paclitaxel (P) (microtubule stabilizer) (also anti-angiogenesis effect, disruption of Ki-Ras function, apoptosis induction by phosphorylation of bcl-2)	Ovarian, breast, and lung cancers (other tumours). Reproducible anti-tumour activity (response rate 15–25%) in platinum-resistant ovarian cancer stimulated further clinical development.	135 (24 h)–175 (3 h) q 3 w. Weekly schedule is under investigation. Combinations: mainly with cisplatin or carboplatin (ovary) and doxorubicin (breast)	Neutropenia, neurotoxicity	Metabolized in the liver. Cisplatin → P: severe neutropenia; P → doxorubicin: more mucositis than the reverse sequence.	Toxicities are sequence- and schedule-dependent. Steroid pre-medication is used to reduce hypersensitivity reactions. Water-soluble analogues and derivatives active in resistant cells of P are under development. Mutations in P53 cell lines confer sensitisation to P. Resistance to P due to PgP and/or alterations in the expression or structure of β-tubulin.

Table 9.1 (*continued*)

Class of spindle poison (mechanism of action)	Useful indications	Drug administration (IV doses in mg/m²)	Main toxicities	Pharmacokinetics and metabolism	Comments of clinical interest
Docetaxel (D) (microtubule stabilizer)	Breast cancer, lung cancer (other tumours) Reproducible anti-tumour activity (response rate 35–50%) in anthracycline-resistant breast cancer stimulated further clinical development.	100 (1 h) q 3 w, 75 q 3 w (if elevated liver function tests). Weekly schedule is under investigation.	Neutropenia, retention syndrome (FRS)	Metabolized in the liver	Steroid pre-medication reduces and delays FRS. Tau and $\beta 4$-tubulin expression correlate with D sensitivity in adenocarcinoma models.
Estramustine phosphate (EP) (binds to the microtubule-associated proteins to promote microtubule disassembly)	Prostate cancer	560 mg × 2/d orally (with meal)	Gastrointestinal	75% of oral EP is absorbed. Terminal half-life: 20–40 h	Most responses observed in prostate cancer were subjective (objective response rate ~ 10%). EP has been combined with other antimicrotubules (P, VBL) and etoposide with a clinical benefit in 30–60% of patients. Overexpression of beta (III & IVa)-tubulin and Tau may play a role in resistance to EP.

which often results in resistance which is really very substantial with concentration variants in excess of 40–100-fold sometimes required to overcome such resistance. It is unclear whether this laboratory-derived resistance correlates with the types of clinical resistance which are outlined above.

Pharmacological resistance

The underlying concept of pharmacological resistance is that the dose of chemotherapy that can be safely given is insufficient to result in an effective concentration of the active drug at its target site. This may be due to:

- Toxicity in other organs
- Enhanced clearance of drugs
- Physical barrier between bloodstream and tumour cells (many tumours have avascular centres)
- *De novo* resistance—tumour does not respond despite full-dose chemotherapy
- Acquired resistance—initial response to chemotherapy, then tumour fails to respond and regrows
- Combination of *de novo* and acquired.

Alteration of target or transport mechanisms

Tumour cells have the ability to mutate such that the drug is either not taken up by the cell or having been taken up is detoxified more rapidly than normal. Alternatively, the actual target of the drug may change by mutation such that it becomes impervious to the form of attack. Or the normal repair mechanisms which are present in all mammalian cells may become more active and repair damage is produced by a cytotoxic agent in a more efficient manner, resulting in overall resistance to the agent.

Classical multi-drug resistance

'Classical' drug resistance has been the most studied form of this phenomenon in the laboratory and results from overexpression of 170 KD glycoprotein known as p-glycoprotein. This spans the outer cell membrane and acts as an energy-dependent drug efflux pump. Thus, as the drug enters the tumour cell, by diffusion or transport, the drug in the interior of the cell is picked up and is effluxed into the extracellular environment. This reduces the effective concentration of the drug within the cell and allows the cell to express resistance to the agent in question.

The development of this form of resistance is most commonly associated with exposure to the anti-tumour antibiotics, the anthracyclines, taxanes and etoposide. In fact, resistance to one of this group of agents usually confers resistance to the other groups in addition, thereby leading to the phenomenon of 'multi-drug resistance'.

P-glycoprotein:

* Found in tissues
  —used for transport e.g. steroids
  —protection against external toxins
* Overexpression leads to drug resistance
* Haematological malignancy
  —early trials of low-molecular-weight inhibitors of P-glycoprotein encouraging
  —but affects normal cells also and therefore more sensitive to chemotherapy

Multi-drug resistance protein (MRP)

This protein is one member of a family of proteins which also act as energy-dependent pumps, in this case resulting in drug efflux or sequestration of the drug, within intracytoplasmic organelles or vacuoles. The most studied member of this family of proteins is 190 kilodalton protein which has a similar substrate specificity to p-glycoprotein but is usually associated with less resistance to the taxanes. The clinical relevance of this form of resistance is less clear than with the p-glycoprotein; clinical trials looking at inhibition of MRP are at an early stage.

Glutathione

Glutathione is the predominant cellular thiol and participates in a complex biochemical pathway which interacts with the alkylating function of some agents (including cisplatin). Glutathione over-expression in cell lines results in relative resistance to alkylating agent attack. In addition, glutathione is able to detoxify free radicals which may be an important pathway of action for some cytotoxics, including doxorubicin. Clinical trials of glutathione depletion have been performed with somewhat equivocal results.

Failure to engage apoptosis

The common final pathway of cell death for many cytotoxics is apoptosis. This is an active process within cells, somewhat akin to 'cell suicide'. The engagement of the apoptosis program is a complex inter-acting pathway. At the centre of this is p53, the so-called 'guardian of the genome'. In cells which are unable to engage apoptosis, the damage done by cytotoxics can be 'ignored' and cell division continues. This results in clinical drug resistance. Gene-therapy approaches to correct this apoptosis failure are being actively investigated.

Summary

Clinical drug resistance is a major problem in oncology and the underlying mechanisms are multifactorial. In any one patient it is unclear to what extent each mechanism contributes. Nevertheless, the potential clinical benefits of mechanisms to circumvent drug resistance are enormous. Undoubtedly, other mechanisms of drug resistance will be found as we come to understand more about the regulation of cell cycle, cell life, and cell death.

Dose intensification

Dose response and dose intensity

The strategy of therapeutic dose intensification in oncology has been largely driven by the incomplete chemotherapy sensitivity exhibited by many tumours. Experimental evidence suggests that the drug resistance of cancer cells is often relative; it can be overcome by exposing the 'resistant' cell to higher concentrations of the drug to which it has become 'resistant'. In most laboratory models, extreme degrees of dose escalation are needed to overcome drug resistance.

The concept of dose intensity takes into account time variables. Thus a regimen might be intensified either by increasing the dose or by abbreviating the inter-treatment interval. The biological impact of these two strategies may be very different.

There is a distinction between maintenance of a standard dose and true dose intensification: the shape of the dose–response curve may not be flat i.e. the mathematical relationship between dose and response may vary at different points. It is possible that dose escalation may increase anti-tumour activity only up to a certain point, after which the dose-response curve 'flattens' and further dose increases will be futile.

Results of studies indicate that arbitrary dose reduction should be avoided, and suggest that clinicians should consider use of prophylactic antibiotics, haematopoietic growth factors, etc. in situations where neutropenia and its complications threaten to undermine timely delivery of potentially curative chemotherapy.

High-dose chemotherapy (HDC) with haematopoietic support

In the clinic, dose escalation within a 'conventional' range has an inconsistent effect on response rates, and with some exceptions, a negligible survival impact. Clinical dose escalation is complicated by a greatly increased toxicity, seen when these relatively non-specific toxins are administered to patients. Substantial advances in haematopoietic support have allowed investigation of very high doses of chemotherapy in the clinic. Autografting, using either autologous marrow or cytokine-mobilized peripheral blood progenitors, is seen to facilitate administration of very high doses of those drugs dose-limited by myelosuppression.

'High-dose chemotherapy' (HDC) is therapy administered in doses clearly outside the standard range and which, with exceptions, require some form of haematopoietic cellular support (some drugs, e.g. cyclophosphamide and etoposide are stem-cell sparing, and it is possible to administer them with growth factors as sole support). For drugs primarily dose-limited by myelosuppression, haematopoietic support allows the clinician to mimic the extreme dose escalation studied in the laboratory. Thus, thiotepa can be dose escalated by 30–40-fold, carboplatin by 4–6-fold, etc.

In early studies of HDC with bone marrow autograft support, high rates of objective response were seen in patients with chemotherapy-resistant lymphomas and solid tumours. Toxicity was also formidable, and up to 20% of patients so-treated died from complications of therapy, especially from infections during the prolonged neutro-penic phase that inevitably occurred, and also from organ-failure syndromes.

The introduction of the haematopoietic growth factors changed high-dose chemotherapy. Administration of these cytokines following bone marrow re-infusion resulted in a dramatic abbreviation of dura-tion of neutropenia. It was also discovered that administration of these factors, either at steady state or following myelosuppressive chemotherapy, resulted in mobilization of haematopoietic pro-genitors from the bone marrow into the peripheral blood. These 'peripheral blood progenitors' (PBP) could be harvested by leuco-pheresis, then re-infused as haematopoietic rescue following sub-sequent HDC. PBP autografting is superior to marrow autografting, with shortened neutropenia and thrombocytopenia, and reduced mortality and morbidity.

Historically, HDC has generally been given as a form of consolida-tion following conventional chemotherapy. Less frequently, it has been studied as primary treatment. It can be administered in single or in multiple cycles.

Role of HDC in the treatment of specific tumours

* Relapsed aggressive lymphoma—proven salvage treatment
* Refractory lymphoma—10% remission
* Poor prognosis NHL—first-line treatment
* Multiple myeloma—first-line treatment
* Relapsed refractory Hodgkin's disease—first-line treatment
* Acute leukaemia—especially if no donor
* Metastatic testicular germ-cell tumours—relapse after second remission
  —failure to achieve complete remission
* Breast cancer—salvage treatment for relapsed metastatic breast cancer
  —(controversial) initial chemotherapy for metastatic disease (50% remission)
  —(controversial) early-stage, poor-risk breast cancer

- Ovarian cancer—early data encouraging
- Small-cell lung cancer—early data encouraging

Future directions

The immediate priority is to determine whether there is a role for HDC in the therapy of breast cancer and other solid tumours. Developmental work is needed to address other important questions e.g. role of late intensification versus primary high dose, graft manipulation, and purging. Newer biological anti-cancer agents may produce maximum impact in the setting of minimal disease, and the proven ability of HDC to produce frequent CRs suggests future investigations may involve both these modalities of treatment.

Chemo-irradiation

Chemotherapy and radiotherapy are complementary; integration of these treatment modalities underpins successful treatment of a number of tumours. Chemotherapy reduces the burden of local diseases and eradicates systemic micrometastases, but effective loco-regional tumour control requires irradiation.

Sequential combined therapy

The traditional approach to combining chemotherapy and radiotherapy has been to attempt to predict whether eradication of systemic disease or local tumour control is of most immediate concern, then deliver the appropriate treatment first; the other treatment is delayed until completion of the first. The main difficulties are the uncertain behaviour of individual tumours and the inevitable delay in delivery of one treatment. Chemotherapy as the first-line treatment has the added potential benefit that in downstaging the tumour it may reduce both the volume of tissue which requires irradiation and the radiation dose required to control the tumour.

Concurrent combined therapy

Problems are avoided by delivering chemotherapy and radiotherapy together. This approach has advantages and some disadvantages (see Table 9.2).

Ideally, cytotoxics chosen for chemo-irradiation regimens will have known activity against the tumour but will not have toxicities that overlap the effects of irradiation of the relevant region. Anthracyclines are avoided because of their effects on skin and mucosa; methotrexate can increase the damage to the normal lung following radiotherapy. Agents such as cisplatin and 5-fluorouracil are particularly attractive

Table 9.2 Benefits and problems of concurrent combined therapy

Advantage	Disadvantage
No delay in either therapy	Increased toxicity
Additive cell kill by two therapies	Compromised dose of one or both treatments
Enhanced cell kill by radiosensitizing effects of chemotherapy	Large volume irradiated
Reduced likelihood of evolution of resistance to either therapy	Pharmacodynamic interactions (e.g. cell-cycle effects)

because of their radiosensitizing effects. At least, *in vitro*, the interactions of chemotherapy and radiotherapy are complex and schedule-dependent: e.g. irradiation of cells may lead to cell-cycle arrest and this may confer relative resistance to subsequent exposure to phase-specific cytotoxics such as taxanes; conversely, exposure to taxanes can lead to radiosensitization.

An attempt must be made to minimize the normal tissue damage of radiation during combined therapy. Treatment times are often a minimum of 6 weeks (to reduce early normal reactions) and the dose per fraction is 2 Gy or less (to reduce late damage).

Anal and bladder carcinomas

For both these pelvic malignancies chemo-irradiation offers the possibility of organ preservation and avoidance of a stoma. There is good evidence that pelvic irradiation with concurrent 5-fluorouracil and mitomycin is the best-established therapy for anal carcinoma. The combination of pelvic radiotherapy and cisplatin-based chemotherapy has proven successful in large phase II studies in muscle-invading transitional cell carcinoma of the bladder.

Small-cell lung cancer and oesophageal cancer

Chemo-irradiation of intra-thoracic tumours is hindered by risk of serious morbidity, in particular pneumonitis and oesophagitis. Nonetheless, small cell-lung cancer is an excellent target for this approach; although chemosensitive local failure is inevitable with chemotherapy alone, and even with conventional consolidation radiotherapy, 40–50% of these patients have locally recurrent disease. The results of combination etoposide, cisplatin, and thoracic irradiation are promising. Toxicity, especially oesophagitis, is considerable.

Chemo-irradiation is superior to radiation therapy alone for oesophageal cancer but local failure rates remain high. Surgery after combined treatment may be the answer to this problem, but the potential for morbidity is increased further.

Ewing's tumour

Chemo-irradiation is incorporated in the regimens under study in EICESS 2, but a major concern in this type of curable cancer is the legacy of treatment-related problems in young patients, in particular the risk of second malignancy.

Pharmacokinetics/ pharmacodynamics of anti-cancer drugs

Terminology

Pharmacokinetics is the study of processes that a drug undergoes between time of administration and time of elimination from the body. The most common pharmacokinetic data is a plot of plasma drug concentration versus time. The administered dose and parameters corresponding to rate and extent of the pharmacokinetic processes determine peak drug concentration, half-life, and drug exposure (the area under the plasma concentration versus time curve or AUC). These processes are:

• Bioavailability, for drug absorption

• Clearance, for elimination

• Apparent volume of distribution, for distribution

Pharmacodynamics describe the relation of both the therapeutic and toxic effects of a drug to the pharmacokinetic parameters.

Pharmacokinetics/pharmacodynamics in clinical oncology

Most drugs have a narrow therapeutic index—dosages required for anti-tumour efficacy usually cause some side-effects and a small increase above the therapeutic dose may be sufficient to cause life-threatening toxicity. Variations in pharmacokinetic parameters of anti-cancer drugs between patients are frequently observed. These variations are caused by diversity in renal or metabolic functions (which are themselves due to advanced disease), drug–drug interactions, and toxic effects of previous chemotherapy on organ functions. These all contribute to variations in drug concentration in patients treated with a similar dose of cytotoxic.

Since the amount of drug reaching the site of action (tumour cells or the tissue expressing toxicity such as bone marrow stem cells) is dependent on the systemic concentration, correlation between pharmacokinetic parameters (e.g. peak concentration, AUC) and pharmacodynamics endpoints is closer than that between administered dose and pharmacodynamics. The ultimate goal of pharmacokinetically-guided dosing will be to maximize the likelihood of producing the antitumour response with minimum normal tissue damage.

Parameters of in pharmacokinetics/ pharmacodynamics relationships

In terms of pharmacokinetic pharmacodynamic relationships of the anti-cancer drugs, the relevant pharmacokinetic parameter is usually the AUC, which represents total systemic exposure of the body to the drug. AUC results from the bioavailable dose (administered dose weighted in case of extravascular administration by the bio-availability) and the patient plasma clearance (CL) which represents the elimination capacity for the drug:

$$AUC = F \times Dose / CL \text{ (F=bioavailability)}$$

Since anti-cancer drugs are administered intravenously, F is equal to 1 and the dose required to provide an optimum AUC may be calculated with knowledge of individual plasma clearance. Then, variability in elimination becomes the more determinant pharmaco-kinetic process involved in pharmacokinetics/pharmacodynamics.

The modified Hill equation, which corresponds to a sigmoidal curve, is frequently used to describe the relationship between a pharmacokinetic parameter (e.g. AUC) and a pharmacodynamic effect (E):

$$E = Emax \cdot AUC^H / (AUC50^H + AUC^H)$$

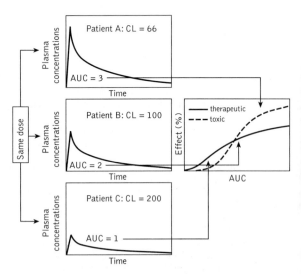

Pharmacokinetic profiles of three individual patients with variation in profile resulting in variable clinical effect (pharmacodynamics).

Emax represents the maximum possible effect and *AUC50*, the AUC that induces 50% of Emax. *H* is Hill's constant (or shape factor) which defines the degree of sigmoidicity of the model.

The relationship between AUC and haematological toxicity is closer than that between pharmacokinetic parameters and clinical outcome. This observation is explained by numerous other causes of variation in tumour-cell response to a drug (cellular metabolism, drug resistance, biochemical and molecular factors, etc.).

Other pharmacokinetic parameters such as duration of concentration above a threshold may be more relevant than AUC, especially for drugs having a schedule-dependent cytotoxicity.

Inter-patient variability in elimination of anti-cancer drugs

The traditional method for individualizing an anti-cancer drug dose is based on body-surface area (BSA), calculated according to the *Dubois formula* using height and weight. In children, morphological criteria (BSA or weight) are a major component of inter-individual pharmacokinetic variability. In adults, clearance of anti-cancer drugs is poorly correlated with BSA, leading to wide variation in drug exposure within patients dosed by this method.

Hepatic and renal functions are the major determinants of drug elimination and have to be explored before administration of anti-cancer drugs. Renal dysfunction is easily assessed by determining serum creatinine, measuring or calculating creatinine clearance, or most accurately, by determining the clearance of radio-labelled EDTA. The impact of hepatic dysfunction on the drug elimination or metabolism is more difficult to estimate. Because of complex pathophysiological mechanisms of liver insufficiency, hepatic enzymes and serum bilirubin levels are often poor indicators of metabolic activity. Alternative hepatic function tests have limited value in predicting pharmacokinetics of chemotherapeutic drugs:

- Indocyanine green (a marker of hepatic blood flow)
- Antipyrine (a substrate marker for cytochrome P450 activity)
- Lorazepam (a substrate marker of hepatic glucuronidation)

Practical considerations make these dynamic liver functions inappropriate for routine clinical practice. When metabolism of a drug is largely dependent on a unique catalytic enzyme, subpopulations of poor metabolizers may result from polymorphism in gene coding for the drug-metabolizing enzyme.

Advancing age also represents a cause of pharmacokinetic variability of many drugs. Ageing is characterized by a combination of various physiological disorders, including reduction of hepatic or renal blood flow, possible declines in microsomal activity, and frequent co-medication.

For some drugs, such as carboplatin, anthracyclines, and docetaxel, close relationships between patient characteristics and drug clearance have been established. Then, *à priori* adaptive dosing based on these characteristics is possible. For other drugs, such as methotrexate, 6-mercaptopurine, and 5-fluorouracil, dose optimization requires determination of plasma concentrations in each patient in order to adjust subsequent doses or to modulate current dose in case of continuous therapy. This approach—'adaptive dosing with feedback control'—requires certain logistics which limit its use for all drugs.

Examples of dosing strategies for individual therapy

Carboplatin

Carboplatin is mainly eliminated by the kidney. Egorin first established two relationships:

- **First**: between carboplatin clearance and measured creatinine clearance.
- **Second**: between the AUC and the percentage decrease in platelets following carboplatin administration as a single agent.

By combining these, a formula was derived for individual dose calculation according to measured creatinine clearance and desired platelet count at nadir. The concept of optimum AUC for carboplatin was demonstrated for treatment of ovarian and testicular cancers.

Calvert developed a formula to allow a dose of carboplatin to be calculated in order to achieve a target AUC:

$$\text{Dose (mg)} = \text{AUC} \times (\text{GFR} + 25 \text{ ml/min})$$

with GFR determined by isotopic measurement of ^{51}Cr-EDTA clearance. The value of 25 ml/min corresponds to the mean non-renal clearance of carboplatin.

The carboplatin target AUC must be chosen with reference to any other cytotoxics given in combination. Drugs (e.g. cyclophosphamide) potentiate the haematological toxicity of carboplatin, but with others such as paclitaxel it is safe to administer an AUC similar to that of carboplatin administered alone. Moreover, patients without prior exposure to chemotherapy may support a larger AUC than those who are heavily pre-treated.

Anthracyclines and taxanes

In the case of impaired hepatic function, guidelines have been proposed for doxorubicin dosage reduction as a function of serum bilirubin level: dose reductions by 50%, 75%, or 100% are recommended when bilirubin exceeds 12, 30, or 50 mg/l. For docetaxel, five covariables (age > 70 years, hypoalbuminaemia, elevation of α1-glycoprotein, and raised ALT and AST) are predictive of reduced clearance. Since correlation was found between docetaxel clearance and risk of severe neutropenia, these parameters may allow prediction of patients with high risk of toxicity and application of rational dose reduction.

Methotrexate

Monitoring of plasma drug concentration in patients receiving high-dose methotrexate is routinely performed. High levels 48 hours after the intravenous infusion and thereafter are associated with a risk of serious toxicity. For these patients with decreased methotrexate clearance and/or a large volume of distribution of the drug (generally due to the presence of a 'third space'—pleural effusion or ascites), folinic acid rescue is administered at a dosage adjusted according to methotrexate plasma levels.

Mercaptopurine

The effect of mercaptopurine is dependent on formation of the active 6-thioguanine nucleotide (6-TGN) metabolites. This anabolic pathway competes with the catabolic pathway mediated by thiopurine methyltransferase. The latter enzyme expression is subject to genetic polymorphism with about 10% of patients having intermediate activity and about 1 in 300 inheriting a deficiency who are exposed to prohibitive toxicity if standard mercaptopurine dosage is administered. The concentration of 6-TGN inside red blood cells has been shown to be an independent and important predictor of treatment outcome of patients taking daily oral mercaptopurine.

Although no definite recommendation on how to individualize treatment can be given, monitoring of erythrocyte 6-TGN should identify patients with a high-risk pharmacokinetic profile (low levels of 6-TGN), allowing assessment of patient compliance.

Summary

Although prospective clinical studies comparing standard (in mg/m^2) versus individualized dosing have yet to be performed, it is likely that individualized dosing of some anti-cancer drugs, based on pharmacokinetics, could increase the probability of tumour response and decrease the probability of major toxicity. In the absence of routine therapeutic drug monitoring, adjustment of the dose of subsequent treatment cycles according to the presence or absence of toxicity should be implemented more systematically.

Further reading

Cleton, F.Y. 'Chemotherapy: general aspects' in Peckham, M., Pinelo, M.M. and Veronesi, V. (eds.) *Oxford Textbook of Oncology*, pp. 445–53.

Chapter 10
Hormone therapy

Introduction

Hormones have been implicated in the development and behaviour of many malignant tumours (including vaginal, ovarian, laryngeal, pancreatic, gastrointestinal, melanomas, and meningiomas). The best evidence that hormones maintain the growth of cancers relates to sex steroid hormones and tumours of their target organs, namely oestrogens and progestins in breast and endometrial cancer and androgens in prostatic cancer.

The effects of endocrine therapy are generally confirmed to target organs, and there are side-effects outside these sites. This accounts for the increased tolerability of this treatment in comparison with cytotoxic chemotherapy. However, many tumours appear resistant to endocrine therapy, even at first presentation, and more become insensitive during the selective pressure of treatment and progression. Thus, most patients with breast and prostate cancers die with hormone-independent disease.

With this background it is important to outline:

- Different types of endocrine strategies and their relative advantages/disadvantages.
- Predictive indices of response.
- Mechanisms of resistance.
- Controversies and future expectations.

Types of endocrine therapy

Ablation of endocrine glands

In men and premenopausal women the major sites of steroid hormone synthesis are the gonads. Castration decreases circulating testosterone in males by over 95% and oestrogens in premenopausal women by 60% (relative to follicular phase levels). These endocrine effects produce benefits in about 80% of men with metastatic prostate cancer and in 30–40% of unselected premenopausal women with advanced breast cancer. Oophorectomy is rarely beneficial in post-menopausal women because the post-menopausal ovary produces little oestrogen.

These response rates represent the gold standard against which to compare other forms of endocrine therapy. Hypophysectomy and adrenalectomy have been used in post-menopausal women with breast cancer. Whilst these may produce benefit in about one-third of cases, the procedures do have significant morbidity and lack specificity, removing other classes of hormones in addition to sex steroids. The irreversible nature of surgical ablation of endocrine organs, when all patients cannot be guaranteed benefits, has provided the impetus to develop alternative drug-based therapies that are specific, reversible, and self-limiting. Thus if therapy proves ineffective, drug withdrawal allows hormone levels to return to normal with amelioration of side-effects.

Agonists/supraphysiological doses of hormone

This approach is epitomized by the use of gonadotrophin-relating hormone agonists (GnRHa or LHRHa). The gonadotrophins LH and FSH provide the stimulus for gonads to produce steroid hormones; in turn their synthesis and release from the pituitary is regulated by the hypothalamic factor GnRH (or LHRH). Highly potent agonist analogues of GnRH have been synthesized by introducing unusual amino acids into the native peptide. When administered for short periods they cause a rapid release of gonadotrophins, but in the long term these agonists down regulate gonadotrophic receptors and desensitize the pituitary. As a result circulating gonadotrophins fall, the trophic drive to the gonads is abolished, and circulating sex hormones are reduced to castration levels. Depot formulations of LHRH agonists are available so that a single injection can maintain effective medical castration over prolonged periods. The use of GnRH analogues in premenopausal women with breast cancer and men with prostate cancer has produced anti-tumour effects equivalent to surgical castration.

A similar mechanism of action underpins the response seen in hormone-dependent cancers following use of pharmacological doses of steroid hormones such as:

- Oestrogen (diethyl stilboestrol).
- Progestogens (medroxyprogesterone and megestrol).
- Androgens (testolactone and fluoxymesterone).

Lower physiological doses of the same hormones may accelerate tumour growth.

While down regulation of steroid hormone receptors occurs in target organs, other non-specific effects can occur, and these agents may be associated with poor toxicity profiles. Also, tumour flare may occur at the start of treatment. Despite this they are of clinical benefit e.g. high-dose progestogens for endometrial and breast cancer.

Inhibition of steroid-producing enzymes

This approach is best illustrated by inhibitors of aromatase or 5α-reductase activity. The aromatase enzyme converts androgens to oestrogens and is the last step of the synthetic cascade. Its inhibition represents the most specific method of blocking oestrogen production. Because oestrogen biosynthesis can occur in non-endocrine tissue such as adipose tissue and malignant tumours themselves (particularly in post-menopausal women), aromatase inhibitors have the potential to suppress oestrogen levels beyond that achievable by surgical ablation of classical endocrine organs. Two major types of inhibitors have been developed:

- **Steroidal or type I inhibitors,** which interfere with the attachment of androgen substrate to the catalytic site.
- **Non-steroidal type II inhibitors,** which interfere with the enzyme's cytochrome p450 prosthetic group.

Early type II inhibitors such as aminoglutethimide were neither potent nor specific, inhibiting other steroid-metabolizing enzymes that had a similar cytochrome p450 prosthetic group. Triazole drugs (anastrozole, letrozole, vorozole) are 2000-fold more potent than aminoglutethimide and have differential affinity towards aromatase cytochrome p450 with highly selective inhibition of oestrogen biosynthesis. These drugs can reduce circulating oestrogens in postmenopausal women to undetectable levels without influencing other steroid hormones.

Amongst type I inhibitors, formestane and exemestane are thought to act as 'suicide' inhibitors, blocking aromatase irreversibly through their own metabolism into active intermediates by the enzyme; oestrogen biosynthesis can only be resumed when aromatase molecules are synthesized *de novo*.

However, aromatase inhibitors may not influence the growth of hormone-dependent tumours. Oestrogenic effects are mediated through non-classical oestrogens such as:

- Adrenal 5-androgens.
- Dietary phyto-oestrogens.
- Industrial pesticides.

In terms of androgens, 5α-dihydrostesterone has much greater biological activity in the prostate than its precursor, testosterone. There has been interest in developing 5α-reductase inhibitors such as finasteride. However, they appear more useful for benign prostatic conditions than for cancer.

Steroid hormone antagonists

These agents block hormone-mediated effects usually at the level of their receptors. Antagonists for oestrogens, progestins, and androgens have been developed. The most extensive experience relates to the use of the anti-oestrogen, tamoxifen, in the treatment of breast cancer. Tamoxifen binds to the oestrogen receptor and blocks the effects of endogenous oestrogens. Responses are more likely to occur in tumours that are oestrogen receptor-positive.

Tamoxifen incompletely blocks the trophic actions of oestrogen and can demonstrate partial agonist activity, especially when endogenous oestrogens are low. More potent 'pure' anti-oestrogens have therefore been developed, such as ICI182780 (Faslodex), which is a 7-alkyl amide analogue of oestradiol and completely blocks the transcriptional activity of the oestrogen receptor (by preventing receptor dimerization and shuttling). This drug produces clinical responses in patients with both acquired and inherent resistance to tamoxifen.

However, pure anti-oestrogens may have more detrimental effects on bones and blood vessels than the partial agonist tamoxifen. Attention has therefore focused on Selective oEstrogen-Receptor ModulatorS (SERMS), such as raloxifine, which have target-site specificity for their anti-oestrogenic activity.

Anti-androgens such as flutamide and casodex have clinical efficacy in the treatment of prostatic cancer. Anti-progestins such as RU-486 and onapristone have been used against breast and endometrial cancer.

Predictive indices of response

Given that hormone therapy is not effective in all tumours, indiscriminate application of treatment exposes patients with resistant cancer to the side-effects of endocrine-deprivation therapy and, more importantly, delays other potentially beneficial treatment.

Currently no marker correlates absolutely with endocrine dependency and the most widely-used predictor is the oestrogen receptor (ER), in relation to breast cancers. Between 60 and 75% of breast cancers are ER-positive by biochemical assay or immunohistochemistry; two-thirds of ER-positive tumours respond to hormone manipulation, compared with 5–10% of ER-negative tumours. The value of other markers such as the progesterone receptor in breast or endometrial cancer is less clear and measurement of the androgen receptor in prostatic cancer has not proved useful.

Previous response to hormone manipulation is a useful clinical predictor for second-line endocrine therapy and suggests that progression on hormone therapy does not equate with acquisition of absolute endocrine resistance.

Resistance to hormone therapy

Resistance to hormone therapy may be primary or acquired during treatment. Two reasons for primary resistance are suggested:

- The tumour may not require hormones for growth.
- The tumour is hormone-dependent but endocrine therapy fails to reduce hormone levels below that needed for growth.

Acquired resistance

- Induction of metabolic enzymes, reduces intra-cellular drug levels.
- Emergence of clones of hormone-dependent cells.
- Production of mitogens.
- Induction of growth factor receptors.
- Second messenger systems allowing transcription in presence of low level of hormones

Controversies

Duration of adjuvant therapy

If hormone deprivation therapy is not cytotoxic but cytostatic, therapy would need to be given indefinitely. The counter argument is that resistance may be accompanied by a change in tumour phenotype induced by the continued presence of the drug. Discontinuation of the treatment followed by another non-cross-resistant regime might be more effective.

Combination therapy

Should endocrine therapies be given sequentially or in combination? Is combination more likely to achieve maximum cell kill and should this be implemented before resistance occurs? Clinical experience suggests that combined treatment may not justify its increased toxicity with the possible loss of second/third-line responses and some evidence of adverse pharmacological interactions between drugs.

Chemo-endocrine therapy

Proponents suggest that endocrine therapy is a form of chemotherapy and since combination chemotherapy is beneficial there is good reason to use chemo-endocrine therapy. However, it can be argued that hormone therapy, by suppressing tumour cell growth, may give protection from chemotherapeutic agents which are most effective against replicating cells.

Immunotherapy of cancer

Introduction

Although new chemotherapeutic agents, increased doses, combinations of drugs, or even high-dose ablative regimens have been used with some success, their use is ultimately limited by their non-specific end-organ toxicity. So, investigators have explored strategies of anti-neoplastic treatment with the potential to specifically kill malignant cells, circumventing tumour-cell resistance and using a different mechanism from conventional chemotherapy. These so-called 'biological' therapies of cancer aim to produce anti-tumour effect through the activation of defence mechanisms of the host or the administration of natural substances. It was the development of molecular biology and hybridoma technology that made available the unlimited supply of appropriate reagents.

The concept of a role for the immune response in the control or even eradication of cancer is not new. In fact, it was as early as in 1891 that William Coley reported tumour regression after stimulation of the patient's immune system by deliberately infecting cancer patients with erysipelas. But it was not until the 1960s that the 'immune surveillance theory of cancer' was introduced by Burnet. According to this theory, immune system cells continuously patrol the body, eliminating newly mutated malignant cells and protecting against the development of cancer. This vigilance would only be circumvented if the immune system was depressed or malignant cells became more aggressive.

This hypothesis provided the background for the development of cancer immunotherapy, which encompasses all the therapeutic manipulations of the immune system, utilizing any immune-related agents, such as cytokines, cellular or humoral products, vaccine preparations, and transfected genes, with or without immuno-potentiation by drugs or other agents.

Active immunotherapy

Active immunotherapy is the immunization of the patient with materials that elicit an immune reaction capable of eliminating/delaying tumour growth. It includes the administration of non-specific stimulators of the immune system, such as the bacillus Calmette–Guérin (BCG) and cytokines.

Unfortunately, cancer usually grows in an immunosuppressed environment and, therefore, non-specific cancer vaccines, with the identification of tumour-associated antigens and the ability to genetically modify tumour cells, offers the promise of a specific, active immunotherapy.

Passive immunotherapy of cancer includes the administration of materials that have the ability to mediate anti-tumour response directly or indirectly. This material could be antibodies, used either native or conjugated to a toxic agent, or cells (lymphocytes or macrophages).

Bacillus Calmette–Guérin (BCG)

The anti-neoplastic effect of the live attenuated tuberculosis vaccine, bacillus Calmette–Guérin (BCG), was reported by Pearl in 1929. Later, Mathe and co-workers demonstrated a survival benefit in animals with haematological malignancies treated with BCG. Unfortunately, the clinical studies that followed did not confirm any effectiveness of BCG systemic administration in patients with various malignancies (lymphocytic leukaemia, melanoma, lung cancer). Currently, only two applications of BCG in cancer patients are successful:

- Intralesional administration into cutaneous metastases in patients with melanoma
- Intravesical instillation for the treatment of patients with superficial bladder cancer

Immunotherapeutic action of BCG

- Activates—macrophages
    —T lymphocytes
    — B lymphocytes
    —natural killer cells
- Induces local type II immunological responses via interleukins (IL-4, IL-1, IL-10)
- Bacterial surface glycoproteins attach to epithelial cells and act as antigens

- Inhibits tumour-cell motility via BCG—fibronectin
—tumour interaction

BCG is the most effective intravesical agent for the prophylaxis of Ta and T1 superficial bladder cancer, with a 38% reduction of recurrence rate. It can also achieve a complete response rate of 60% or more in stage Ta or T1 residual bladder cancer, although it is generally preferable to resect all visible tumours when possible, prior to beginning treatment.

Immunotherapy, in the form of BCG, is the only approved intravesical treatment for CIS (carcinoma *in situ*), with an average complete response rate of 72% (vs < 50% for chemotherapy).

The optimal dose and schedule of administration of BCG varies from patient to patient: the proposed intravesical dose is between one hundred million (1×10^8) and one billion (1×10^{10}) colony forming units (CFU), but responses have been reported with doses as low as 10 million CFU or 1 mg BCG.

Many patients (up to 90%) experience symptoms of cystitis, with dysuria, haematuria, mild fever, and urinary frequency. It is advisable to withhold BCG administration to patients with gross haematuria, because the risk for absorption and major systemic BCG toxicity is increased. The most serious complication of BCG therapy is sepsis. It is mediated by traumatic catheterization with bleeding, severe cystitis, bladder biopsy, or transurethral resection of bladder tumour. Sepsis from gram-negative bacillae may occur following instrumentation of the genitourinary tract.

Nevertheless, treatment must be initiated on the basis of medical history of BCG instillation and of clinical suspicion: patients typically, but not invariably, develop:

- High fever
- Rigors
- Hypertension
- Mental confusion
- Disseminated intravascular coagulopathy
- Respiratory failure
- Jaundice
- Leukopenia

Identification of BCG DNA with techniques of molecular biology may prove useful in the future.

Cytokines

Cytokines are soluble proteins that mediate the interactions between the cells and their extracellular environment, in both an autocrine and paracrine manner. They exert their biological effect in a wide range of tissues, but mainly on cells of the haematopoietic and immune lineage.

Although several cytokines have been identified and characterized, their biological role is not fully understood because their physiology is particularly elaborate, since a given cytokine can both promote and inhibit tumour growth. How the cytokine will act depends on its concentration, the type of the tumour, and the temporal stage of the tumour–host relationship.

Several cytokines promise to be of therapeutic importance in oncology, including:

- Interleukins (IL)
- Tumour necrosis factor (TNF)
- Erythropoietin
- Colony-stimulating factor (CSF) and interferons (IFNs)

Interferons

The interferons (IFNα-, β, and γ) are a family of proteins that are produced by the immune system in response to viral infection. They have anti-viral, anti-microbial, anti-proliferative, and immuno-modulatory activity.

Anti-tumour effects of IFNs:

- Direct cytostatic activity
- Interfere with cell metabolism proliferation
- Modulate oncogene expression
- Enhance tumour-associated surface antigens
- Enhance cytotoxicity of natural killers (NK), macrophages, and T lymphocytes
- Reduce tumour neovascularization
- Promote differentiation of malignant cells to less aggressive types.

Interferon–α (IFN-α)

IFN-α is the treatment of choice for hairy-cell leukaemia (HCL), with a 90% response rate in the peripheral blood and 40% normalization of the bone marrow. The standard dose is 2×10^6 U/m^2 given three times a week, for 6–12 months, either intramuscularly or subcutaneously. It may induce partial or, less frequently, complete remission. Patients who relapse can be successfully retreated. The combination of IFN-α with the purine analogue 2-chlorodeoxyadenosine may be more effective for HCL patients.

IFN-α also has a first-line role in the management of chronic myeloid leukaemia (CML): IFN-α (5×10^6 U/m^2 daily) exerts a marked effect on the white blood count, with 50–75% haematological remission, while prolonged administration can induce complete cytogenetic eradication, suppressing the Philadelphia chromosome-positive clone. IFN-α monotherapy increases the median survival from 3 to 5 years, while its combination with other treatment modalities increases further the clinical response.

Several phase III studies have demonstrated progression-free and overall survival when IFN-α (3–10 MU/m^2 subcutaneously)was added to conventional chemotherapy to multiple myeloma patients. Up to 50% of patients with nodular (follicular) non-Hodgkin's lymphoma, refractory to conventional chemotherapy, may respond to IFN-α. Cutaneous T-cell lymphoma is another malignancy where responses of >50% can be achieved with IFN-α (6 × 10^6 U/m^2 daily).

With regard to solid tumours, responses can be seen in 10–20% of patients with renal cell carcinoma (RCC). They usually are partial and last for 6–8 months, although complete remissions have also been reported. Responses are more often in patients with a low tumour burden, good performance status, and lung metastases only. Relatively high doses of IFN-α (10–20 × 10^6 U/m^2 three times per week) have to be given.

IFN-α monotherapy has a moderate anti-tumour activity in malignant melanoma patients, but when combined with chemotherapy (dacarbazine) response rates are as high as 20%. Responses are usually partial, but they provide a survival benefit. IFN-α, alone or combined with zidovudine, may induce tumour responses in Kaposi's sarcoma patients, while IFN-α monotherapy has been used in carcinoid tumours. IFN-α has also been given intravesically, intraperitonally, intrapleurarly, and intralesionaly for the loco-regional treatment of cancer.

Clinical uses of IFN-α:

- Hairy-cell leukaemia (HCL)
- Chronic myeloid leukaemia (CML)
- Multiple myeloma
- Non-Hodgkin's lymphoma
- Cutaneous T-cell lymphoma
- Renal cell carcinoma
- Malignant melanoma
- Kaposi's sarcoma
- Carcinoid tumours

IFN-β and IFN-γ

Despite the fact that only IFN-α is currently in routine clinical use, IFN-β and IFN-γ have also some anti-tumour effect. Clinically, they have been used in patients with:

- Multiple myeloma
- HCL
- CML
- Renal cell carcinoma

* Melanoma
* Ovarian cancer
* Bladder cancer

There is not enough data to support any advantage over IFN-α, or with the concomitant administration of more than one IFN.

IFN-α, alone or in combination with tamoxifen, has been used also in breast cancer patients, with poor results.

However, the combination of IFN-α and TNF has been shown to be particularly effective in preclinical models. Clinically, this combination has been used in the treatment of melanoma and sarcoma using isolated limb perfusion. IFN-α has been used also in combination with IL-2, in patients with peritoneal carcinomatosis, and with 5-fluorouracil, in patients with advanced colorectal cancer. It synergistically enhances LAK cell activity of IL-2. Phase I/II clinical trials are currently ongoing.

Toxicity of IFNs

The major side-effects include flu-like symptoms (fever, chills, headache, malaise), which can be relieved with paracetamol or prednisolone. Other toxicities include:

* Anorexia
* Fatigue
* Rashes
* Gastrointestinal complaints
* Lethargy
* Thrombocytopenia
* Elevation of liver function tests

Tolerance to IFN-α increases with prolonged administration and all side-effects are reversible when treatment is discontinued.

IFNs represent an anti-neoplastic agent, effective for some malignancies resistant to conventional chemotherapy.

Interleukin-2 (IL-2)

IL-2, a lymphokine produced by activated T cells (Th1), plays a pivotal role in immune modulation, enhancing the growth of activated T cells, the proliferation of lymphoid cells, and the migration of lymphocytes from the peripheral blood. Anti-tumour activity of IL-2 includes the capacity to lyse fresh tumour cells, the regression of distant metastases in murine models, and the *in vivo* release of other members of the cytokines family.

IL-2 has been widely applied in the management of patients with advanced cancer. The systemic administration of high doses of IL-2, alone or in combination with lymphokine-activated killer (LAK) cells, activated *ex vivo*, may induce objective responses in a small proportion of patients with renal cell carcinoma (5–15%) or metastatic melanoma (<15%). Responses have also been demonstrated in patients with acute myeloid leukaemia. These studies were performed in patients of poor prognosis, with advanced and refractory disease.

IL-2 can be given intravenously at doses from 72 000 to 720 000 IU/kg every 8 hours. Toxicities associated with IL-2 administration include:

- Flu-like syndrome
- Capillary leak syndrome
- Severe hypotension
- Arrhythmia
- Angina
- Respiratory distress
- Somnolence
- Anaemia
- Thrombocytopenia
- Multi-organ malfunction
- Toxic fatalities in up to 10% of patients

In melanoma, administration of IL-2 alters the biodistribution of dacarbazine due to enhanced capillary permeability, resulting in synergy. IFN-α enhances IL-2 lymphocyte proliferation and IFN-α /IL-2 combination therapy is undergoing clinical assessment in patients with renal cell carcinoma and melanoma.

Tumour necrosis factor (TNF)

TNF is an important mediator of the inflammatory response, being involved in stress conditions, cachexia, and endotoxin shock. It is mainly produced by monocytes, activated macrophages, and T cells. It induces the expression of MHC class I and II antigens, as well as adhesion molecules responsible for leukocyte migration and accumulation.

TNF (mainly TNF-, has been used in various clinical trials, mostly in patients with advanced melanoma and sarcoma. Results have been disappointing, with <5% response rate. Loco-regional administration (intraperitoneally, intravesically, intralesionally) seems more promising, but its clinical use is limited by the severe side-effects which include:

- Acute fever
- Anaemia
- Thrombocytopenia
- Hepatotoxicity

- Cytochrome P450 depression
- Transient impairment of renal function
- Central nervous system toxicity, especially in the elderly

Local administration of rTNF and of TNF encapsulated liposomes could be used in the future to circumvent the problems of toxicity.

Data show synergy between TNF and conventional chemotherapeutic agents such as cyclophosphamide, doxorubicin, and cisplatin. TNF may reverse cisplatin resistance. On the other hand, cisplatin and cyclophosphamide may act as biological modulators by increasing TNF binding to the cell surface.

Monoclonal antibodies

Although the management of cancer by exploiting properties distinguishing neoplastic and normal cells has always been an attractive concept, it was the development of hybridoma technology and the resulting tumour-associated monoclonal antibodies (mAbs) that offered new prospects for this strategy. Some of the applications of mAbs in oncology are now part of everyday diagnosis (i.e. immunohistochemistry, radio-immunodetection).

With regard to cancer therapeutic modalities, unconjugated or native mAbs can activate components of the complement and of cytolytic cells and result in tumour lysis, with a mechanism known as Antibody-Dependent Cellular Cytotoxicity (ADCC). Several studies have been conducted, mainly in patients with haematological malignancies. The responses achieved were generally poor and of short duration: circulating malignant cells were reduced, but with little effect on lymph node or bone marrow disease.

Since the cytotoxic effect of the mAbs was minimal, they have been used as carriers of more potent agents such as conventional cytotoxic drugs, radionuclides, liposomes, and toxins, to achieve specific delivery at the tumour sites and therefore reduced host toxicity. Another approach is to use mAbs-enzymes conjugates to catalyse various substrate conversions at the tumour. The pro-drug is administered after the conjugate has localized to the surface of the malignant cells and cleared from the circulation.

These approaches are currently undergoing clinical evaluation; the major problem seems to be in the immune response elicited by murine antibodies, known as HAMA (Human Anti-Mouse Antiglobulin response). Nevertheless, it is expected that the evolution of genetic engineering and the subsequent production of single-chain, chimaeric and humanized antibodies and of fusion proteins will overcome this problem. Other limiting factors are the low antibody uptake by the tumour, the antigenic heterogeneity of the tumour, the poor tumour penetration, and the poor stability of the immuno-conjugates *in vivo*.

In conclusion, the use of mAbs as targeting devices for cytotoxic agents is a very attractive approach for tumour immunotherapy. However, there are still several complex issues to be resolved before they become part of the routine practice in oncology.

Adoptive immunotherapy

The demonstration that the cell-mediated immune response is crucial in the rejection of allogeneic and syngeneic tumours has prompted the use of cells with anti-tumour activity in patients with malignancies—an approach known as *adoptive immunotherapy* of cancer.

Several strategies have been applied to generate cells with reactivity to tumours, the most common being the production of lymphocyte-activated killer (LAK) cells that can lyse fresh tumour cells, by incubating human peripheral blood lymphocytes with IL-2, *ex vivo*. The exact mechanism of recognition and destruction of tumours by LAK cells is not fully understood. Trials in renal cell carcinoma and melanoma patients did not reveal any therapeutic advantage in the administration of LAK plus IL-2, compared to monotherapy with IL-2.

In an alternative approach of adoptive immunotherapy, tumour-infiltrating lymphocytes (TILs), that can recognize tumour-associated antigens, have been isolated from human tumours and administered to patients with advanced melanoma, with a response rate (PR + CR) of 25–35%. Recently, genetically manipulated TILs have been produced, with the transduction of the gene encoding either the neomycin phosphotransferase or tumour necrosis factor.

Tumour vaccines

Hepatitis B virus (HBV) vaccine is a widely used, very effective vaccine against hepatocellular carcinoma, while studies are in progress to develop vaccines against Epstein–Barr virus, which is closely linked to the development of:

- Burkitt's lymphoma
- Nasopharyngeal carcinoma
- Non-Hodgkin's lymphomas

Other obvious candidates for development of an anti-tumour vaccine are the human papilloma virus (HPV) and the human retrovirus, HTLV, which are causative agents for several human malignancies.

While the development of a vaccine is obvious in a virally-induced tumour, in non-virally-induced tumours, the concept of a vaccine is more complicated. In this case, tumour cells or tumour cell extracts are used as cancer vaccines intending to enhance a humoral or cell-mediated immune response to relevant tumour antigens, rather than to induce prophylactic immunity. The antibodies produced may kill the tumour cells by complement fixation or antibody-dependent cellular cytotoxicity, while the activation of cytotoxic T cells that recognize antigens on the tumour cell surface may induce specific cytolysis. This approach was expected to reduce tumour-induced immuno-suppression and selectively augment long-lasting humoral and cellular anti-tumour immunity but, in general, it seems to have only minimal clinical significance.

More promising is the vaccination with anti-idiotype antibodies, directed against determinants expressed on the variable regions of anti-tumour antibodies. However, this strategy is limited by the fact that anti-idiotypic antibodies have to be produced individually and are thus expensive and labour-intensive.

Several vaccines for melanoma, colorectal, breast, prostate, and lung cancers are currently under clinical evaluation. Preliminary data support the concept that active immunization will be effective to patients with high-risk recurrent disease, after surgical removal of the tumour, when the tumour burden is small. Unfortunately, most of the clinical trials have been in patients with advanced, extensive disease, refractory to conventional therapies and probably already immunosuppressed.

Gene therapy

Gene therapy is the therapeutic strategy in which a functioning gene is inserted into a cell to provide a new function or to correct a genetic error. Since cancer is the result of 'misbehave' genes, it provides an ideal candidate for gene-therapy interventions.

Two requirements exist for successful genetic manipulations: first, a method to transfer the gene into the correct cell and second, a way to adequately control its expression.

Techniques to introduce DNA into cells

- Lipid complexed with DNA
- DNA in lipid vesicles
- DNA in red blood cell ghosts
- Direct micro-injection of DNA
- Exposure of cells to high voltage
- Use of viruses

The non-viral methods are convenient and have an obvious safety advantage, but they have low efficiency and result in transient gene expression. On the contrary, viral (retroviruses, adenoviruses, poxviruses) vectors represent the most efficient, stable manner of integrating DNA into large numbers of target cells.

Based on the knowledge gained from other approaches of cancer immunotherapy, several strategies have been proposed for using gene therapies in patients with malignancies. Genes encoding for cytokines can be transferred *in vivo* to the tumour or to TILs. Alternatively, tumour cells or antigen-presenting cells (APC) can be genetically engineered *ex vivo* and re-injected in the patient to enhance tumour immunogeneity. Furthermore, genetic modification of immune effector cells may enhance their survival and increase their tumour recognition and anti-tumour efficacy, *in vivo*.

Clinical trials are being conducted in patients with pancreatic, lung, breast, prostate, and bladder cancer. These trials have demonstrated the feasibility and safety of genetic manipulations in cancer patients, although the clinical benefit from gene therapy is not clear. Attempts are currently focused on the development of techniques that would warrant the efficient gene delivery to selected tissues and control its expression, anticipating the mobilization of an effective anti-tumour immune response.

Summary

Molecular biology has opened new frontiers for the understanding of tumour immunology. Biological therapies of cancer are based on sound scientific rationale and show promising preliminary results. Immunotherapy in particular is based on the breaking of the host's immunological tolerance to the tumour. This would allow the immune system of the patient to recognize the tumour as non-self and mediate an effective anti-tumour response directly or indirectly.

To date, immunotherapy has failed to bring radical improvements in patients' care. Nevertheless, several complete and partial remissions have been induced in some cancer patients, mainly those with minimal tumour burden, indicating a potential role for immunotherapy in the armentarium against cancer.

The main challenge for tumour immunologists in the near future is to carry out properly controlled studies of the safety and efficacy of the immunotherapy approaches, in order to identify the individuals most likely to benefit from them.

Further reading

Berd, D. (1998) Cancer vaccines: reborn or just recycled? *Semin Oncol* **24**, 605–10.

Efraim, B. (1999) One hundred years of cancer immunotherapy: a critical appraisal. *Tumour Biol.* **20**, 1–24.

Gore, M. and Riches, P. (ed.) (1996) *Immunotherapy in cancer.* John Wiley & Sons, London.

Rosenberg, S.A. (1998) New opportunities for the development of cancer immunotherapies. *Cancer J Sci Am* **4**, 1–4.

Syrigos, K.N. and Epenetos, A.A. (1999) Antibody directed enzyme prodrug therapy (ADEPT): a review of the experimental and clinical considerations. *Anticancer Res* **19(1A)**, 605–14.

Syrigos, K.N., Deonarian, D., and Epenetos, A.A. (1999) Use of monoclonal antibodies for the diagnosis and treatment of bladder cancer. *Hybridoma* **18(3)**, 219–24.

Syrigos, K.N., Karayiannakis, A.J. and Zbar, A. (2000) Mucins as immunogenic targets in cancer. *Anticancer Research* **20**, 420–6.

Part 3
Principles of prevention and care

Chapter 12
Cancer prevention and screening

Prevention strategies

Chemoprevention is the use of chemical agents or dietary compounds to reduce the incidence of cancer. The chemical compounds could be trace elements or hormones or other medicaments, the dietary compounds could be fibre, nutrients, vitamins, etc. This field of medical oncology brings together the discipline of:

- Epidemiology
- Carcinogenesis
- Toxicology
- Pharmacology
- Molecular biology
- Genetics

Burkitt observed that colorectal cancer was almost unknown in numerous tribes in Africa, possibly due to their high-fibre diet. Migration studies of these African tribesmen moving into townships showed that within a generation, bowel cancer increased in incidence, approaching that of the city dwellers. This had been accompanied by a preceding change of diet to include less fibre, more fat, and more sugar. Similarly a number of studies associated breast cancer with obesity and numerous studies have subsequently attempted to explore the relationship of fat in the diet and the onset of breast cancer.

There are numerous risk factors for breast cancer including:

- Delayed puberty
- History of nulliparity
- Lack of breast feeding
- Contraceptive pill in early life
- Hormone replacement therapy around the menopause

Interventions with hormones based on breast tumour biology are therefore tempting but the biological mechanisms need first to be defined.

Biochemical alterations have been shown in population studies of cancer patients' blood. Low levels of retinoids such as vitamin A and β carotene and elements like selenium have been associated with cancer. Whether these biochemical alterations are cause or effect is perplexing. It is clear that a number of carcinogens stimulate resting cells to proliferate and grow under the influence of oncogenes such as ras, raf, Bcl2. This process should be inhibited by tumour suppressor genes such as Rb or p53 or substances such as TGFβ.

Another possible route for cells to become immortal is to avoid apoptosis. The apoptopic pathway involves at least a dozen known mediators, including p53. Cancer cells classically will have either an increase of the proliferation genes or anti-apoptopic signals or defective tumour suppressor genes.

Having understood the cancer process and the predisposing factors it is easier to identify which patient group might be at highest risk and might benefit from an intervention either in change of diet or addition of a medicine.

Genetic risks

Patients with certain genetic defects are more likely to get cancer—either they have overexpressed oncogenes such as Kras or a mutated tumour suppressor gene such as p53 or Rb. In the aetiology of colorectal cancer Kras is one of the first of six or more genetic alterations known to accumulate in the malignant progression from normal mucosa through adenoma or polyp to carcinoma. p53 mutations are associated with the last and critical stage. Injection of wild-type p53 into human cultured colorectal cells bearing several genetic alterations leads to reversion to a benign phenotype.

Environmental risks

A number of environmental factors are known to cause pre-malignant lesions e.g. chewing tobacco frequently causes leucoplakia, which progresses to oral carcinoma. This is an ideal situation for testing interventions, including many retinoids. Metaplasia of the oesophagus is known to herald frank carcinoma and high-risk populations, such as those found in China, are the subject of chemoprevention trials of drugs.

Smoking and lung cancer is a clear-cut cause and effect, but trials of intervention require large numbers of smokers to be randomized. Two-tail analyses are mandatory as evidence from two such trials indicate that β carotene increases lung cancer incidence.

Viruses have been incriminated in the aetiology of:

- Hepatoma (hepatitis viruses)
- Burkitt's lymphoma
- Nasopharyngeal carcinoma (Epstein–Barr viruses, EBV)
- Cervical carcinoma (human papilloma virus 16).

Vaccines are available against each of these agents but only the first has been tested for long enough to show efficacy. Studies in Taiwan and West Africa have indicated a decreased incidence of hepatoma as well as a marked protective effect on hepatitis.

Helicobacter pylori has been linked to gastric carcinoma and early claims of eradication of the organism by antibiotics and subsequent protection from cancer are being validated. These examples could also be categorised as chemoprevention.

The association of ultraviolet light with skin cancer is well-established, as is the increase of malignant melanoma in the UK (approximately 10% per annum). Primary intervention is the obvious solution. A recent randomized trial of a retinoid showed adequate protection from new squamous carcinomas but no effect on basal carcinomas.

Clinical trials

The rules of intervention in prevention trials in normal people are very different from the classical therapy trials known to oncologists. The disciplines come together, for instance in breast cancer, with the observation made in the therapeutic trials of tamoxifen used as an adjuvant in early breast cancer that the incidence of second primary breast cancer in the contralateral breast was less with tamoxifen than with placebo. It led to the notion that tamoxifen might be a preventive agent as well a cytotoxic drug. There followed a series of trials leading to the landmark publication of the Breast Cancer Prevention Trial (BCPT) from the United States in 1998, which showed that tamoxifen could halve the number of breast cancers observed in normal women at high risk by virtue of previous benign lesions in the breast or a positive family history. However, in two further trials no proven benefit was observed in different patient populations.

The tamoxifen illustration is important because it highlights a number of problems. First is the duration of administration of tamoxifen—presumably those at risk from breast cancer, for instance due to mutated BRCA1 or BRCA2 genes, have a lifetime risk. Indeed it is measured to be around 80% for breast cancer and 50% for ovarian cancer in BRCA1 mutation carriers. How long should tamoxifen be given and when should it be started? The second issue is the incidence of side-effects, which may be tolerable in a cancer therapy trial but not in 'non-patients' in a prevention trial.

It is known that the effectiveness of tamoxifen as a therapeutic agent plateaus after five years, but the risk of uterine cancer does not. The risk of the latter is of the order of 1 in 500 women. The notion of giving a chemopreventive drug that is also a carcinogen, presents a dilemma, so second-generation tamoxifen agents have been developed to remove the moiety of the drug which is associated with the carcinogenic effect on the uterus.

Phase I/II trials

The main objectives of early trials of chemopreventive agents that have been proven to be effective in laboratory tests, either in cell lines or in animal models, is to establish tolerance and side-effects. The major difference between the early trials of these agents, compared to cytotoxic agents, is that the duration of administration of the preventive agent will be much longer than a cytotoxic, so chronic side-effects are as important as acute side-effects. It is important to show proof of principle where possible, so if a particular drug is designed to show target-cell differentiation, then the endpoint would be a histological one. If the endpoint were to increase apoptosis where this had been defective, then measurement of apoptosis would be important.

A major side-effect would be either fatality or problems requiring intervention by a physician or long-term disability. Major side-effects would automatically rule out any further development of an agent. Dose and duration of administration of the new agent are essential endpoints, but escalation of dose would not necessarily be carried out to the level at which toxicity is produced. Rather a dose might be defined as ideal which achieves the biological effect as described.

An important part of Phase III trial evaluation is compliance and it is also important to get some sort of measure of this in the early clinical trials. Clearly this is frequently related to appearance of toxicity, but can also be influenced by the ease and route of administration. The target population will frequently be those at highest risk, for instance cancer patients who are cured but at high risk of a second malignancy.

A Phase II trial will frequently be of longer duration with more emphasis on compliances; it may well be randomized with a placebo control and may also, as in Phase I, evaluate further multiple-dose levels. Duration may be one to five years and the sample size could be anything from one hundred to many thousands of 'patients' or potential patients.

Again the use of intermediate endpoints is extremely important for cost-efficient studies, though there is a paucity of good candidates for these biomarkers that are of proven value. Ease of recruitment is important because 'high risk' may be clear to a physician but not so clear to a normal individual.

These parameters are important for calculating the Phase III trial size and the statistical power, by which is measured.

Phase III trials

Studies of chemopreventive agents in randomized Phase III design require to be very large and very lengthy. For instance, a study of smokers randomized to retinoids needs to recruit thousands of smokers for a follow-up period of up to twenty years to detect any impact on lung cancer rate or survival. As it is impossible to afford, in terms of time or money, to test each new agent with the classical Phase II design, two solutions are being tested. One is the concentration on high-risk groups of individuals and the other is the development of intermediate biomarkers. Individuals can be at high risk because of a genetic predisposition or a previous treatment or by having had a previous cancer.

The Euroscan trial was designed to be cost-effective, as it tested patients who had been cured of one smoking-related cancer either in the lung, head, or neck. The primary endpoint was the appearance of a second smoking-related cancer, genotypically different from the first, anywhere in the aerodigestive tract. 'Ex-patients' were randomized to receive retinol or n-acetyl cysteine.

Retinol induces differentiation and inhibits malignant transformation. It acts at the promotion stage of carcinogenesis and there is evidence that it antagonizes a number of growth factors. It is an immune stimulant and it may actually be cytotoxic (transretinoic acid has been shown to be effective in the treatment of acute myelomonocytic leukaemia). N acetyl cysteine has been used widely in chronic bronchitis in Europe and works in a totally different way from retinol. It is a potent anti-oxidant and increases intracellular glutathione. It has been shown in laboratory animals to be an anticarcinogen.

In order to test the possible advantages in combining two chemopreventive agents, which have different mechanisms of action, the third arm of the Euroscan trial includes both agents and the fourth arm, neither. This allows two questions to be answered with half the number of patients by analysis of the data at the end of the study by factorial methods. As second primary tumours are seen within seven years in 15% of this cohort, the study only requires 2500 individuals to be randomized.

Summary

Chemoprevention is in its infancy. New methodologies are being evaluated and new surrogate endpoints and novel candidate interventions are emerging rapidly from the revolution in molecular biology and genetics. It is an extremely promising and exciting branch of oncology.

Cancer chemoprevention

Many human cancers are preventable, because their causes have been identified in the human environment. Wattenberg first suggested that regular consumption of certain constituents of fruits and vegetables might offer protection from cancer. He coined the term 'cancer chemoprevention', which can be defined as 'the use of specific diets, or natural or synthetic chemicals, to reverse, suppress, or prevent carcinogenic progression to invasive cancer'.

Minimization of exposure towards carcinogens in the environment (primary prevention) is an effective strategy in cancer prevention. However, most environmental factors that initiate cancer remain to be identified and, once identified, the avoidance of such factors may necessitate difficult lifestyle changes.

Epidemiological data suggesting that cancer is preventable by intervention with chemicals are based on:

- Time trends in cancer incidence and mortality
- Geographic variations and effect of migration
- Identification of specific causative factors
- Lack of simple patterns of genetic inheritance for the majority of human cancers

Chemopreventive agents and their molecular targets

Epithelial carcinogenesis proceeds via multiple, discernible steps of molecular and cellular alterations, culminating in invasive neoplasms. These events can be separated into three distinct phases:

- **Initiation** (rapid; involves direct carcinogenic damage to DNA; and the resulting mutation is irreversible).

- **Promotion** (follows initiation and is generally reversible; involves the clonal expansion of initiated cells induced by agents acting as mitogens for the initiated cell).

- **Progression** (results from promotion in the sense that cell proliferation caused by promoters allows cellular damage inflicted by initiation to be further propagated).

During tumour progression, genotypically and phenotypically altered cells gradually emerge. Both promotion and progression phases are prolonged. Depending on which phase of carcinogenesis they affect, chemopreventive agents can be divided into tumour 'blocking' agents, which counteract cancer by interfering with initiation, and tumour 'suppressing' agents, which intercept promotion or progression. The synthetic dithiolethione compound, oltipraz, and the organic selenium compound, selenomethionine, are examples of blocking agents. 13-cis retinoic acid, a member of the retinoid family (which are natural and synthetic compounds related to vitamin A), is a tumour-suppressing agent.

Blocking agents such as oltipraz, which prevent metabolic activation of carcinogens or their subsequent binding to DNA, probably play a significant role in reducing the accumulation of initiating mutations. The fact that initiation can occur very early in life confounds clinical chemoprevention strategies based only on anti-initiation. Suppression of the development of the initiated cell to a malignant tumour is probably the strategy of choice in human cancer chemoprevention.

Altered states of cell and tissue differentiation are characteristic of pre-malignant lesions long before they become invasive and metastatic. This pathology of differentiation (dysplasia) offers a defined target for pharmacological intervention because, in some circumstances, it is possible to reverse abnormal differentiation with a hormone-like non-toxic agent. Two other approaches to the control of pre-neoplastic lesions are to block their expansion with non-toxic agents that suppress cell replication, or to induce an apoptotic state in cells which ordinarily would be programmed to die but may have undergone carcinogenic mutations providing an extended life span.

Although in the past, cancer chemopreventive agents have been discovered serendipitously or developed empirically, recent advances in the molecular biology of carcinogenesis suggest that it will be possible to develop new and better agents by a more mechanistic approach. A good example is colon cancer—the recent discovery that over-expression of the gene coding for inducible cyclo-oxygenase (COX-2), a key enzyme in the formation of prostaglandins from arachidonic acid, is an early and central event in colon carcinogenesis now provides an important target for new drug development. Recently, the novel specific COX-2 inhibitors, celeoxib, was approved by the FDA for the reduction of polyps in familial adenomatous polyposis (FAP) patients.

Tumour-suppressing compounds such as the retinoids, genistein, an isoflavonoid constituent of soya, and curcumin (the pigment which gives curry its characteristic colour) affect, in a complex fashion, several biochemical and physiological cell parameters potentially associated with carcinogenesis. Some of these agents not only suppress tumour formation but also possess a tumour-blocking component.

Information about the pharmacokinetic behaviour of chemopreventive agents is scarce. It is therefore not yet possible to assess whether the concentrations at which these agents are known to elicit biochemical responses are achieved *in vivo* after eating foods that contain them.

Clinical cancer chemoprevention

The substance under test has to be innocuous from a toxicological standpoint, as it is likely to be administered over a considerable period of time and to healthy individuals. Foodstuffs are attractive sources of tumour-suppressive substances, as the effects of long-term exposure are well-documented.

Currently, more than 60 randomized trials of potential chemopreventive agents have been reported. Only a few of these trials constituted 'definitive trials'. A primary chemopreventive trial with a significantly positive outcome is the retinol study that showed protection against squamous cell skin carcinoma. Tamoxifen has been approved in the US to reduce the risk of breast cancer in high-risk women.

Two definitive trials of β-carotene were significantly negative. In these trials lung cancer incidence was studied in 50 000 individuals. The outcome of these trials made headlines, suggesting that in high-risk groups of smokers and/or workers occupationally exposed to asbestos, β-carotene increases rather than decreases the risk of developing lung cancer. Subgroup analyses of these two trials revealed that the risk of lung cancer was highest among those individuals who continued to smoke at least 20 cigarettes per day and those in the highest quartile of alcohol consumption. It is conceivable that β-carotene suppresses tumours only in those individuals from whom the initiating stimulus has been removed, but not in those who continue to be subjected to it.

These results underline the importance of understanding how chemopreventive agents exert their effects and under which conditions they are beneficial or indeed detrimental, prior to extensive clinical evaluation.

Several trials were 'classically' negative—the investigational agents (among them β-carotene, 13-cis retinoic acid, retinol, selenium, and α-tocopherol) failed to prevent a variety of cancers. Analyses of subsets of populations in some of the trials yielded intriguing positive or negative results. For example, a nutritional supplement of selenium reduced total cancer mortality and incidence of prostate, lung, and colorectal cancer, and recently, α-tocopherol was reported to protect against prostate cancer.

Whenever possible, trials of agents for 'primary prevention' should be preceded by clinical evaluation of their efficacy for 'secondary prevention' of cancer in specific epithelial target sites. These studies are aimed at the reversal or arrest of pre-malignant lesions, or the prevention of second primary tumours in patients cured of an initial cancer. Secondary prevention trials are more cost-effective than large and long-term primary prevention trials. The burden of carcinogenic stimuli on the patient is high and a meaningful endpoint can be measured in a reasonable time frame in a smaller number of patients. Such trials have furnished important leads concerning the benefit of retinoids to prevent pre-malignant lesions and secondary primary malignancies of the head and neck, lung, skin, and liver, and of the non-steroidal anti-inflammatory drug, sulindac, in the prevention of the development of tumours in familial adenomatous polyposis.

Summary

Clinical and laboratory-based research in cancer chemoprevention is expanding in an attempt to prevent or postpone the disease. Definitive, clinical, Phase III trials include the current studies of tamoxifen. But equally important are the mechanism of action studies which will furnish better methods of designing and testing chemopreventive agents, and the identification of specific biomarkers of carcinogenesis that can serve as surrogate endpoint markers.

Table 12.1 Mechanisms of tumour suppression and examples of cancer chemopreventive agents

Scavenging oxygen radicals	Polyphenols (curcumin, genistein), selenium, tocopherol (vitamin E)
Inhibition of arachidonic acid metabolism	N-acetylcysteine, NSAIDs (sulindac, aspirin), polyphenols, tamoxifen
Modulation of signal transduction	NSAIDs, retinoids, tamoxifen, genistein, curcumin
Modulation of hormonal/growth factor activity	NSAIDs, retinoids, curcumin, tamoxifen
Inhibition of oncogene activity	Genistein, NSAIDs, monoterpenes (D-limonene, perillyl alcohol)
Inhibition of polyamine metabolism	2-Difluoromethylornithine, retinoids, tamoxifen
Induction of terminal differentiation	Calcium, retinoids, vitamin D_3
Induction of apoptosis	Genistein, curcumin, retinoids, tamoxifen

NSAIDs = non-steroidal anti-inflammatory drugs

Screening for cancer

Introduction

The strongest evidence that early detection increases the chance of cure comes from randomized trials of screening, but there is also evidence that survival after diagnosis is related to duration of symptoms. This has led to public awareness campaigns to persuade individuals to seek advice regarding suspicious symptoms at an early stage. There is, however, no evidence as yet that this strategy can improve survival.

Screening is the process whereby asymptomatic individuals are tested in order to detect a disease that has yet to declare itself. For this to be effective in a population there are certain criteria that must be met by the disease in question, the screening test, and the screening programme.

The disease

- Its natural history is well understood
- It has a recognizable 'early' stage
- Treatment at an early stage is more effective than at a later stage
- It is sufficiently common in the target population to warrant screening

The test

- Sensitive and specific
- Acceptable
- Safe
- Inexpensive

The programme

- Adequate facilities for diagnosis in those with a positive test
- High quality of treatment for screen-detected disease
- Screening repeated at intervals if the disease is of insidious onset
- Benefit must outweigh physical and psychological harm
- Benefit must justify financial cost

It is crucial that treating the disease to be screened at an early stage is more effective than treating at a later stage. To justify a screening programme one cannot compare the outcome of screen-detected disease with that of symptomatic disease, because three biases operate in favour of screen-detected disease:

- **Lead-time bias** arises from the fact that if early diagnosis advances the time of diagnosis of a disease, then the period from diagnosis to death will lengthen irrespective of whether or not treatment has altered the natural history of the disease. Screening will only be of value if it shifts the survival curve upwards.

- **Length bias** operates as slow-growing tumours are more likely to be detected by screening tests when compared to fast-growing tumours which are more likely to present with symptoms before a screening test can be applied or between tests. Thus, screen-detected tumours will tend to be less aggressive and associated with a relatively good prognosis.

- **Selection bias** results from the type of person who accepts an invitation to be screened. Such a person is more likely to be health conscious than one who refuses or ignores screening and is therefore likely to survive longer, irrespective of the disease process.

These three biases make patients with screen-detected tumours appear to have a better prognosis than when tumours present with symptoms. For the true effect of screening to be revealed, screening research must take these biases into account. The only way to do this is to carry out randomized, controlled trials in which mortality from a specific disease is compared between a population offered screening (including those who present with symptoms before screening can take place or between screens and those who refuse to be screened) and a population not offered screening. Such trials have been done in breast and colorectal cancer.

Screening

In screening it is also important to have a target population to avoid large numbers of fruitless tests. In screening for the common cancers, where the incidence is highly age-dependent, the age range should be that in which the disease is relatively common and in which the patients are likely to be fit enough for treatment.

There are other high-risk groups, however, and family history is becoming important in this respect, particularly as it is now possible to detect specific genetic mutations from blood samples and to use these to screen close relatives. Examples of this are mutations in the APC gene in familial adenomatous polyposis, in the DNA mismatch repair genes in hereditary non-polyposis colorectal cancer, and in the BRCA 1 and 2 genes in familial breast and ovarian cancer.

A screening test must be acceptable and safe, so that it will be adopted by the target population. It must also be sensitive and specific. Sensitivity is the proportion of individuals with the disease who have a positive test, and specificity is the proportion of individuals without the disease who have a negative test. Thus the ideal test would be acceptable to everyone, have no associated morbidity or mortality, and have 100% sensitivity and specificity—but this ideal has never been realised and any screening test has to be a compromise between these factors.

Screening programme

When a screening programme is established, it is important that the diagnostic facilities are adequate—this usually requires additional start-up funding. It is also essential that the diagnosis is of the highest quality to avoid patient dissatisfaction and the litigation that can result from missed disease or misdiagnosed benign pathology. Similarly, treatment of early disease must be associated with minimal morbidity and mortality.

It must also be remembered that screening does cause psychological morbidity, and along with any physical morbidity caused by investigation and treatment, this represents part of the cost of screening. The benefits gained must outweigh such morbidity, and society must make a decision whether or not the health gain justifies the financial cost.

Randomized trials have been done in breast and colorectal cancer, and in both instances screening has been shown to reduce mortality. In the former condition, the screening test studied was the mammogram, and efficacy of screening proved highly dependent not only on the quality of the X-rays but also on the quality of the reporting. In colorectal cancer, the test investigated was the faecal occult blood test, followed by colonoscopy when positive. Here, it is the secondary investigation (i.e. the colonoscopy) where quality control is of the utmost importance.

Breast screening is currently available for all women aged 50–65 years in the UK, but provision of colorectal cancer screening is still under discussion. Cervical cancer screening using cervical cytology is established but has never been subjected to a randomized trial.

Further reading

Benner, S.E., Lippman, S.M., Hong, W.K. (1994) Chemoprevention of second primary tumours: a model for intervention trials. *European Journal of Cancer* **30A, No 6,** 727–9.

Goodman, G.E. (1992) The clinical evaluation of cancer chemoprevention agents: defining and contrasting phase I, II and III objectives. *Cancer Research (Suppl.)* **52,** 2752–7.

Kelloff, G.J., Boone, C.W., Steele, Y.E., Crowell, J.A., Lubet, R., and Sigman, Ca.C. (1994) Progress in cancer chemoprevention: perspectives on agent selection and short-term clinical intervention trials. *Cancer Research (Suppl.)* **54,** 2015–24.

Lippman, S.M., Benner, S.E., and Ki Hong, W. (1994) Cancer chemoprevention. *Journal of Clinical Oncology* **12, No 4** 851–73.

Lippman, S.M., Lee, J.J. and Sabichi, A.L. (1998) Cancer chemoprevention: progress and promise. *Journal of the National Cancer Institute* **90, No 20,** 1514–28.

Meyskens Jr. F.L. (1992) Biomarker intermediate endpoints and cancer prevention. *Journal of the National Cancer Institute Monographs* **No 13,** 177–81.

Nixon, D.W. (1994) Special aspect of cancer prevention trials. *Cancer (Suppl.)* **$474, No 9,** 2683–6.

Sporn, M.B. (1993) Chemoprevention of cancer. *The Lancet* **342,** 1211–12.

Stewart, B.W., McGregor, D., and Kleihues, P. (1996) *Principles of chemoprevention. IARC Scientific Publication No 139.*

Chapter 13
Clinical trials

Methodology in cancer

Introduction

Clinical trials can be classified as:

- Phase I studies
- Phase II studies
- Phase III studies

In addition, some Phase III studies are sometimes referred to as Phase IV or post-marketing studies.

No study should be started without a protocol that describes in detail:

- Aim of the study
- Patient eligibility criteria
- Screening and follow-up studies
- Treatment
- Criteria to score toxicity and activity

In addition, rules for informed consent procedures should be specified.

All of these criteria have been specified in guidelines produced by the International Conference for Harmonisation for Good Clinical Practice (ICH-GCP).

Phase I studies

Phase I studies are human toxicology studies. Their endpoint is *safety* and they usually include 15–30 patients. They are designed to define a feasible dose for further studies. These studies begin at a dose that is expected to be safe in man. This dose is projected from toxicology studies in animals, most frequently rodent studies (although other species are used).

If there is no difference in the sensitivity between species, the starting dose of the study in humans is frequently 10% of the LD_{10} (the dose that is lethal to 10% of the animals exposed to it) in mice. Once this dose is found safe, it is escalated. Dose escalation is usually between cohorts and infrequently in individual patients. It can be:

- According to the Fibonnaci method (dose is escalated in decreasing percentages of the previous dose i.e. 100%, 66%, 50%, 33%, 25%).
- According to pharmacokinetics (Pharmacokinetically Guided Dose Escalation or PGDE), using a method that combines statistics with the experience and expectations regarding side-effects (continuous reassessment method).
- Variation on these methods.

The aim of the Phase I study is to describe the side-effects that limit further dose escalation (dose limiting toxicities or DLTs) and to recommend a dose for further studies with the drug or the new administration method (maximal tolerated dose or MTD). Most often the MTD is the dose level just below that that induces DLTs.

This approach assumes that there is a linear relationship between drug dose and therapeutic effect. For studies with biological agents the MTD may be different from the optimal dose due to a bell-shaped efficacy curve.

Phase II studies

In Phase II studies anti-tumour activity of a new drug or method is the endpoint. There are various statistical designs, including 14–60 patients on average. In the case of new drugs, where the exposure of patients to potentially inactive agents should still be avoided, the design is aimed to exclude activity with a level of certainty, instead of showing activity.

With the emergence of drugs that create tumour dormancy rather than cell kill, the endpoint of time to progression becomes important. This is the time from the start of treatment until the first evidence of tumour progression. In addition, Phase II studies can provide information on side-effects related to cumulative drug dose.

Phase III studies

Phase III studies have either time to progression or survival time as the endpoint. Phase III studies always include randomization against a standard form of therapy (although this may be 'best supportive care' in some situations), where the randomization is included to avoid bias. Toxicity is never a major endpoint in Phase III trials which can involve between 50 and several thousands of patients.

Study monitoring

Long-lasting accrual periods have clearly hampered the quality of data and the enthusiasm of investigators has been shown to colour the results they report. Therefore it is important that protocols do optimally define issues such as:

- Measurability of the disease (e.g. minimum size of lesions still considered measurable).

- Criteria to use for toxicology reporting (e.g. the WHO or NCI Common Toxicity Criteria (CTC) grading systems) and monitoring of data which relate to both the anti-tumour response and side-effects.

To improve quality of data from clinical trials the implementation of systemic treatment checklists has proven to be of value.

Quality of life

Introduction

Most cancer treatment produce unwanted toxicities that interfere with the patient's quality of life. In many cancers the benefits of new treatments over existing approaches have been modest. Thus there have been few examples of new treatments for common cancers that afford a dramatic improvement in cure rate; rather, small but incremental improvements in overall survival have been made.

As new cancer treatments are developed, randomized, controlled trials are conducted to evaluate them, and a common problem is the comparison of a novel intensive treatment regimen against a relatively less toxic standard. In such circumstances, if the survival gain from the new treatment is reliably established but of modest magnitude, then it may be questioned whether the gain is worthwhile for individual patients. Does a small improvement in median survival compensate for additional discomfort (and risks) experienced by the patient?

The discomfort referred to here will be a compound of items comprising features of the treatment itself (e.g. surgery, radiotherapy, or chemotherapy). It will include aspects associated with:

- Duration of treatment
- Length of hospital stay
- Number of clinic visits
- Short- and long-term toxicities
- Less clinical aspects (perhaps less well-appreciated) summarized as quality of life (QoL) Just as treatment-related toxicity must be documented and compared between therapeutic regimens, it is also mandatory to compare QoL in randomized, clinical trials.

Assessing health-related QoL

Several questionnaires for completion by patients have been developed. The EORTC Quality of Life Study Group have developed a core questionnaire, the EORTC QLQ-C30, to which are added disease-specific modules. The core questionnaire contains 30 questions and, for example, the associated lung cancer module, QLQ-LC13, contains 13 further questions. To simplify the analysis of QoL scores, some of the items on these instruments are combined. For the QLQ-C30 there are five function, three symptom, and one global health-status scales. A patient who scores high for global health-status/QoL is deemed to have high QoL.

Frequency of QoL questionnaires

- Baseline QoL after consent but before randomization
- Not too frequent to burden patient
- Frequent during active treatment period
- Assess multiple scores for statistical analysis

Difficulties in QoL assessment

- Compliance declines as patient becomes terminal
- Compliance may also be poor if patient feels well
- Surrogate, relative, nurse, physician can fill in form?

'Missing' data

The missing response may result from an oversight by the patient but alternatively may be due to ambiguity in the question or the patient's reluctance to answer the particular item. It is often important to the investigator to collect information on the impact of treatment on psycho-sexual aspects of the patient's QoL, but patients may regard items relating to sexuality as embarrassing or not relevant. In such cases, the fact that such data is 'missing' will need to be reported. However, a trial nurse who is sensitive to the patient's wishes for privacy will often facilitate the collection of complete data.

Clinical trials

In planning a clinical trial it is fundamental to consider the number of patients required to demonstrate the anticipated change in treatment outcome. When survival is the primary endpoint of the study, this may be expressed as the anticipated improvement in median survival time or reduction in hazards ratio for the test group over the control. In trials comparing treatments in terms of QoL, it is difficult to quantify the 'gain' (or 'loss') that may be anticipated with the test therapy. In addition, there will be many aspects of QoL that are measured and it may be difficult to predict which of these should be the primary endpoint variable that is required for sample size calculations. In practice, QoL data are rarely used as the primary determinant of trial size.

There are important challenges in reporting QoL outcomes in clinical trials. These include the description of compliance, summarizing longitudinal data in a complete yet clinically meaningful way, balancing the multiple endpoints under consideration, and perhaps, most importantly, relating the findings with regards to QoL to other treatment outcomes such as patient survival and treatment-related toxicity.

Attempts have been made to integrate QoL and survival data into quality-adjusted life years (QALY). The duration of survival is adjusted according to periods of different levels of QoL before summing to give the overall survival time for analysis. Thus, a month during which the QoL is high will contribute more to the QALY than will a month with a lower score. The final QALY can then be used for a comparison between treatments, embracing both survival effects and changes in QoL. However, this integration process has not been readily accepted—its application is clearly limited by the arbitrary choice of weights or values put onto different levels of QoL.

It should be recognized that including the measurement of QoL into cancer clinical trials adds a considerable burden. This burden is felt immediately by the trial team as it may affect the basic trial design, the content of the protocol, and patient follow-up schedules. It may impact on patient numbers. Implementing the trial will burden the patients themselves and the clinical team. It will increase the volume of data to be collected and may adversely affect the overall data quality. It will certainly increase the complexity of analysis and reporting. All this adds to overall trial costs.

It is important to give due consideration to these factors when considering whether or not assessment of QoL is an essential part of a trial. In general however the difficulties are justified in cancer studies.

Chapter 14
Principles of palliative care

Pain control

Introduction

Roughly 80–90% of pain due to cancer can be relieved relatively simply with oral analgesics and adjuvant drugs in accordance with World Health Organisation (WHO) guidelines. WHO guidelines should be used in combination with interdisciplinary management. Relief of pain at the expense of side-effects is unacceptable to most patients; therefore a variety of treatment modalities is required.

Failure to control pain can result in many other problems e.g. fatigue, anorexia, depression, anxiety, constipation, nausea, and hopelessness. It is more difficult for the patient with pain to continue with demanding cytotoxic treatment and hospital visits. Pain control is an obvious priority for patients with cancer, whether embarking on curative or palliative treatment.

The commonest causes of uncontrolled cancer pain are:

• **Lack of sophistication** in patient assessment, resulting in misdiagnosis of cause and type of pain and failure to detect general distress, which lowers the pain threshold.

• **Lack of a systematic approach to analgesia.** 'Panic prescribing' is more likely to result in unacceptable side-effects.

• **Lack of knowledge of opioid pharmacology** and of evidence for adjuvant analgesics and non-steroidal anti-inflammatory drugs.

• **Lack of sophistication in use of opioids and adjuvant analgesics,** in particular, failure to prevent or treat drug side-effects.

An accurate patient assessment underpins appropriate analgesic choice. If pain distress is greater than pain severity and this is not identified it means:

• The patient is especially susceptible to opioid toxicity (pain is the physiological antagonist to the side-effects of opioids).

• The 'pain' will never be adequately dealt with if pyschological distress is treated as a physical pain.

• Appropriate strength of analgesic cannot be chosen.

Principles of the WHO ladder

• Strength of analgesic chosen (i.e. step of ladder) depends on *severity of pain*, not stage of disease.

• Adjuvant analgesic is chosen according to cause and type of pain.

• Opioids should generally be used in combination with non-opioids.

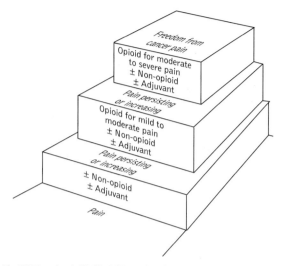

The WHO analgesic 'ladder'. (Reproduced with permission.)

The prototype analgesics for each step of the analgesic ladder are:

- **Step 1**: paracetamol or non-steroidal anti-inflammatory drug (NSAID).
- **Step 2**: codeine or dextropropoxyphene + paracetamol or NSAID.
- **Step 3**: morphine or diamorphine + paracetamol or NSAID.

Opioids should be prescribed at regular intervals. Therapeutic doses should be given and codeine preparations with sub-therapeutic doses of codeine (<30 mg) should be avoided (e.g. codydramol, cocodamol, cocodaprin).

Prescribed doses and indications for the common adjuvant analgesics are listed in the table. There is evidence for the tricyclic antidepressants and carbamazepine in neuropathic pain but the former generally have fewer side-effects and should usually be used first.

There is strong evidence for the effectiveness of NSAIDs as analgesics; however, their use will depend on the individual risk:benefit ratio. Those at high risk of side-effects are:

- age >60 years
- past history of peptic ulcer
- smokers
- concomitant steroid use

Table 14.1 Adjuvant analgesics (drugs with a primary indication other than pain)

Drug	Dosage	Indications	Side-effects
NSAIDs e.g. ibuprofen, diclofenac naproxen	See prescribing information for specific guidance	Bone metastases; soft tissue infiltration; liver pain	Gastric irritation; fluid retention; headache; vertigo; caution in renal impairment
Steroids e.g. dexamethasone	4–16 mg/day po, sc, iv	Raised intracranial pressure; nerve compression; soft tissue infiltration; liver pain	Gastric irritation if together with NSAID; fluid retention; confusion; Cushingoid appearance
Amitriptyline	25 mg nocte (starting dose) Titrate according to response and tolerability	Nerve pain — any type	Sedation; dizziness; dry mouth; constipation; urinary retention
Carbamazepine	200 mg nocte (starting dose) Titrate according to response and tolerability	Nerve pain — any type	Vertigo; constipation; rash

There is no evidence as yet of the superiority of the selective Cox 2 inhibitors available. Sulindac has been favoured for patients with renal impairment needing a NSAID.

Effective use of morphine

The keystone to using morphine for moderate to severe pain is in proper prescribing, patient reassessment, patient information, and prevention of side-effects.

Ideally start with a quick-acting morphine preparation. This has onset of analgesia in 20–30 minutes, which peaks at 60 minutes, and, when the required dose for the individual's pain is reached, will last four hours. This information should be given to the patient.

Morphine may relieve pain completely, partially, or not at all. It was previously thought that some pains, especially neuropathic pain, were unresponsive to opioids. Clinical practice and evidence from clinical trials tells us that opioid responsiveness is a continuum and no pain can be predicted as opioid-unresponsive. It is true that neuropathic pain often requires larger doses of opioids and titration is limited because at higher doses unacceptable side-effects, especially sedation, are problematic.

It is obvious that if side-effects of opioids are not prevented or minimized, especially sedation, then titration of opioids and subsequently pain control is not achieved. Review and rationalization of all drugs, especially drugs with sedative side-effects, is mandatory for successful titration of opioids. Monitoring of symptoms of opioid toxicity as part of regular patient review will prevent much distress and also save on resources such as unnecessary hospital admissions with confusion, cerebral imaging, and blood analysis. Opioid toxicity is a spectrum, which includes vivid dreams, shadows at the periphery of visual fields, nightmares, hallucinations, agitation and confusion. These features can be associated with myoclonic jerks or even generalized seizures.

The management of opioid toxicity is to reduce the dose of the opioid and reassess the pain syndrome, psychological factors, and

Table 14.2 Preventing opioid toxicity

Side-effect	Management
Constipation	Regular codanthramer or codanthrusate
Dry mouth	Frequent sips of cool water and regular mouth washes
Nausea/vomiting	Haloperidol 1.5–3 mg nocte or metoclopramide 10 mg 8-hourly
Sedation	Explanation very important. Expect to settle in about 2–3 days. Avoid other sedating medication where possible

Table 14.3 Management of difficult pain

Bone pain	Palliative radiotherapy; NSAIDs with opioids titrated to control pain; consider bisphosphonates
Neuropathic (nerve) pain	Titrate through analgesic ladder, remembering adjuvants (amitriptyline, carbamazepine, or steroids); consider nerve block
Rectal/vaginal/bladder pain	Use standard analgesic ladder approach (+ nifedipine amitriptyline, steroids); consider nerve block, local anaesthetic gel, steroid enemas
Bed sores	NSAIDs

biochemistry as appropriate. Haloperidol (1.5–3 mg po/sc, repeated as necessary) may be required to manage the altered sensorium in the acute situation. Rehydrate as appropriate—patients who are opioid-toxic are usually dry-mouthed.

Often pain is still controlled on the reduced dose of opioid. Sometimes an adjuvant drug may be needed. If the patient was using the opioid as an anxiolytic, another approach to anxiety is needed.

Occasionally opioid toxicity heralds renal dysfunction. In renal failure, a reduction in opioid dose may need to be accompanied by a reduction in dosing frequency. Liver dysfunction usually has to be severe before opioids accumulate. Methadone is safer than morphine in severe liver dysfunction.

NMDA antagonists

N-methyl-D-aspartate (NMDA) antagonists have a role in some pains, especially neuropathic pain and difficult inflammatory pains. Unfortunately, a convenient preparation is missing. However, SC or IV ketamine may be considered after seeking advice from a palliative care or pain team.

Alternative opioids

There are second-line opioids for moderate to severe cancer pain. The potential benefit in a switch from one opioid to another is a better balance between analgesia and unwanted effects. There are no controlled trial data at present to indicate definite benefits of one opioid over another. However, the following is suggested:

• **TTS-Fentanyl**—may cause less constipation than morphine. Suitable for stable pain. Time to peak blood levels is 12 hrs (up to 48 hrs in some patients) and terminal half-life after patch removal is up to 24 hrs. It is usually unsuitable in uncontrolled pain. The manufacturer's conversion chart is about right.

- **Hydromorphone**—useful if patient has cognitive impairment or hallucinations on morphine. May be useful in renal dysfunction because no known accumulation of active metabolites. Available as quick-acting and controlled-release capsules. Hydromorphone is about seven times as potent as morphine.

- **Oxycodone**—similar benefits to hydromorphone. It is about equipotent with morphine (2:3). Available as quick-acting and controlled-release preparations.

- **Phenazocine**—useful if dysphoria with morphine. Size of tablets limits use (5 mg tablet is equivalent to 20 mg morphine).

- **Methadone**—alternative to morphine. However, for the non-specialist, difficult to titrate. Equianalgesic dose is variable; methadone can be up to 10 times as potent as morphine.

When switching from one opioid to another, the equi-analgesic doses are not always easily predictable because the relative potencies of the two drugs are the result of the complex variables. Equi-analgesic doses are just for guidance and careful reassessment is required after an opioid switch.

Incident pain

Bone pain is, in fact, responsive to opioid analgesia. However, bone pain on movement can be difficult to control with opioids alone. Pain is a physiological antagonist to the side-effects of opioids, and intermittent pain allows less titration of opioids since the patient is unacceptably sedated at rest. NSAIDs and radiotherapy are usually essential adjuncts where possible. It is appropriate to try a breakthrough dose of quick-acting oral morphine 20–30 minutes before movement. However, surgical intervention (e.g. for spinal stabilization or anaesthetic block techniques) should be considered sooner rather than later.

Bisphosphonates

Bisphosphonates should be considered in bone pain secondary to breast carcinoma an to multiple myeloma; intravenous pamidronate, in doses ranging from 60–90 mg, 2–4 times weekly, is used. Work to assess the role of bisphosphonates in other cancers, such as prostatic carcinoma, is underway. Whilst intravenous pamidronate is successful in some acute-pain situations, there is no way at present of predicting for whom it will be effective.

Anaesthetic techniques

In a minority of patients, carefully managed drug treatment, with or without palliative radiation or chemotherapy or hormonal therapy, fails to provide acceptable pain relief or does so only at the cost of intolerable side-effects. In these cases anaesthetic techniques should be considered. Anaesthetic techniques should also be considered in acute situations e.g. pathological fracture awaiting internal fixation. Consider the early use of anaesthetic techniques if:

- **Failure of pharmacological management** due to side-effects in the presence of opioid-responsive pain; this may benefit from spinal opioids
- **Pancreatic pain**—coeliac plexus block
- **Nerve infiltration**—brachial plexus block or epidural local anaesthetic/steroids if lumbosacral nerve pain
- **Unfixed/unfixable fractures** or unstable bones

Non-drug methods

These should be used in conjunction with drug treatment and include:

- Occupational therapy
- Physiotherapy
- Relaxation therapies
- Transcutaneous electrical nerve stimulation (TENS)
- Acupuncture

Control of other symptoms

Introduction

Symptom control requires accurate assessment and history taking, with individualized treatment and a holistic approach. Good symptom control enhances quality of life and trust in the carers. The aim should be to integrate active symptom control with anti-tumour therapy through the whole course of the patient's illness.

Nausea and vomiting

Nausea occurs in 40–70% of patients with advanced cancer. Its appropriate management is dependent on establishing the probable cause and mechanism.

- Raised intra-cranial pressure
- Acute abdominal pathology
- Constipation
- Renal failure
- Hypercalcaemia
- Drugs

A first-line anti-emetic is selected according to the most likely cause and administered via a suitable route. If vomiting prevents oral administration, other options include sublingual and rectal routes, as well as IV/IM/SC. If symptoms persist after 24 hours, second-line or combination therapy should be introduced.

Breathlessness

Breathlessness is commonly multifactorial in origin. Simple reversible causes (pleural or pericardial effusion, anaemia, fluid overload, asthma) must be corrected. A multidisciplinary approach is helpful, with consideration given to non-pharmacological strategies such as breathing exercises, relaxation therapy, massages, and other complementary therapies. Patients should be helped to adjust their lifestyle and expectations.

The following treatments may be used singly or in combination:

- Nebulized saline for tenacious secretions.
- Morphine eases the sensation of breathlessness—current evidence of nebulized morphine does not support its use.
- Benzodiazepines—bring relief through anxiolytic and sedative effects and, possibly, muscle relaxation. Concerns about respiratory depression are usually unfounded.

Table 14.4 Selection of antiemetics

Cause of nausea/vomiting	Antiemetic	Dose schedule	Class of drug
Gastric stasis	Metoclopramide	20–30 mg qid	Prokinetic
Gastric irritation (drugs, abdominal radiotherapy)	Metoclopramide; ondansetron; granisetron	20–30 mg qid, 8 mg bd, 1 mg bd	Prokinetic and dopamine antagonist; 5HT$_3$ antagonist
Bowel obstruction	Cyclizine; haloperidol, dexamethasone	50 mg tds, 2–5 mg bd, 2–4 mg bd	Antihistaminic and anticholinergic; dopamine antagonist; corticosteroid
Chemical (chemotherapy, radiotherapy)	Haloperidol; ondansetron; granisetron; dexamethasone	2–5 mg bd, 8 mg bd, 1 mg bd, 2–4 mg bd	Dopamine antagonist; 5HT$_3$ antagonist; corticosteroid

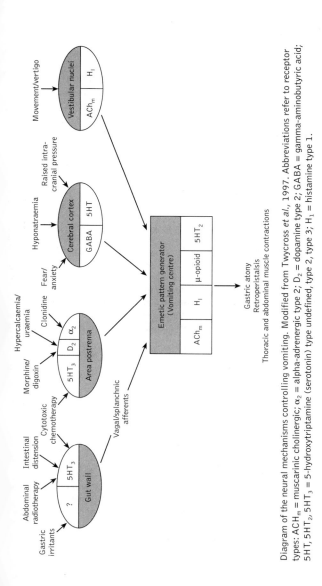

Diagram of the neural mechanisms controlling vomiting. Modified from Twycross et al., 1997. Abbreviations refer to receptor types: ACH$_m$ = muscarinic cholinergic; α$_2$ = alpha-adrenergic type 2; D$_2$ = dopamine type 2; GABA = gamma-aminobutyric acid; 5HT, 5HT$_2$, 5HT$_3$ = 5-hydroxytryptamine (serotonin) type undefined, type 2, type 3; H$_1$ = histamine type 1.

* Oxygen therapy should be considered on an individual basis. A trial of continuous or intermittent oxygen accompanied by some form of subjective assessment by the patient and oximetry may be helpful.

Constipation

The aim should be to anticipate and prevent this ubiquitous problem. Constipation may result in nausea, colic, overflow diarrhoea, urinary retention, or an acute confusional state. Common causes in malignancy are:

* Drugs (particularly analgesics)
* Immobility
* Dehydration
* Hypercalcaemia
* Spinal cord compression
* Pelvic or abdominal tumour

If well enough, patients should be encouraged to increase fluid and fibre intake and mobilize. When opiate analgesics are prescribed, a laxative (usually a softener and a stimulant) should routinely be added.

Drug therapy is straightforward. A softener laxative such as sodium docusate is prescribed if the stool is hard; a stimulant laxative (e.g. senna), if unable to expel stool; and a combination preparation (e.g. codanthramer/codanthrusate) for a mixed picture. Lactulose can cause troublesome wind. Rectal examination is required to identify faecal impaction and this may require suppositories, enemas, or digital evacuation.

Lymphoedema

Failure of lymph drainage is commonly due to tumour infiltration of lymphatics and/or compromise of these channels by surgery, radiotherapy, or both. It is important to exclude venous occlusion as a cause of limb swelling and oedema. Prevention is the best strategy, with attention to massage and exercise, and avoidance of, and vigorous therapy for, cutaneous infection, in patients at risk e.g. following axillary lymph node clearance for breast cancer.

Treatment of established lymph oedema requires daily skin care, self-massage, exercise, and the use of fitted compression garments. Refractory oedema may require pressure bandaging before compression garments can be fitted. The value of mechanical devices such as the flowtron pump is uncertain. In selected patients, a therapeutic trial of corticosteroids or diuretics may be appropriate.

Anorexia/cachexia

The precise mechanisms by which cancer causes anorexia and weight loss are still poorly understood, although circulating cytokines such as tumour necrosis factor clearly play a role.

This may be compounded by physical obstruction of the GI tract by tumour, therapeutic interventions, and depressed mood. Control of nausea should be optimized and attention paid to pain control, mouth care, and constipation. Simple dietary advice and the use of alcohol can help.

While enteral/parenteral feeding may be appropriate during active anti-cancer therapy, it is less appropriate as the disease progresses. Judicious prescription of progestagens or corticosteroids can aid appetite but will not usually influence cachexia.

Psychological distress

Assessment of psychological problems and the provision of psychological support must be an integral part of the package of care for patients with malignant disease. Presentation may be in the form of denial, anger, anxiety, or depression. All health care professionals should be aware of the frequency with which psychological problems are overlooked and all patients should be given time and space to voice their distress. Patients should be given control over their management and helped to set realistic goals and develop coping strategies. Medical staff should recognize when drug therapy (antidepressant or anxiolytic) or referral to a psychologist/liaison psychiatrist and/or specialist palliative care team is required.

Supporting cancer patients

Introduction

For cancer patients, the trauma of diagnosis, protracted and sometimes toxic curative treatments, possible disease relapse, with progression to incurable and increasingly disabling or terminal disease, provokes intense, often distressing emotional and psychological reactions. These may include:

+ Fear
+ Anxiety
+ Anger
+ Confusion
+ Sense of loss
+ Alienation
+ Sadness/depression

The cancer not only impacts on the patient personally, but also on family, friends, their work, and finances. Up to one-third of cancer patients suffer significant psychological morbidity. Appropriate support interventions can help alleviate much of their distress.

Palliative care is synonymous with good supportive care, at every stage of a cancer illness. Palliative care ameliorates all distressing symptoms, whether physical, psychological, social, or spiritual in an integrated approach, as essential in achieving the best of quality of life for patients and families. For patients with a terminal diagnosis, it strives to enable them to live as actively as possible until death, while offering support of the family during the patient's illness and in their own bereavement.

Detecting patients in need of support

All patients benefit from support but assessment of the following can identify patients at particular risk:

+ Degree of physical disability
+ Internal resources of the patient
+ Past history of functioning
+ Social supports—family (marital status, living arrangements, number of family members in the immediate geographical area and their capacity and willingness to provide support), friends, community/church links
+ History of substance abuse

Use a standardized measure of psychological morbidity and quality of life such as:

- Hospital Anxiety and Depression Scale (HADS)
- Functional Assessment of Cancer Therapy (FACT)
- Functional Living Index–Cancer (FLIC)
- Cancer Rehabilitation Evaluation Systems (CARES)
- European Organisation for Research and Treatment Quality of Life Questionnaire (EORTC QLQ-C30)
- The Schedule for Evaluation of Individualised Quality of Life (SEIQoL)—allows patients to nominate the aspects of life they consider important in the evaluation of QoL, and they are scored on these

Providing support

We can all offer support to cancer patients. Cancer patients tell us that they need to find meaning and hope in the midst of deterioration, distress, and despair. Our challenge is to find the balance in providing hope and alleviating fears throughout the cancer journey.

Communication

Effective communication is the cornerstone of good supportive care. Patients should be able to participate in decisions about their care, allowing them to retain some control over their lives. Doctors are not legally or ethically obliged to provide treatments that are futile or prolong life (and sometimes the distress of dying) at all costs. Competent patients are entitled to refuse life-prolonging or life-sustaining treatments. Potential conflict about such decisions can be avoided by good communication. Patients need honest, compassionately delivered information.

Poor communication and breaking of bad news are consistently mentioned by patients and families as a cause of stress and dissatisfaction. Good communication builds trust, reduces uncertainty, and allows appropriate adjustment (practical and emotional) by patient and family, thus reducing psychological morbidity. Breaking bad news is not a single, isolated event. The process is ongoing and recurring, involving telling the diagnosis, updating the patient and family on changes and, possibly, preparing them for death.

Breaking bad news—a ten-step approach

This approach can be used as a general framework and adapted for specific situations. *Remember*, a patient has a right but not a duty to hear bad news.

1. Preparation: (know the facts; arrange the meeting; find out who the patient wants present).

2. Establish what the patient already knows (both doctors and family generally underestimate the level of patient's knowledge).
3. Establish whether the patient wants more information.
4. Allow denial (denial is a defence and a way of coping). Allow the patient to control the amount of information.
5. Give a warning shot (allows patient time to consider their own reactions and whether they feel able to ask for more information).
6. Explain (if requested—be clear and simple; avoid harsh statements; avoid medical jargon; check understanding; be as optimistic as possible).
7. Listen to concerns (avoid premature reassurance or excessive explanations).
8. Encourage ventilation of feelings (the key phases, as it conveys empathy).
9. Summarize and make a plan (reduces confusion and uncertainty; fosters hope).
10 Offer availability (communicating bad news is an ongoing process).

Formal counselling/psychological therapies

Some patients will need more formalized support—trained counsellors, social workers, hospital chaplains may provide this. Cognitive–behavioural and brief psychotherapeutic interventions are effective for more significant levels of anxiety or depression e.g. adjuvant psychological therapy.

Psychiatric interventions

When psychological interventions are inadequate, psychotropic medication may help. Drug therapy benefit 20–25% of cancer patients suffering significant anxiety and depression.

Support groups and information services

These can help to reduce the sense of alienation and isolation sometimes associated with cancer. They facilitate the sharing of experiences, the ventilation of feelings in a supportive environment, and the exchange of information about the physical, psychological, and social consequences of cancer and its treatment (e.g. Bristol Cancer Help Centre, Cancer BACUP, Cancerlink).

Support in death

Often it is the actual mode of death that patients fear rather than the fact of dying e.g. 'What will it be like?' or 'I'm afraid of dying in agony'. Patients need reassurance that any physical distress can be alleviated and that death is normally peaceful. Issues of spirituality may be important for individual patients and religious ritual should be facilitated where possible. Doctors need to be sensitive to psychological distress (a sense of hopelessness, despair, meaninglessness; questions such as 'why me?') as it often masks intractable, distressing, physical symptoms (e.g. pain).

During final hours, patients should never be left alone to feel isolated or abandoned. Families need to be involved, and this includes children; they need to be kept updated on changes and encouraged to be present. Good care of a patient's family will reduce the likelihood of complicated bereavement. If the family can't be there, a member of staff should sit with the patient.

Staff stress

Supporting cancer patients is stressful to the health professionals involved. Staff also need support structures (including training in communication skills, as well as direct supportive measures such as counselling and relaxation therapies).

The 'holistic' approach to cancer

The holistic approach is typified by the emphasis placed on the role of 'mind, body, and spirit' in health and illness management, either by the individual themselves or by those caring for them. In cancer medicine this approach is implemented in three settings:

- **Psychosocial care** given within hospitals, hospices, voluntary sector support groups, or within the community via health visitors, social workers, or the Church.

- The **palliative care** setting, where there is increasing use of complementary therapies, particularly by nurses, for symptom control, comfort, and support.

- The **patient self-help** movement, where a mixture of self-help approaches, complementary and alternative therapies, nutrition, and psychological approaches are used with the aim of improving health, well-being, and treatment outcome.

The holistic model

The purist model is health-based in which individuals and therapists work in partnership to achieve the best levels of health, energy, and emotional and spiritual well-being, whether as a preventive measure or to promote health in the presence of illness. The holistic model is integrative, with the states of mind, body, and spirit inextricably linked—an individual's spirit or will to live, mental state, level of stress, self-expression, lifestyle, and emotional state are all seen as relevant in terms of the illness and potential to improve health. The physical state, in terms of nutrition, fitness, energy levels and oxygenation are also given key attention.

The holistic approach for individuals who are seeking to improve their health is ideally divided into two phases:

- Therapeutic
- Self-help

During the therapeutic phase, help is sought from:

- **Holistic doctors and nurses** for medical counselling, needs and lifestyle assessment, symptom control with stress reduction and natural remedies (herbal and homeopathic), and specific nutritional advice.

- **Counselling, psychotherapy, and group work** aimed at promoting emotional expression, for examination of lifestyle, stress, and self-stressing attitudes, for re-orientation and rehabilitation of individuals towards more authentic and meaningful personal values and

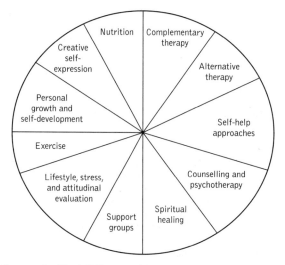

Components of the holistic approach.

goals, and for learning self-help techniques of visualization, meditation, and relaxation.

- **Nutritional approaches** based on replacing high-fat, high-protein, high-salt, high-sugar, highly-processed Western diets with a wholefood, vegan, preferably organic diet, supplemented with antioxidant vitamins and minerals (A, β-as carotene, C, and E, plus the minerals selenium and zinc). Nutritional changes should be supervised by qualified nutritional therapists to avoid weight loss and an inappropriate diet.

- **Complementary therapies** which include acupuncture, shiatsu, and homeopathy (which may increase energy levels and improve well-being and symptom control) and body work, such as massage and aromatherapy (which can reduce fear, tension, isolation, and the alienation felt by cancer patients towards their diseased or disfigured bodies).

- **Spiritual healing** which lifts underlying energy, improves coping, is calming, and has emotional and spiritual benefits.

- **Support groups** aimed at giving encouragement, social contact, and support.

- **Alternative cancer therapies** that are reputed to have 'anti-cancer' activity, and in this sense are more like allopathic medicines than holistic, health-based therapies. These fall into the categories of:

—**Herbal remedies** e.g. Rene Caisse herbs (Essiac), Iscador (mistletoe therapy), or Carnivora (Venus flytrap).

—**Metabolic approaches,** which may be immuno-stimulant.

—**Dietary approaches,** which are based on fasting to 'detoxify' the body, followed by 'super nutrition' with very pure, plant-based juice, raw food, or other 'spring cleaning' diets.

—**Alternative remedies** e.g. shark's cartilage, that has some anti-angiogenesis activity.

—**Hormonal therapies** aimed at inhibiting tumour growth e.g. melatonin, somatostatin, and bromocryptine 'cocktails'.

Self-help approaches

A point will come when, through the application of holistic therapies, the patient feels sufficiently strong to embark upon self-help approaches. It is important not to encourage patients to take up self-help approaches before they are strong enough to do so, because if they are unable to implement this advice they will blame themselves and feel they have failed. Key self-help strategies include:

• **Mind/body approaches** aimed at calming the mind and inducing states of well-being and happiness (e.g. regular practice of relaxation and meditation). Visualization promotes a positive mental state using pictures or words, in an attempt to affect disease outcome and morale. Visualization is divided into guided imagery, where therapists guide individuals or groups with the sequential use of pleasant visual images into happier states of mind, or personal imaging, where a cancer patient creates images of their cancer being destroyed or images of themselves as completely recovered.

• **Holistic forms of exercise** such as yoga, tai chi, or chi gong, which again promote emotional, physical, and spiritual well-being.

• **Healthy eating,** where once the patient has been taught and guided through dietary changes, healthy eating can be incorporated into their lifestyle.

• **Creative self-expression,** in which patients are encouraged to live a more balanced, expressive life with more emphasis on recreation, self-expression, and the fulfilment of personal goals and ambitions.

Psychological approaches

These overlap with interventions undertaken in traditional cancer centres and typically involve:

• Counselling and psychotherapy
• Support groups
• Use of creative therapies

Benefits of the holistic approach

Individual patients report significant benefits from the use of these approaches including:

- Reduction in fear, anxiety, isolation
- A sense of control, involvement, and partnership with health care professionals
- Improvement in physical state, energy levels, and sleep
- Improved symptom control and tolerance of treatment
- Improved quality of life

Use of the holistic approach

During the 1990s, studies showed that up to 35% of cancer patients were using complementary therapies, and up to 75% would use them if they were available on the NHS. Currently, use of complementary therapies within palliative care has become accepted, but mainly within the passive/dependent context of patient care. The current challenge in oncology is whether the model of holistic self-help can be incorporated into the spectrum of options available within conventional healthcare settings, or whether at the very least information about, and access to such resources are made routinely available to patients.

Further reading

Kaye, P. (1995) *Breaking bad news – a ten-step approach*. EPL Publications, Northampton.

Zech, D.F.I., Grond, S., Lynon, J., *et al.* (1995) Validation of World Health Organisation Guidelines for cancer pain relief: a 10-year prospective study. *Pain* **63**, 65–76.

McQuay, H. and Moore, A. (1998) *An evidence-based resource for pain relief*. Oxford University Press. *Oxford Textbook of Palliative Medicine*.

Twycross, R. (1996) *Symptom management in advanced cancer*. Radcliffe Medical Press, Oxford.

Chapter 15
Psychosocial aspects of cancer

Cancer and its treatment impose a severe threat to a patient's sense of well-being and quality of life. People tend to overestimate the numbers of deaths, underestimate cure rates, and see cancer as the single most alarming disease.

Distress

A cancer diagnosis provokes considerable psychological, social, and sexual difficulties for most people. Estimations vary, depending on the measurement used, but 20–35% of patients, irrespective of disease site or stage, experience psychological problems which merit intervention with anxiolytics and antidepressants or referral to a liaison psychiatrist or oncology counsellor.

There are several studies showing that oncologists are not very good at detecting psychiatric morbidity among their patients. In a study examining the ability of doctors to identify distress when patients were being given confirmation of a cancer diagnosis or recurrence, only one out of six senior oncologists behaved above chance level. Recent meta-analysis of 62 randomized trials of psycho-educational interventions with adult cancer patients demonstrated positive effect, suggesting that such interventions should be an integral part of cancer services, not just an optional extra.

Decision making

Once the diagnosis has been confirmed, decisions about treatment must be made. Innumerable studies show that patients are manifestly unhappy with much of the communication that takes place at this time. Too many leave their consultations uncertain of the precise diagnosis and prognosis, unclear about the likely therapeutic benefits of treatments, and wanting more information than is usually provided. A study of women with breast cancer showed those who were unsatisfied with the information given at this time failed to adjust to the fact of their cancer and its treatment. They suffered twice as much anxiety and depression up to three years post-diagnosis than women who felt well-informed.

Research has shown that the number of patients who genuinely prefer to have little information and leave everything up to the doctor is less than 5%. The large number of calls from patients and their families to charitable information services such as Cancer BACUP, attest to the difficulties some have in getting sufficient, understandable information to enable them to make decisions and give informed consent to treatment.

There has been some confusion about patients' preference for more information and their desire to participate in decision making. Surveys have shown that lay populations without cancer believe that they would wish to play an active role in decision making if they themselves were to get cancer but that patients with cancer usually desire a more passive role or an offer of joint decision making. In a study of women with breast cancer, perceived adequacy of the information given, and not merely being offered choice of treatment, influenced psychological distress.

Dealing with uncertainty

Uncertainty in any situation is one of the most difficult problems for the psyche to bear. It is a state in which most patients with cancer remain from the time that they discover sinister symptoms and undergo diagnostic tests until they complete treatment. Doctors are also faced with a dilemma when trying to offer reassurance to an anxious patient and be honest about an enigmatic disease which has an uncertain outcome. This can be especially problematic when discussing clinical trials where uncertainty about the efficacy of treatment is inherent and must be discussed in order to gain informed consent. Some doctors find it useful to attend specialist courses in communication to learn ways of dealing with these issues more appropriately.

Discomfort, disfigurement, and disability

Treatments for cancer are unpleasant and cause considerable distress. Surgery can be mutilating and may cause losses of function, body image, self-esteem, and libido. Radiotherapy can induce:

* Anxiety and depression
* Nausea and vomiting
* Fatigue
* Skin irritation

Chemotherapy probably has the worst reputation for side-effects, in particular:

* Alopecia
* Sore mouth
* Neurotoxicity
* Cardiotoxicity
* Nausea and vomiting

The advent of the $5HT_3$ antagonists in the past decade has made many toxic treatments more tolerable, but clinicians should be aware of the need to prevent emesis occurring at the beginning of treatment to avoid classically conditioned responses developing. One study of patients successfully treated for lymphoma showed that they continued to experience nausea and vomiting in response to any stimuli associated with the hospital many years after the cessation of treatment.

Disruption to lifestyle

Cancer treatment inevitably means a considerable disruption to a patient's life. Some manage to continue working through their radio-therapy and chemotherapy, but others require lengthy periods of hospitalization with its associated effects on social, family, sexual, and occupational functioning. After initial therapy, even if this has been successful, the months and years of follow-up visits and tests can continue to make it difficult for patients to ever see themselves in the same way as they did prior to diagnosis. Individuals may describe themselves as living 'under the sword of Damocles', never sure when the disease will reappear, anxiously monitoring aches and pains as signs of recurrence.

Paradoxically, it is when treatment ends that patients may be more in need of support and help from a trained counsellor in re-appraising their lives and coping with survivorship.

Dependence on others

The advanced technology of modern cancer treatment, as well as its potential dangers, renders patients extremely vulnerable and dependent on others. For many this loss of control is overwhelming and contributes significantly to psychological distress. This is especially true for adolescents who may already be struggling with the challenges of establishing their own identity. Helping these people and their families cope with the stresses of treatment for a life-threatening disease at such a crucial time in their development is a vital part of their care if normal social, intellectual, and personal growth is to be achieved.

Deleterious impact on quality of life

Although many cancers can be cured and the survival rate in some cancers is good, psychological, social, sexual, and physical dysfunction caused by both the diagnosis and treatment exerts a deleterious impact on the quality of most patients' lives. The range of possible treatments may have very similar outcomes in terms of response and survival but can produce very different effects on psychosocial well-being.

Monitoring quality of life is now more frequent in clinical trials but has failed to be used routinely in clinical assessment. Some groups are attempting to rectify this by introducing user-friendly touch screens that provide clinicians with a 'print out' of current and past scores, together with normal ranges which are adjusted for age and disease state.

Data derived from studies of quality of life can help the doctor and patient in management decisions and identify those patients who might profit from psychosocial interventions. Generic tests are available and valid and reliable tests exist for the measurement of quality of life in relation to most of the common cancer sites.

Summary

For many, the diagnosis of cancer is a major emotional catastrophe; for others, it is yet one difficulty to overcome in the midst of other social iniquities and disadvantages. Some may see their cancer as a challenge, offering an opportunity to completely reappraise attitudes to relationships, work, and life in general. Many people display extraordinary courage, resilience, and fortitude during the course of their illness, while others find that it exposes or magnifies the limits of their ability to cope. The doctor can do much to prevent or ameliorate their burden by good communication and preparedness to discuss psychosocial concerns.

Chapter 16
Thoracic cancer

Lung cancer

Epidemiology

Lung cancer is now the most frequent cause of cancer mortality in both men and women in the UK and US. Its incidence is continuing to rise worldwide, in particular in developing countries, where smoking is increasing.

It is estimated that 80% of cancer deaths are due to smoking. The risk of lung cancer relates to the number of cigarettes smoked, the number of years of smoking, early age of starting to smoke, and the type of cigarette (greater risk with unfiltered and high-nicotine).

While health education has had some success in reducing tobacco consumption in men, smoking in women and adolescents is increasing.

Much less frequent causes of lung cancer are exposure to:

- Asbestos
- Radon
- Polycyclic aromatic hydrocarbons
- Nickel
- Chromate
- Inorganic arsenicals

Pathology

There is evidence that lung cancers may arise in pluripotent stem cells in the bronchial epithelium, and this would certainly offer an explanation for the mixed histology that is fairly commonly seen. The WHO pathological classification is:

A   Squamous cell carcinoma (30%)

B   Small cell carcinoma (20%)

C   Adenocarcinoma (40%):

   1   acinar

   2   papillary

   3   bronchoalveolar

   4   mucinous

D   Large cell carcinoma

E   Mixed

For the purposes of management, lung cancers are grouped as non-small cell (NSCLC) or small cell (SCLC), but within the former certain patterns of disease do relate to histological subtype. For example, squamous cancers typically arise in proximal segmental bronchi and grow slowly, disseminating relatively late in their course. Adenocarcinomas are often peripheral in origin and even small resectable lesions carry a risk of occult metastases.

However the risk of dissemination is greatest in SCLC, where it is estimated that >90% of patients have either overt or occult metastases at presentation. These aggressive tumours most frequently arise in large airways but can rarely present as a small peripheral nodule. Some have suggested that the latter presentation is in fact indicative of a different pathology with an inherently better prognosis.

Non-small cell lung cancer

Introduction

Surgical removal of non-small cell bronchogenic carcinoma continues to offer best possibility of a cure. Consequently, each patient should be considered where possible for surgical treatment, although advanced stage and significant co-morbidity will preclude this option in many patients. The aim of surgical treatment is cure; in patients where this is not possible suitable alternative treatments should be considered.

Before embarking on surgery all cases should undergo careful and detailed pre-operative assessment to establish:

- Histological proof of disease
- Staging of disease
- Fitness for surgery

Histological/cytological proof of non-small cell lung cancer

Pre-operative proof of malignancy is possible in the majority of patients suffering from lung cancer. Main methods of diagnosis continue to be:

- Sputum cytology
- Bronchoscopy with biopsy
- Bronchial brushings
- Washings

These methods have a high yield of positive diagnosis, particularly in more centrally placed bronchogenic tumours. In more peripherally situated tumours percutaneous fine-needle aspiration for cytology or trucut-needle biopsy performed under fluoroscopic screening or guided by CT are preferred.

In a few patients pre-operative proof of malignancy may not be possible and surgery may be offered on radiological evidence (a mass lesion that has grown on sequential imaging).

Staging of disease

- Bronchoscopy
- CT — chest and abdomen
  - size of tumour
  - site

- — relationship to chest wall, fissures, mediastinal structures, diaphragm
- — lymph nodes >1 cm suggestive of tumour
- Mediastinoscopy
- Thoracoscopy
- Mediastinotomy
- Pleural aspiration, pleural biopsy
- Nodes may be enlarged due to reactive change
- CT liver and adrenals for metastases
- Bone scan and brain scan—only if symptoms

Fitness for surgery

In patients undergoing surgery for non-small cell lung cancer, pre-operative assessment is vital. Age alone should not be considered a contraindication to lung resection. Patient's performance status can be a useful indicator of ability to withstand major lung resection. Weight loss is an indicator of poor prognosis in lung cancer.

Table 16.1 TNM staging of lung cancer

T1	Tumour 3 cm or less in diameter, surrounded by lung or visceral pleura, distal to the main bronchus
T2	Tumour >3 cm diameter; or involving main bronchus 2 cm or more distal to carina; or invading visceral pleura; or associated with atelectasis which extends to the hilum but does not involve the whole lung
T3	Tumour invading chest wall, diaphragm, mediastinal pleura, or pericardium; or tumour in main bronchus <2 cm distal to carina; or atelectasis of the whole lung
T4	Tumour invading mediastinum, heart, great vessels, trachea, oesophagus, vertebra, or carina; or intralobar tumour nodules; or malignant pleural effusion
N0	No regional node metastases
N1	Ipsilateral peribronchial or hilar node involvement
N2	Ipsilateral mediastinal or subcarinal nodes
N3	Contra-lateral mediastinal nodes; scalene; or supraclavicular nodes

Stage grouping

I	T1–2 N0
II	T1–2 N1; or T3 N0
IIIa	T1–2 N2; or T3 N1–2
IIIb	T4 any N M0; or any N3 M0
IV	Any M1

Pulmonary function tests are essential—as well as demonstrating adequate respiratory reserve they are useful in post-operative management. Other investigations include haematological and biochemical screening to exclude significant co-morbidity and electrocardiogram, with or without an exercise test.

NSCLC—surgery

Thoracotomy and major lung resection continue to carry significant morbidity and mortality. Surgery for lung cancer should be carried out in a unit with the appropriate level of experience and expertise. Unnecessary delay may result in a previously operable lung tumour becoming inoperable by progression of disease. In the majority of patients, general anaesthesia with use of double lumen endotracheal tube is desirable to allow one-lung anaesthesia during thoracotomy.

Surgical resection

The essential procedures involved include:

- Lobectomy
- Bi-lobectomy
- Pneumonectomy

Segmental or wedge resection is generally not advisable because of the risk of incomplete resection due to the presence of satellite tumour foci within the surrounding lung. In a few patients with poor lung function, segmental or wedge resection may be appropriate.

In addition to the removal of all primary tumour with clear margins, regional lymph node sampling is essential to guide the planning of any adjuvant therapy. In cases where histological proof of malignancy is not available pre-operatively, every effort should be made to obtain histology at operation by frozen section before resection is undertaken.

In a minority of cases where the tumour is sited at the origin of the upper lobe bronchus, and is essentially confined to it, an upper lobectomy with sleeve resection of the main bronchus, followed by reconstruction by end-to-end anastomosis, will be possible, thus preserving the remainder of functioning lung.

Involvement of the chest wall (T3) or pericardium, including the phrenic nerve, in the absence of significant mediastinal lymph node involvement, does not necessarily constitute inoperability. Resection of the involved chest wall should be considered. A significant portion of pericardium can be removed *en bloc* in patients with pericardial involvement. Similarly removal of an involved section of the diaphragm is technically feasible.

Post-operative management

Patients should be nursed in an intensive care or high-dependency unit with adequate monitoring of:

- ECG
- Pulse rate
- Blood pressure
- Central venous pressure
- Respiratory rate
- Oxygen saturation

Adequate pain control is essential following thoracotomy and can be provided by thoracic epidural anaesthesia, intravenous opiates administered by patient-controlled analgesia (PCA), intercostal nerve block prior to wound closure, or opiates administered by intermittent intra-muscular injection.

Oxygen therapy is required in the early post-operative stage, preferably through a nebulizer, and in patients with significant airways' obstruction, a bronchodilator should be added. Regular chest physiotherapy is essential.

Post-operative complications

Early (within days)

- Haemorrhage (particularly when there has been widespread pleural adhesions) that may result in a substantial haemothorax
- Respiratory failure due to drug-induced respiratory depression, pneumothorax with or without surgical emphysema, and retained bronchial secretions leading to significant atelectasis
- Prolonged air leak following lobectomy
- Cardiac arrhythmias, particularly atrial fibrillation
- Chest infection
- Wound infection
- Broncho-pleural fistula (particularly on the right following pneumonectomy)
- Empyema

Late (within weeks to months)

- Post-thoracotomy pain
- Late broncho-pleural fistula with empyema
- Tumour recurrence

Results of lung resection

Post-operative mortality rate should be less than 3% following lobectomy and less than 5% following pneumonectomy. Five-year survival is influenced by a number of factors, the most important of which is pathological staging, post-resection (see Table 16.2). Overall five-year

Table 16.2 Five-year survival by stage

Stage	Five-year survival
I	60–80%
II	25–40%
IIIa	10–30%
IIIb and IV	<5%

survival for patients undergoing resection may be as high as 40%, approaching 70% in cases without nodal involvement (N0). However, when mediastinal nodes are involved (N2) only 15% of patients will survive five years.

NSCLC—radiation therapy

Introduction

Radical radiotherapy is indicated for patients with stage I–II NSCLC who are unfit for surgery, or have good performance status and stage III disease which can be encompassed in a radical volume.

Patients with inoperable non-small cell lung cancer (NSCLC) have a 20–30% chance of surviving two years if fit for radical radiotherapy and a similar chance of surviving one year if not. No randomized trial has examined the role of radical radiotherapy in these outcomes.

Dose and fractionation

The standard international dose is 60 Gy in 30 fractions over 6 weeks. Attempts to increase dose by hyperfractionation without acceleration have not shown any benefit. CHART, delivering 54 Gy in 36 fractions over 12 days has afforded a 9% survival advantage at two years compared with standard therapy. No trial has compared these regimes with shorter 3–4 week schedules (e.g. 50–55 Gy in 20 fractions), which remain popular in the UK.

CHART is logistically difficult to deliver because of weekend treatment; its modification to exclude weekends, CHARTWEL, delivers 60 Gy in 40 fractions over 17 days. Modification has not yet been compared to other schedules.

Treatment volume

No randomized trials have examined what volume should be irradiated. The standard in most of the world is the primary tumour and hilar and mediastinal lymph nodes, with a 1–2 cm margin. Retrospective comparisons have not demonstrated any advantage over volumes encompassing tumour and involved lymph nodes only. In dose escalation studies with conformal therapy, adjuvant nodal irradiation constrains the radiation dose delivered to the primary tumour. Omitting uninvolved nodal groups does not appear to increase local relapse rate.

Chemo-radiation

The Non-Small Cell Lung Cancer Collaborative Group (1995)[1] overview suggested a 2% increase in 5-year survival when cisplatin-based chemotherapy is added to radical radiotherapy. The RTOG 88-08 study reinforces these conclusions, with a 4-year survival advantage of 5% with combined therapy.

Chemotherapy delivered synchronously with radiotherapy has not yet been shown to increase survival in randomized trials and certainly adds to toxicity. A recent review of the RTOG database reported a significant increase in morbidity in combined regimes. Over one-third of patients receiving chemotherapy and hyperfractionated radiotherapy experienced severe oesophagitis.

Future developments

Even with CHART, long-term local control is poor. Dose escalation with conformal therapy is being explored to improve this. Using normal tissue complication probabilities to estimate a 'safe' dose of radiotherapy, up to 92.4 Gy has been delivered to small volumes without significant morbidity.

Post-operative radiotherapy

A meta-analysis of randomized trials of post-operative radiotherapy for completely resected NSCLC has shown impaired survival following irradiation in patients with N0 and N1 disease. There is evidence that radiotherapy affords an improvement in local control for patients with N2 disease. The best results have been reported in an American trial delivering 50 Gy in 25 daily fractions.

Palliative radiotherapy

For many patients with advanced NSCLC, radiation therapy is a key component in symptomatic treatment. Palliative radiotherapy is effective for:

• Haemoptysis
• Chest pain
• Dyspnoea
• Cough

Radiotherapy can also ameliorate systemic symptoms such as anorexia and weight loss.

MRC trials have shown equivalent survival and symptom control for 1-, 2-, and 10-fraction regimes, establishing the shorter courses as the treatment of choice for symptom control in advanced NSCLC. However, these short schedules are associated with pain and flu-like symptoms in up to 40% of patients. A transient reduction in peak expiratory flow rates may occur. Most patients receiving two fractions suffer moderate to severe oesophagitis.

A third MRC trial suggested that higher-dose palliative therapy (39 Gy in 13 daily fractions) did offer modest survival advantage for good performance status patients with large tumours; comparable to that seen with cisplatin-based combination chemotherapy.

NSCLC—chemotherapy

Introduction

Initial studies with alkylating agents in advanced NSCLC showed decreased survival with chemotherapy, and until recently no agents were available with objective response rates in excess of 20%. UK clinicians' attitudes to chemotherapy for NSCLC have remained negative, despite now wide acceptance of such treatment for small cell lung carcinoma. Recent developments indicate pessimism is misplaced.

Metastatic disease

Tumour response and survival

It is now established that cisplatin-based therapy significantly improves survival and quality of life. In the UK, the most studied regimen is MIC (mitomycin C, ifosfamide, and cisplatin)) which, when compared with best supportive care, has been shown to improve median survival (by ~2 months), 1-year survival (from 18% to 28%), and quality of life.

New drugs have emerged with enhanced activity in NSCLC as single agents and in combination with carboplatin or cisplatin. The majority of combination regimens have yet to be tested in randomized Phase III studies, though paclitaxel/cisplatin proved superior to standard therapy in terms of tolerability and improvement in quality of life in an EORTC trial, and had a significantly superior 2-year survival (14.1% v. 11.3%) in an Eastern Co-operative Oncology Group study.

In a Phase III study by the South Western Oncology Group, response rate and 1-year survival were improved when vinorelbine was added

Table 16.3 New agents for NSCLC[†]

Drug	Patient no.	1-year survival (%)	Median survival (Weeks)	Response rate (%)
Vinorelbine	621	20	32.5	24
Gemcitabine	572	21	40.6	39
Paclitaxel	317	26	37.3	41
Docetaxel	300	26	41	52
Topotecan	119	13	38	35

RR = response rate; MS = median survival

[†] From Bunn, P.A Jr and Kelly, K. (1998) New chemotherapeutic agents prolong survival and improve quality of life in non-small cell lung cancer: a review of the literature and future directions. *Clin Cancer Res* 5, 1087–100.

Table 16.4 New platinum-based combination therapies for NSCLC†

Drug combination	Patient nos.	RR (Weeks)	MS (%)	1-year survival (%)
Paclitaxel + C	333	46	38	40
Vinorelbine + P	328	41	38	35–40
Paclitaxel + P	286	42	42	36
Docetaxel + P	255	35	35	58
Gemcitabine + P	245	47	57	61
Topotecan + P	22	22	32	26

P = cisplatin; C = carboplatin; RR = response rate; MS = median survival

† From Bunn, P.A. Jr and Kelly, K. (1998) New chemotherapeutic agents prolong survival and improve quality of life in non-small cell lung cancer: a review of the literature and future directions. *Clin Cancer Res* 5, 1087–100.

to cisplatin. A large, ongoing American study is making direct comparison in advanced NSCLC of platinum complexes in combination with taxol, gemcitabine, or vinorelbine.

Quality of life

Although established cytotoxic regimens provide objective tumour response rates of the order of 20–30% in advanced NSCLC, symptomatic improvement can be achieved in a greater proportion of patients:

- Cough, haemoptysis, and pain are relieved in 70%
- Anorexia in 40%
- Dyspnoea in 30%

Despite this, use of chemotherapy in this setting is limited in UK, and it has been questioned whether the cost of non-surgical treatment for NSCLC (both financial and in terms of treatment-related toxicity) can be justified. However, a Canadian health economic analysis suggests that the cost of gaining a year of life for these patients is between $500 and $7000—small compared with $30 000 basic cost of diagnosis and supportive and terminal care.

Stage III disease

- 33% of NSCLC present in Stage III
- Trials difficult to interpret
- Combination chemotherapy and radiotherapy gives better survival than radiotherapy alone in unresectable disease—3-year survival, 13–23% v. 6%
- Poor performance status patients do badly with chemotherapy

Cisplatin, and some of the new drugs like gemcitabine and the taxanes, are potent radiosensitizers and there is interest in concomitant delivery of chemotherapy and radiotherapy to take advantage of potential synergy. As in SCLC there is evidence that concurrent radiotherapy may be more effective than sequential, but toxicity remains a problem and an optimum chemotherapy regimen and fractionation schedule for radiotherapy is yet to be determined.

Where Stage III disease is technically resectable (Stage IIIA disease, where only ipsilateral mediastinal nodes are involved) surgery cures less than 10% of patients, because of a combination of unresected loco-regional disease and occult systemic disease. Chemotherapy improves survival over surgery alone, but timing of this remains to be defined. Several small studies have suggested a survival advantage for pre-operative or neo-adjuvant chemotherapy (with or without radiotherapy) in Stage III disease. Five-year survival rates up to 40% have been reported, but this has been achieved in small, selected groups of patients. Two recent randomized studies have shown significantly improved relapse-free and overall survival for patients given cisplatin-based treatment before and after surgery.

Overall, the data are not dissimilar from that seen with chemotherapy followed by radiotherapy in unresectable disease, and it is not clear if surgery has a role in this situation. On the other hand, only 5–15% of patients undergoing neo-adjuvant therapy have a pathological complete response at surgery, demonstrating the importance of further local treatment if cure is the aim. Large Phase III trials of chemo-radiotherapy pre-surgery (Intergroup) and of chemotherapy followed by radiotherapy or surgery (EORTC) are in progress to help clarify this issue. Other groups are testing efficacy of newer drug combinations in this setting.

Adjuvant therapy

Meta-analysis of adjuvant chemotherapy trials in NSCLC has shown a 5% improvement in 5-year survival for patients treated with a cisplatin-based regimen after surgical resection. This benefit held for patients across Stages IB–IIIA. Such treatment has not however been widely adopted in the UK.

While neo-adjuvant strategies offer potential downstaging of disease, increasing the likelihood of a complete resection and theoretical reduction in risk of tumour dissemination at surgery, no studies have yet shown pre-operative chemotherapy to be superior to post-operative adjuvant therapy.

Conclusion

Chemotherapy for inoperable NSCLC offers benefits similar to those obtained with chemotherapy in SCLC in terms of survival. Results of adjuvant treatment also suggest that a survival benefit comparable to that observed in breast and colorectal cancer can be achieved. Grounds for the current nihilistic view of NSCLC chemotherapy are diminishing, but patients still need to be entered into clinical trials wherever possible in order better to refine current approaches.

Small cell lung cancer— radiotherapy

Background

Patients with small cell lung cancer (SCLC) are usually treated by primary chemotherapy because of its chemo-responsiveness and frequent dissemination at time of diagnosis. SCLC is, however, also the most radio-responsive variety of bronchial carcinoma and radiotherapy has an important role in its management. In patients with a localized tumour, thoracic irradiation (TI) and prophylactic cranial irradiation (PCI) improve disease control at these sites and lead to prolongation of survival when compared to chemotherapy alone. In addition, radiotherapy is a useful palliative treatment for patients relapsing after, resistant to, or refusing chemotherapy.

Thoracic irradiation (TI)

+ 60% of relapses after chemotherapy are in the thorax
+ TI reduces risk by 50% and improves survival
+ Survival improves from 9 to 14% at 3 years
+ Schedule is uncertain
+ Early and concurrent with chemotherapy—best results but more side-effects

Prophylactic cranial irradiation (PCI)

+ SCLC has propensity for brain metastases
+ 20% have brain involvement at diagnosis
+ 80% have brain involvement at death
+ Blood–brain barrier limits effectiveness of chemotherapy (sanctuary site)
+ Median survival once CNS disease develops is 3 months; 50% only have reasonable palliation with chemotherapy or radiotherapy
+ Low-dose PCI halves risk of brain metastases
+ Low-dose PCI—small improvement in survival
+ Dose and schedule of PCI is uncertain
+ Not given concurrently with chemotherapy

Palliative radiotherapy

A short course of irradiation to either the primary tumour or the site of metastases can provide useful symptom control. The choice of dose and radiation schedule is similar to that used in NSCLC and should follow the basic principles of using the lowest effective dose with minimal additional toxicity. In most situations a single fraction or up to five fractions of treatment will suffice.

Radiotherapy administration

Decisions about use of combined modality treatment for individual patients are based on assessment of their prognostic factors. This approach brings increased risks of toxicity and overall demands on patients and should be reserved for those with a realistic prospect of long-term survival. Exact timing of administration, dose, and fractionation schedule of TI and PCI will be determined by individual protocols and may be subject of study in a randomized clinical trial. Hyperfractionated schedules and concurrent administration of chemotherapy and irradiation remain investigational. For routine use outside clinical trials, the following are commonly used:

> TI—50 Gy in 2 Gy daily fractions or biological equivalent
> PCI—24 Gy in 8 fractions, 30 Gy in 10 fractions,
> or 36 Gy in 18 fractions

Treatment volume of TI will depend on time of administration and on local practice. It is common practice to irradiate the mediastinum even in the absence of lymphadenopathy because of frequency of occult nodal metastases.

Pre-chemotherapy CT and chest radiographs are important to ensure that pre-chemotherapy sites of disease are encompassed by radiotherapy fields. Mega-voltage irradiation is used and sophisticated approaches to field placement and dosimetry are necessary to ensure optimal trade-off between preserving spinal cord tolerance and minimizing radiation dose to the surrounding normal lung. This often means a 'shrinking field' or phased approach.

For PCI planning it is important to encompass all meningeal surfaces, particularly the cribriform plate and middle cranial fossa.

Follow-up

This is designed to detect recurrences and monitor side-effects of treatment. Treatment of recurrent disease is always palliative in intent. Late effects of TI on lung and PCI on cognitive function are important limitations and need to be formally assessed by the team responsible for administration of radiotherapy. Follow-up chest radiographs will show mediastinal fibrosis in all patients. Associated functional impact depends on volume, previous respiratory reserve, and patients' activity levels.

Mediastinal fibrosis makes interpretation of follow-up radiology difficult and may lead to concerns about recurrence that can only be resolved by sequential radiology. Thoracic CT gives better definition of cross-sectional anatomy, but still needs to demonstrate a change to reliably confirm recurrence.

Following PCI about 30% of patients will develop 'somnolence' as a classical, self-limiting effect, 2–3 months after treatment. With longer follow-up patients may complain of recent memory loss, but formal neuropsychometric evaluations have failed to demonstrate significant deterioration attributable to PCI.

Future research

The question of optimal scheduling of TI needs to be resolved. Current evidence suggests early introduction may be more effective than traditional consolidation therapy. This approach may not be suitable for patients with bulky mediastinal disease or with tumour involvement outwith a safe size of radiation field. Further research needs to address the use of hyperfractionated or accelerated radiation techniques and use with concurrent chemotherapy. Similar uncertainties exist for radiation timing, dose, and optimal schedules of PCI.

SCLC—chemotherapy

Introduction

SCLC accounts for 16–20% of all lung cancers and its incidence is rising in the developed world, particularly in women. It is a rapidly growing tumour that is now recognized as a systemic disease making surgery inappropriate for the vast majority of patients.

Prior to the introduction of systemic treatment with chemotherapy in the 1970s, the outlook for patients diagnosed with this disease was dreadful, with a median survival of six weeks for patients with extensive disease and three months for those with limited disease. Combination chemotherapy is now the standard treatment for both categories of disease.

Overall survival has been extended significantly in recent years—5–10% of selected patients with limited disease can survive long term. Unfortunately, the vast majority of patients die of their disease, and patients with extensive disease only have a median survival of 7–11 months.

Staging and prognostic factors

A much simplified staging system is used for SCLC as the vast majority of patients are initially treated with chemotherapy irrespective of disease extent. A two-stage system was drawn up by the Veterans Administration Lung Group:

- **Limited-stage disease**: tumour confined to one hemithorax and regional nodes that may be encompassed within tolerable radiation therapy fields.

- **Extensive-stage disease**: disease beyond these bounds.

Within these broad categories, subgroups may be defined according to one or more of the following prognostic factors:

- Performance status
- Sex (females fare better)
- LDH
- Alkaline phosphatase
- Hyponatraemia

A number of drugs have been found to have activity as single agents and a variety of combination regimens have been developed (see Table). CAV and EP have similar efficacy. EP causes more nausea and vomiting but less myelosuppression, neurotoxicity, and cardiac toxicity. The substitution of ifosfamide for EP has shown a modest improvement in survival in extensive disease.

Table 16.5 Commonly used combination regimens in SCLC

EP	Etoposide	115 mg/m² i.v. days 3–5 q. 3 weeks
	Cisplatin	60–80 mg/m² i.v. day 1 q. 3 weeks
CAE	Etoposide	50 mg/m² i.v. days 1–5 q. 3 weeks
	Doxorubicin	45 mg/m² i.v. day 1 q. 3 weeks
	Cyclophosphamide	1000 mg/m² i.v. day 1 q. 3 weeks
CAV	Cyclophosphamide	1000 mg/m² i.v. day 1 q. 3 weeks
	Doxorubicin	50 mg/m² i.v. day 1 q. 3 weeks
	Vincristine	2 mg/m² i.v. day 1 q. 3 weeks

These combination regimens produce response rates of over 80%, with complete responses in 30–40% of patients with limited disease and 10–20% with extensive disease. Many patients with SCLC are elderly, with co-morbid conditions, and it was hoped that single-agent oral etoposide would be effective and better tolerated by this group. However, in two randomized trials oral etoposide was found to be detrimental to quality of life and less effective than the standard regimens.

Chemotherapy alone is not entirely responsible for improvement in survival, with developments in thoracic and cranial irradiation taking place in tandem. The wide range in survival rates between different clinical trials can be explained in part by differences in selection criteria. Intrinsic and emergent drug resistance are thought to underlie ultimate treatment failure in SCLC and a number of strategies have been investigated in an attempt to overcome this.

Alternating chemotherapy regimens

Goldie *et al.*[2] proposed a hypothesis, based on a mathematical model, that drug resistance could be overcome by using alternating regimens, provided that each regimen was capable of producing high rates of complete remission and that the two regimens were not cross-reactive. However, several trials have failed to show clinically significant improvement in survival with this approach.

Dose intensification

This can be achieved by decreasing the interval between treatments or by increasing the dose at each treatment. Modest increases in the doses of CAV and EP regimens have been achieved but failed because of increasing haematological toxicity. An improvement in median survival was found in patients with limited stage disease when a combination of ifosfamide, carboplatin, etoposide, and vincristine was given in a three-weekly compared to a four-weekly schedule.

If there is a role for dose intensification it is likely to be in patients with limited disease. Failure to achieve planned dose intensification as a result of toxicity may actually result in shorter survival for patients in the intensified arm.

The addition of colony-stimulating factors to facilitate dose escalation has been shown to decrease haematological toxicity in some trials but not to affect survival. Their routine use is not therefore currently recommended. High-dose therapy with autologous haemopoietic cell support has again failed to show an increase in survival and currently is not recommended for use outwith a clinical trial.

Maintenance chemotherapy

It was postulated that extending the period of chemotherapy might delay relapse. Several trials have assessed the benefit of following standard induction treatment with maintenance chemotherapy. Overall, though they have shown longer times to progression with maintenance treatment, there has been little impact on survival.

Biological therapies are always more likely to be effective in cancer patients with a low tumour burden, and for this reason their use has been explored in patients with SCLC in complete remission following standard treatment. However, trials of maintenance interferon in such patients have failed to show any survival advantage.

New drug development

The demonstration of activity with novel chemotherapeutic drugs in SCLC is difficult since most patients with the disease will have received first-line chemotherapy, and there is a danger that active agents may be dismissed because they fail to show activity as second-line agents. However, it has been observed that patients relapsing longer than three months from the completion of chemotherapy have a much greater chance of responding to the same treatment, suggesting continued drug sensitivity. Patients in this clinical situation are appropriate candidates to receive investigational combinations. Similarly, patients who relapse within three months, and who are, therefore, thought to have disease refractory to conventional therapy, test non-cross-resistant drugs with novel modes of action.

Docetaxel, paclitaxel, topotecan, irinotecan, and gemcitabine have all been found to be active in SCLC. Whether they are incorporated into standard regimens will depend on a number of factors including toxicity, cost-effectiveness, and the demonstration of non-cross-resistance with current standard drug. Other novel treatments under development include:

- Drugs interfering with autocrine growth-factor loops
- Matrix metalloproteinase inhibitors
- Anti-angiogenic factors
- Gene transfection approaches

Mesothelioma

Epidemiology and incidence

Malignant pleural mesothelioma (MPM) is an aggressive tumour arising from the serosal lining of the chest and abdomen with survival rates of less than one year reported following diagnosis.

* Rare—3000 cases per year in UK; the incidence is expected to rise over the next decade before peaking
* Age—60–70 years
* Male:female ratio, 5:1
* Caused by asbestos exposure
* Other causative agents include
  — radiation
  — thorium dioxide
  — silicate fibres
  — Simian Virus 40 (SV40), discovered as a contaminant of early poliovirus vaccines

Pathology

Mesothelioma may present as a benign or malignant process. Benign mesothelioma usually presents as an asymptomatic solitary mass and is not typically associated with asbestos exposure. Malignant tumours may be localized or diffuse and are more commonly associated with asbestos exposure and symptoms such as chest pain and dyspnoea. Three distinct malignant subtypes have been identified microscopically:

* Epithelial (approx. 50% of all cases)
* Sarcomatous
* Mixed histologies

Distinguishing mesothelioma from other intra-thoracic malignancies such as adenocarcinoma, requires the assistance of an experienced pathologist. Frequently, light microscopy and standard histochemical stains are inadequate alone. Therefore pathologists use techniques such as electron microscopy and immunohistochemistry to facilitate this distinction.

Clinical and radiological presentation

Mesothelioma can be insidious in its onset with a median time from first symptoms to diagnosis of 2–3 months. Symptoms at presentation commonly include non-pleuritic chest pain and dyspnoea. Constitutional symptoms such as fever, fatigue, and weight loss are seen in

30% of patients. Physical examination frequently demonstrates decreased breath sounds and dullness to percussion due to a pleural effusion or diffuse pleural tumour. Signs of advanced disease are:

* Chest wall mass
* Hoarseness
* Superior vena cava syndrome
* Horner's syndrome
* Ascites—heralding abdominal involvement
* Lymphadenopathy—an infrequent finding

Laboratory results in mesothelioma are usually unremarkable with no serological tumour marker reproducibly isolated. The radiological presentation of mesothelioma is non-specific. Pleural effusion is common and may be associated with pleural thickening and nodularity. The extent of the pleural mass and encasement of the lung is well demonstarted by CT. However, this imaging modality is less sensitive in detecting mediastinal or transdiaphragmatic involvement.

Magnetic resonance imaging (MRI) of the chest and upper abdomen provides superior definition of tissue planes, in addition to sagittal and coronal views of the diaphragm and thorax apices, and is an important adjunct to staging.

Diagnosis

Thoracoscopy remains the procedure of choice to obtain a pathological diagnosis of malignant mesothelioma, with an 80% diagnostic yield. Thoracocentesis and percutaneous pleural biopsy has a yield of only 30–40%. When thoracoscopy is not possible due to obliteration of the pleural space by the tumour, an open pleural biopsy may be performed. Careful planning of the incision site is essential because mesothelioma has a propensity to implant within chest wall wounds. Exploratory thoracotomy should be avoided.

Table 16.6 Brigham Staging System for malignant pleural mesothelioma

Stage	Description
I	Disease completely resected within the capsule of the parietal pleura without adenopathy; ipsilateral pleura, lung, pericardium, diaphragm, or chest wall disease limited to previous biopsy sites
II	All of Stage I with positive resection margins and/or intrapleural adenopathy
III	Local extension of disease into the chest wall or mediastinum, heart, or through diaphragm into peritoneum; or with extrapleural lymph node involvement
IV	Distant metastatic disease

Staging

In 1976, Butchart proposed a staging system based on the extent of tumour involvement within the chest, but this system correlated poorly with survival. Subsequently, alternative staging systems have been proposed, several based on a TNM concept, although none have gained universal acceptance.

The Brigham staging system provides a straightforward characterization method, based on key disease characteristics, that stratifies survival. In a series of 183 patients treated in a multimodality setting, median survival for patients with stage I, II, and III disease was 25, 20, and 16 months respectively.

Accurate pre-operative pathological staging is best achieved by thoracoscopy for pleural evaluation, mediastinoscopy for mediastinal nodal involvement, and laparoscopy to rule out peritoneal seeding or diaphragmatic involvement when indicated.

Treatment

Without treatment, the average patient with MPM survives less than one year from the time of diagnosis. As a result of this poor prognosis various therapeutic options have been explored including:

- Radiotherapy
- Chemotherapy
- Immunotherapy
- Surgery

Individually, each of these modalities has been disappointing when compared to single-modality treatment results. Current experience has shown multimodality therapy to offer improved survival in selected patient groups. Multimodality therapy should be carried out in the context of an approved study protocol by thoracic surgeons experienced in treating this disease.

At Brigham and Women's Hospital, Boston, extrapleural pneumonectomy followed by chemotherapy (carboplatin and paclitaxel) and radiotherapy (40.5 Gy) is being used. Recently, 183 patients have been reviewed, demonstrating an overall median survival of 17 months and 2- and 5-year survival rates of 36% and 14% respectively. Positive predictors for improved outcome were epithelial histology, negative resection margins after operation, and negative extrapleural nodal status. Patients with all three positive predictors enjoyed a 51-month median survival with 2- and 5-year survival rates of 68% and 46% respectively.

The following novel therapeutic approaches are currently undergoing active clinical investigation in an effort to improve treatment survival outcome:

- Intracavitary, hyperthermic chemotherapy
- Gene therapy
- Immunotherapy
- Photodynamic therapy

Thymic tumours

Introduction

Tumours derived from the thymus (thymomas) comprise approximately 20% of all mediastinal tumours and are the most common tumour in the anterior mediastinum. Thymomas occur at any age but are rare before the age of 20 and peak between 40–60 years. The incidence varies somewhat in different countries with high values in the Far East. The average in Europe is around 0.5 new cases per year per 100 000. Aetiology of these tumours is unknown; a possible relation to Epstein–Barr virus infection has not been proven.

Pathology

Most thymomas are slow-growing 'low-grade' malignant tumours. It is believed that they derive from epithelial elements, but the tumours retain the capacity for production of T cells. The T cells are generally of normal phenotype. According to the relative abundance of epithelial and lymphocytic cells, histological subgroups have been described:

- Epithelial
- Lymphocytic
- Mixed or lympho-epithelial type

These cellular characteristics have no clear influence on prognosis. In contrast, the gross appearance of the tumour is related to clinical prognosis. The presence or absence of an intact capsule is of prognostic importance and local invasiveness remains the most consistent factor in predicting outcome.

The metastatic potential of thymomas is difficult to assess on the basis of histology and cytological features.

A 'benign' thymoma has been defined as a tumour that is well encapsulated and does not invade adjacent mediastinal structures; 50–65% of thymomas fit this definition. The differentiation between benign and malignant thymoma is, however, difficult and thymomas should in general be regarded as potentially malignant. In all cases where residual tumour is left after surgery, adjuvant therapy should be considered.

Presentation and clinical features

- 30%—no local symptoms
- Produce paraneoplastic syndromes
- 70% associated with an immunological phenomenon

- Antibodies target acetylcholine receptor causing myasthenia gravis
- Myasthenia occurs in 10–15% of patients with thymoma
- 10–25% of patients with myasthenia have a thymoma
- Red-cell aplasia occurs in 5% of thymomas
- 30–50% of patients with red-cell aplasia have a thymoma
- In 30%, low platelets or low white-cell count occur
- Hypogammaglobulinaemia occurs in 5–10% of patients with thymoma
- 10% of patients with hypogammaglobulinaemia have a thymoma

Many of the patients with autoimmune disorders belong to the older age group and removal of the thymoma results in remission in only approximately one-third of these patients. As these symptoms can arise also in small tumours, the possibility of curative treatment may be better when paraneoplastic syndromes prevail. In the absence of paraneoplastic effects, thymomas are often large before they give rise to local symptoms such as cough, dyspnoea, dysphagia, stridor, and chest pain. Superior vena cava obstruction (SVCO) may result.

Thymomas are most commonly located within the anterior mediastinum but half will extend to the superior mediastinum. CT or MR scanning is necessary to:

- Direct surgical intervention
- Plan radiotherapy treatment
- Evaluate treatment response
- Monitor recurrence of disease

Treatment and staging

Surgery is the treatment of choice for localized disease. Median sternotomy is the preferred incision for thymectomy, since it provides excellent exposure of the thymoma and the adjacent organs. The staging of disease is based on the surgical findings as well as radiology:

Stage I: tumour confined within intact capsule
Stage II: pericapsular growth into the mediastinal fat tissue
Stage III: invasive growth into the surrounding organs
Stage IV: disseminated disease

The most effective therapy of thymoma is complete removal, and modern techniques have made it possible to resect even invasive thymomas. The superior vena cava can be removed and reconstructed and parts of the lung or pleura can be resected when required.

In Stage I disease adjuvant treatment is not applied. In all other cases, additional antineoplastic treatment is recommended after surgery. In local disease with or without residual tumour, radiotherapy is recommended in doses of 50–60 Gy given in 20–30 fractions. The treatment is delivered via a linear accelerator often using an anterior and two oblique fields, minimizing the dose to the normal lung and the spinal cord.

The reported series are not big enough to have sufficient statistical power to show significant survival benefits of adjuvant treatment. Radically resected invasive thymomas have 5- and 10-year survival rates of 80% and 73% respectively. This should be compared with the results after subtotal resection followed by radiotherapy—59% and 54%. The rate of recurrence is 3% with Stage I, 13% with Stage II, 27% with Stage III disease, and 54% with Stage IV disease.

Paraneoplastic effects such as myaesthenia gravis improve after thymectomy in 30–50% of cases. Patients with persistent myaesthenia require medical treatment with anticholinesterase agents and/or immunosuppressants.

Recurrent and metastatic thymoma should be treated with systemic treatment. The reported series are small, but a commonly used active regimen is cisplatin, doxorubicin, cyclophosphamide. The response rate with combination chemotherapy is 50–70%. This relatively high efficacy has given rise to Phase II studies of adjuvant chemotherapy and neo-adjuvant chemotherapy followed by surgery and radiation, with promising results.

Summary

The contemporary standard of treatment of thymoma is radical surgery whenever possible. Total resection alone is adequate therapy for Stage I thymoma. Adjuvant therapy should be used for local disease with demonstration or suspicion of invasion. Locally advanced, relapsing, or disseminated disease should be treated with combination chemotherapy including corticosteroids. Cisplatin-based regimens are recommended.

Further reading

1. Non-Small Cell Lung Cancer Collaborative Group (1995) Chemotherapy in non-small cell lung cancer: a meta-analysis using updated data on individual patients from 52 randomized clinical trial. *British Medical Journal* **311**, 899–909.
2. Goldie, J.H., Goldman, A.J., and Gudanuskas, G.A. (1982) Rationale for the use of alternating non-cross resistant chemotherapy. *Cancer Treat Rep* **66**, 439–49.
3. Gregor, A., Cull, A., Stephens, R.J. *et al.* (1997) Prophylactic cranial irradiation is indicated following complete response to induction therapy in small cell lung cancer. *Eur J Cancer* **33**: 11, 1752–8.
4. Healy, E.A. and Abner, A. (1995) Thoracic and cranial radiotherapy for limited-stage small cell lung cancer. *Chest* **107**, 249S–54S.
5. Pignon, J.P., Arriagada, R., Ihde, D.C. *et al.* (1992) A meta-analysis of thoracic radiotherapy for small cell lung cancer. *N Eng J Med* **327**, 1618–24.
6. Steward, W.P., Von Pawel, J., Gatzemeier, U. *et al.* (1998) Effects of granulocyte-macrophage colony-stimulating factor and dose intensification of V-ICE chemotherapy in small cell lung cancer: a prospective randomised study of 300 patients. *J Clin Oncol* **16**, 642–50.
7. Sugarbaker, D.J. and Garcia, J.P. (1997) Multimodality therapy for malignant pleural mesothelioma. *Chest* **112** (**Suppl**), 272S–5S.

Chapter 17
Breast cancer

Much effort has been invested in this most common solid tumour occurring in women. The study of breast cancer has rewarded us with lessons in many aspects of oncological practice:

- Population screening
- Medical genetics
- Adjuvant therapy
- Meta-analyses
- Clinical guidelines

The benefits of this industry are now visible, with a fall in breast cancer deaths over the last decade.

Epidemiology

- Commonest female cancer in Europe (200 000 cases per year)
- 20% of all malignancies
- Incidence is increasing by 1% per year
- Rate of increase is increasing especially in low-risk populations
- Lifetime risk in USA is 1 in 10
- Risk of breast cancer correlates with income per capita
- Mortality in Western Europe and USA, 15–25 per 150 000 women
- In UK—35 000 new breast cancers diagnosed per year
     —14 000 breast cancer deaths per year
- Breast cancer deaths in UK is highest in world
- In UK, recent decrease in breast cancer mortality by 20%

Several risk factors have been identified by epidemiological studies:

- **Age**: breast cancer is very rare before the age of 20 and rare below 30 years. The incidence of breast cancer doubles every 10 years until the menopause, when the rate of increase slows and in some countries plateaus.

- **Geography**: there is a seven-fold variation in incidence between countries, with low rates in the Far East. Migrants from low-incidence countries assume the risk in the host country within two generations.

- **Age at menarche and menopause**: early menarche and late menopause increase the risk. Ovarian ablation before 35 years reduces the risk of breast cancer by 60%; menopause after the age of 55 years doubles the risk.

- **Age at first pregnancy**: nulliparity and late age at first pregnancy increase the risk. A woman whose first pregnancy is at 30 years has double the risk of breast cancer compared with first pregnancy at <20 years.

- **Family history**: genetic predisposition accounts for around 10% of breast cancers.

- **Exogenous oestrogens**: use of oral contraceptives for >4 years before first pregnancy increases the risk of pre-menopausal breast cancer. The use of unopposed oestrogens in hormone replacement therapy for 10–15 years is associated with an increase in breast cancer. Combined preparations also increase the risk, but the magnitude of effect is uncertain.

- **Diet:** associations have been shown with high dietary fat intake, obesity, and alcohol consumption.

- **Benign breast disease:** previous breast surgery for severe atypical epithelial hyperplasia is associated with a four-fold increase in risk.

- **Radiation:** exposure to ionizing radiation at an early age e.g. treatment of Hodgkin's. Mammographic screening is associated with a decrease in breast cancer deaths but the effects of screening younger women are uncertain.

Male breast cancer is rare (0.7% of all male cancers) with a peak incidence 10 years later than women. It may occur in association with Klinefelter's syndrome.

Genetics of breast cancer

It is estimated that 5–10% of female breast cancer is due to inheritance of a mutated copy of either *BRCA1* or *BRCA2*. Women who inherit a mutated copy of either gene have an elevated lifetime risk of breast cancer—up to 87% by the age of 70 years. There is particular risk of pre-menopausal breast cancer, often before the age of 40 years; there is an associated risk of ovarian cancer (greater with *BRCA1*); and male carriers are at risk of prostate cancer. Some ethnic groups are at particular risk for carriage of these mutations (estimated 2% of US Ashkenazi Jews).

Other genes contribute less frequently to familial breast cancer. It is hypothesized that ataxia telangiectasia heterozygotes are at risk, but this is as yet unproven. Breast cancer occurs with mutation in PTEN (Cowden disease), MSH1 or MSH2 (HNPCC), and p53 (Li Fraumeni syndrome).

The management of hereditary breast cancer is essentially that of non-hereditary disease. Less clear is how to manage asymptomatic female members of these families. Guidelines suggest referral to medical genetic clinics for counselling, advice on risks, consideration of testing for mutations of *BRCA1* and *BRCA2*, and referral for appropriate further management. Currently, the options open to these women are:

- **Prophylactic surgery**: bilateral subcutaneous mastectomy does reduce the incidence of breast cancer in these women but its impact on survival is uncertain.

- **Screening**: is of unproven benefit in this setting, with uncertainty about the age of first testing, frequency of testing, and the value and risks of frequent mammography.

- **Breast cancer prevention trials**.

Table 17.1 Eligibility criteria for referral to breast cancer families' clinic

♦ Mother or sister developed breast cancer aged <40 years

♦ Mother or sister developed breast cancer aged <50 years and another maternal relative had cancer of the breast, ovary, endometrium, or a sarcoma <65 years

♦ Mother or sister developed breast cancer aged 50–65 years and another maternal relative had cancer of the breast, ovary, endometrium, colorectum, or a sarcoma <50 years

♦ Mother or sister developed double primary cancer (breast plus any of ovary, endometrium, colon, or sarcoma) with at least one tumour before age 50 years and breast cancer before 65 years

♦ Dominant history of breast cancer—4 or more cases of breast or ovarian cancer on same side of the family at any age

♦ Cancer of colorectum, ovary, endometrium, or sarcoma in mother or father before age 50 years, and at least one first-degree relative with breast cancer age <50 years

♦ Two or more cancers of breast, colorectum, ovary, endometrium, or sarcoma in close relatives of father with at least one before age 50 years

Pathology

Breast cancer is more common in the left breast and around 50% arise in the upper outer quadrant. The commonest pathology is ductal carcinoma.

Ductal carcinoma *in situ* (DCIS)

90% of breast carcinomas arise in the ducts of the breast. They begin as atypical proliferation of ductal epithelium that eventually fill and plug the ducts with neoplastic cells. As long as the tumour remains within the confines of the ductal basement membrane it is classified as DCIS. Localized DCIS is impalpable but often visible on mammography as an area of microcalcification. Not all DCIS will inevitably progress, but the probability of development of invasive cancer is estimated at 30–50%.

Lobular carcinoma *in situ*

These pre-invasive lesions carry a risk not only of ipsilateral invasive lobular carcinoma but also of contralateral breast cancer. They typically are neither palpable nor contain microcalcification.

Invasive ductal carcinoma

This accounts for 75% of breast cancers. The malignant cells are associated with a fibrous stroma which can be dense (scirrhous carcinoma). The tumour invades through breast tissue into the lymphatics and vascular spaces, to gain access to the regional nodes (axillary and, less often, internal mammary) and the systemic circulation.

Table 17.2 Histological types of breast malignancy

◆ Invasive ductal carcinoma
No special type
Combined with other type
Medullary carcinoma
Mucinous carcinoma
Paget's disease
◆ Invasive lobular carcinoma
◆ Mixed lobular and ductal carcinoma
◆ Sarcoma (various)
◆ Lymphoma
◆ Metastases (e.g. breast cancer, small cell lung cancer)

The histological grade of the tumour is assessed from three features (tubule formation, nuclear pleomorphism, and mitotic frequency) and predicts the behaviour of the tumour. Oestrogen and progesterone receptor status is commonly assessed by immunocytochemistry. Other biological markers (e.g. c-erbB2) may be of value both as a predictor of prognosis and as a guide to therapy.

Ductal carcinoma of special type

A number of pathological variants are identified with relatively good prognosis, namely medullary carcinoma, tubular carcinoma, and mucinous carcinoma. Paget's disease of the breast is ductal carcinoma of the excretory ducts with involvement of the skin of the nipple and areola.

Invasive lobular carcinoma

Lobular carcinomas account for 5–10% of breast cancers. About 20% develop contralateral breast cancer.

Prognostic factors

Survival after a diagnosis of breast cancer is dependent upon:

- Eradication of the primary tumour
- Loco-regional disease, particularly axillary and/or internal mammary nodes
- Any systemic metastases

The latter determines the prognosis for the vast majority of women and is closely correlated with a number of recognized prognostic factors:

- Tumour size
- Number of involved axillary nodes
- Tumour grade
- Oestrogen receptor status (ER)

The usefulness of other biological factors (c-erbB2, markers of angiogenesis, cathepsin D, etc.) is currently being explored.

Breast cancer screening

There have been at least seven randomized controlled trials of mammographic screening over the last 30 years. The HIP study of New York and the Two Counties Study from Sweden both showed a 30% reduction in mortality in the >50-year-old age group who were screened with mammography. Meta-analysis of all the published trials confirms a significant benefit for the over-50s.

None of the trials published so far have shown a mortality benefit for women under the age of 50 years, although two meta-analyses report a 14% but non-significant reduction in mortality. Screening the under-50 age group remains a controversial area and in the UK a current trial is recruiting over 200 000 women to address this question.

Imaging modality

The aim of screening for this disease is to identify pre-invasive disease or invasive disease before dissemination (through the lymphatics or blood). There is no evidence that simple breast self-examination is an effective means of screening for breast cancer. X-ray mammography is the most sensitive technique for detecting breast cancer and is also the most specific. Mammography is most sensitive once involution of the breast tissue has occurred (i.e. once the menopause has taken place). The test is less sensitive in women with dense breasts—that is those with predominantly glandular tissue or residual stromal tissue.

Breast ultrasound, useful for focal abnormalities, is also useful in detecting impalpable lesions. Telediaphanography (infrared scanning of the breast tissue) has both low sensitivity and specificity. Magnetic resonance imaging with dynamic intravenous contrast is a very sensitive technique but variable specificity has been reported.

Mammographic technique

The breast is compressed to flatten the breast tissue to reduce movement, overlapping shadows, and radiation dose. The uniform thickness of the tissue improves image quality and contrast. Low-energy radiation is passed through the breast, resulting in a high-contrast image. The image is recorded on X-ray film presently, but in the future will be digitally recorded, with display on a high-resolution computer screen.

Two views of each breast are performed—one in the lateral oblique position diagonally across the chest, the other in the cranio-caudal position. Some 7% of women find the examination very painful, and a large proportion find it uncomfortable. The compression of the breast tissue lasts only a few seconds.

Table 17.3 Indications for referral to breast clinic

◆ Screen-detected breast cancer

◆ Breast lump

—any new discrete lump

—new lump in pre-existing nodularity

—asymmetrical nodularity persisting after menstruation

—abscess/inflammation which does not settle after one course of antibiotics

—persistent or recurrent cyst

◆ Pain

—associated with a lump

—intractable pain which interferes with the patients life and fails to respond to simple measures (well-supporting bra, simple analgesics, abstention from caffeine, evening primrose oil)

—unilateral persistent pain in post-menopausal women

◆ Nipple discharge

—in any women age >50 years

—in younger women if blood-stained, persistent single duct or bilateral, sufficient to stain clothes

◆ Nipple retraction, distortion, or eczema

◆ Change in breast skin contour

Radiation dose

A low radiation dose of approximately 2 mGy per examination is used. The radiation risk is 1–2 excess cancers per million women screened after a latent period of 10 years in the post-menopausal age group but is higher in women under 30 years. The dose to the breast is approximately five times that of a chest X-ray.

Organization of the UK Breast Screening Programme

In the UK, women aged 50–64 years are invited through their GP, to attend either a breast screening centre or a mobile van for mammography every three years. Women aged over 64 years can self-refer every three years. It was thought that the over 64-year-old age group would be less likely to take up screening, but this has not been substantiated in European screening programmes. The 65–69-year-old age group will in the future be formally invited for screening as there is a higher yield of cancers in this older age group. The under-50 age group will not be invited until the UK CCCR age trial, screening 40–49-year-olds, is completed.

The mammograms are read by a consultant radiologist. If an abnormality is seen which is thought to be suspicious, the woman is recalled to an assessment clinic at the breast screening centre. A clinical examination is performed at the recall visit with further X-rays, an ultrasound examination, and a needle test for cytology or core biopsy if appropriate. Women thought to have cancer are referred promptly to a breast surgeon who will arrange appropriate treatment.

An average of 72% of women accept the invitation to be screened and approximately 5% of women are recalled for further tests; 5 cancers per 1000 women screened are found.

The quality of the UK programme is monitored rigorously, with regular checks on all aspects of screening. Performance data on breast screening centres, as well as individuals within the centre, are monitored annually.

Interval cancers

These are cancers that occur in the interval between two screening episodes. They fall into five categories:

• **True interval cancer**: where a cancer appears in the 3-year interval and was not present on the previous screening mammogram.

• **False negative**: where the lesion was present on the previous screening mammogram.

• **Technical**: where the cancer was not on the film due to its position.

• **Mamographically occult**: where the cancer is not visualized on either the screening mammogram or at the time of diagnosis.

• **Unclassifiable**: no mammogram taken at the time of diagnosis.

There are approximately 12 interval cancers per 10 000 women screened in the first two years after screening and 13 interval cancers appear in the third year.

One- or two-view screening

The UK NHS Breast Screening Programme was initially funded for one X-ray (lateral oblique view) of each breast. A large trial comparing one-view with two-view mammography has shown that the second view results in a 24% increase in detection rate compared with single-view mammography.

All women attending screening for the first time have two views performed and screening centres are encouraged to perform two-view mammography on all women. The additional radiation dose for the second view is very low.

Frequency of mammography

Many European countries offer screening every two years, whereas the UK service is currently funded to perform screening every three years. There is a large ongoing UK trial looking at the question of frequency of screening. Although there is almost certainly increased detection o cancers when screening every two years, it may be that the large costs associated with more frequent screening will outweigh the benefit.

Screening for high-risk groups

Women thought to have strong family history of breast cancer are recommended to have genetic counselling and not assessment. If they are found to be at more than 16% risk, then mammographic screening is recommended. Meta-analysis of screening data of 40–50-year-olds suggests there is a non-significant benefit of mammography. At present, annual mammography is performed, with data being systematically collected. The MRC have funded a multi-centre trial to determine the place of magnetic resonance imaging in the detection of asymptomatic breast cancer. Women who are *BRCA1*, *BRCA2*, or p53 gene carriers, or at 50% risk of being a gene carrier, are being recruited into this study of annual MRI and mammography.

Features of screen-detected breast cancer

The expected outcome of breast cancer screening is a reduction in breast cancer deaths. Other useful measures are the pathological features of screen-detected tumours, which should reflect earlier disease compared with symptomatic women. This has been confirmed in a number of studies that show:

- 10–20% screen-detected disease is non-invasive
- >30% invasive cancers are less than 10 mm diameter
- <20% cancers are Grade 3 tumours
- 70–80% of patients are node negative

Breast cancer—presentation and staging

The diagnosis of breast cancer is made by 'triple assessment':
- Clinical examination
- Bilateral mammography
- FNA cytology or core biopsy

This combined approach to assessment has >90% sensitivity and specificity. The axilla is staged surgically. In the absence of locally advanced breast cancer or symptoms of metastatic disease or biochemical abnormality, routine radiological staging with CXR, CT scan, and isotope bone scan has not been found useful. The TNM staging system is commonly used.

Table 17.4 TNM staging system

Tis	Carcinoma *in situ*, non-infiltrating intraductal carcinoma, or Paget's disease of the nipple with no demonstrable tumour
T0	No evidence of primary tumour
T1	Tumour <2 cm
T2	Tumour >2 cm but <5 cm
T3	Tumour >5 cm
T4	Any size with extension to chest wall or skin
T4*a*	Fixation to chest wall only
T4*b*	Oedema, infiltration, or ulceration of skin
	Ipsilateral satellite nodules
T4*c*	Both *a* and *b* present
NX	Regional nodes cannot be assessed
N0	No regional node metastases
N1	Mobile ipsilateral axillary node metastases
N2	Fixed ipsilateral axillary node metastases
N3	Ipsilateral internal mammary node metastases

Management of non-invasive breast cancer

DCIS and LCIS are rarely symptomatic although extensive pre-invasive disease may present with a mass or thickening of breast tissue.

Treatment options

+ Simple mastectomy

  95% cure rate

  Rarely relapse, due to micro-invasive cancer

  No need for axillary dissection
+ Wide excision alone—30% recurrence at 5 years
+ Wide excision + radiotherapy—15% recurrence at 5 years

The management of LCIS is controversial; Bilateral breast excision of LCIS should be followed by close surveillance. Few surgeons would instead advocate bilateral subcutaneous mastectomies and immediate reconstruction.

Management of early breast cancer

Early breast cancer is defined as disease that can be completely extirpated by surgery, that is T1–3, N0–1 tumours. The management of this disease comprises:

- Treatment of the breast and axilla
- Pathological staging to direct adjuvant therapy
- Adjuvant therapy—endocrine, chemotherapy, radiotherapy
- Follow-up

Breast surgery

All patients require removal of the primary tumour with either wide local excision or mastectomy. Halsted mastectomy was the operation most extensively applied to breast cancer patients during the first half of the twentieth century, but it has gradually been replaced by a variety of less radical operations.

Total mastectomy and axillary dissection is a less mutilating operation preserving the pectoralis major muscle and its neurovascular bundle. Quadrantectomy, introduced at the beginning of the 1970s, is a breast-conserving operation that removes the primary cancer with a margin of 2.0 cm of normal breast tissue. Lumpectomy is an operation that provides for the removal of the tumour mass with a limited portion of normal tissue (1 cm).

Randomized trials comparing breast-conserving surgery followed by radiotherapy with mastectomy alone have demonstrated similar local control rates and survival. Breast conservation is not always suitable for women with multifocal disease and large tumours in small breasts. Some patients simply prefer mastectomy, not least because of the possible avoidance of radiotherapy. Either treatment should afford a local recurrence rate of <10% after 10 years.

Breast reconstruction can be done either at the time of primary surgery or at a later date—TRAM flap, latissimus dorsi flap, and implants all have a role.

Treatment of the axilla

- Clinical assessment is inaccurate
- 30% of involved nodes are impalpable
- Surgery—axillary node sampling (>4 nodes) (diagnostic)
  —axillary clearance levels, I, II, and III (therapeutic); lymphodema and arm pain are complications

—sentinel node biopsy:
—removal of first node which contains secondary deposit
—ongoing UK trial
—use either blue dye or ^{99M}Tc colloid
—negative sentinel node avoids clearance

Loco-regional radiotherapy

Breast irradiation has been shown to reduce the risk of local recurrence after breast-conserving surgery from about 30% to <10% at 10 years. Typically, the whole breast is treated with tangential fields to a dose of 50 Gy in 25 fractions (or an equivalent dose-fractionation regimen), with care taken to minimize the volume of lung and heart irradiated. Although a boost of 10–15 Gy is commonly delivered to the tumour bed, using electrons or ^{192}Ir implant, its benefits are unproven.

- Older techniques—cardiac side-effects
- Modern techniques—safe
  —may improve survival
- Irradiation of axilla—not required if clearance performed
- Radiation to axilla may cause lymphodema and brachial neuropathy

Adjuvant systemic therapy

Breast cancer patients who remain disease-free after local and regional treatment may eventually relapse and die of overt metastases. The current hypothesis ascribes the failure to obtain a cure to occult micrometastases in distant organs, already present at the time of first surgery. The risk of harbouring occult metastases is low in cases with a small carcinoma and negative nodes and increases with the size of the primary carcinoma and number of axillary metastatic nodes.

There have been many trials among women with operable breast cancer, examining the effects of systemic treatment, either endocrine manoeuvres or chemotherapy or both, on the survival of these patients. The basis of all these therapies is the reduction or eradication of microscopic systemic metastatic disease in women in whom all macroscopic local tumour has been effectively removed. In 1992 the Early Breast Cancer Trialists' Collaborative Group published an overview of 133 randomized trials involving 75 000 women with early breast cancer[1–3]. This has had major impact, setting standards of care for adjuvant therapy for this disease.

Adjuvant endocrine therapy

- 60% of breast cancers are oestrogen receptor positive
- Ovarian ablation—improves survival in women under 50 years
  —morbidity of vascular disease and osteoporosis

- Tamoxifen—improves disease-free and overall survival
  - all women, especially post-menopausal
  - little benefit if ER negative
  - 5 years is sufficient: better than 2 years; no need for longer
  - 10% increase in survival for node-positive disease
  - 5% increase in survival for node-negative disease
- Side-effects of tamoxifen—menopausal symptoms
  - endometrial cancer, 4-fold increase in risk
  - decreases contralateral breast cancer risk

Adjuvant chemotherapy

- Combination chemotherapy reduces recurrence and mortality
  - absolute 10-year survival benefit: 7–11% women <50 years; 2–3% women >50 years
- CMF (cyclophosphamide, methotrexate, 5FU) used in most trials
- Anthracycline regimes may be better
- Used most often in node-positive, large, Grade 3, ER-negative, pre-menopausal tumour patients
- Used in some ER-negative, node-positive, post-menopausal patients

Neo-adjuvant therapy

Primary chemotherapy or hormone therapy for operable breast cancer provides early systemic treatment and allows assessment of the response to treatment; by definition this is impossible with adjuvant therapy. Its disadvantages are the delay in definitive local surgery and the risk of over-treatment with chemotherapy in the absence of pathological staging (e.g. post-menopausal, ER-positive, node-negative tumour).

A large randomized trial (NSABP-B18) has shown no difference in survival when pre- and post-operative chemotherapy (doxorubicin and cyclophosphamide) was compared. Pre-operative treatment does downstage the primary tumour and, in some women, facilitates breast-conserving surgery where mastectomy would otherwise be required.

Management of locally advanced breast cancer

Locally advanced disease is defined by the presence of infiltration of the skin or the chest wall or fixed axillary nodes. The probability of metastatic disease is high (>70%) but long-term survival is possible and the median survival of these patients exceeds two years.

Local control of the tumour and the prevention of fungation are of major importance to the quality of life of these women. A combination of primary systemic treatment and radiotherapy is commonly used. Many of these patients are elderly and have indolent ER-positive disease that responds to endocrine therapy with tamoxifen, aromatase inhibitors, or progestins. In younger women, particularly with aggressive 'inflammatory' breast cancer, primary chemotherapy is preferred. In patients with a good response to systemic treatment surgery may be feasible.

Management of metastatic breast cancer

* Aim is palliation
* If hormone-sensitive, bony disease—may survive years
* 20% survive 5 years
* visceral ER-negative disease has bad prognosis
* Usual sites—lung, liver, bone, brain
* Rare sites—choroid, pituitary

Endocrine therapy

Treatment with tamoxifen, ovarian ablation, progestins, or aromatase inhibitors will provide an objective response in 30% of women with advanced disease, and in 50–60% of those with ER-positive tumours. Disease that responds to endocrine therapy and then progresses has a 25% response rate with second-line treatment; the response to a third agent is 10–15%.

Chemotherapy

Advanced breast cancer is moderately chemosensitive. Active agents include:

* Anthracyclines
* Alkylating agents
* Antimetabolities

Combinations such as FAC (5-fluorouracil, doxorubicin, cyclophosphamide) produce response rates of 40–60%, with a median time to progression of around 8 months. Despite the toxicity of such combinations (alopecia, nausea, mucositis, lethargy, myelosuppression) it has been shown that the quality of life of women improves as they respond to treatment.

25–50% of women respond to second-line chemotherapy with a taxane and studies are currently evaluating the promising combination of anthracycline plus taxane as first-line chemotherapy. Although Phase II studies have suggested that high-dose chemotherapy may produce durable remissions from metastatic breast cancer, no survival benefit has yet been proven for such treatment.

Radiotherapy

Low-dose radiotherapy provides effective palliation for painful bone metastases, soft tissue disease, and spread to sites such as the brain and choroid.

Bisphosphonates

These agents are the mainstays of treatment for malignant hypercalcaemia. In addition, they can produce healing of some osteolytic metastases and prolonged treatment with bisphosphonates for bone metastases from breast cancer reduces osteolysis, improves bone pain, and prevents hypercalcaemia and fractures. Recent data suggest that prophylactic treatment with these agents may prevent the future development of bone metastases in women with high-risk early breast cancer.

Prevention of breast cancer

The initial results of three tamoxifen studies in the prevention of breast cancer in 'high-risk' well women are controversial. An American study has shown a significant reduction in breast cancer with tamoxifen, but a UK and an Italian study have not confirmed this. The groups of women in each study were different, and it may be that the US study was positive because of the preponderance of older women (in whom tamoxifen may be more effective).

Fenretinide, a derivative of retinoic acid, appears a good candidate for chemoprevention as it has been shown to reduce the risk of contralateral and ipsilateral breast carcinomas in menopausal women. Other agents such as raloxifene have also shown promise.

1. Early Breast Cancer Trialists' Collaborative Group. (1992) Systemic treatment of early breast cancer by hormonal, cytotoxic or immune therapy—Parts I and II. *Lancet* 339, 1–15, 71–85.
2. Early Breast Cancer Trialists' Collaborative Group. (1998) Tamoxifen for early breast cancer: an overview of the randomized trials. *Lancet* 351, 1451–67.
3. Early Breast Cancer Trialists' Collaborative Group. (1998) Polychemotherapy for early breast cancer: an overview of the randomized trials. *Lancet* 352, 930–42.

Chapter 18
Colorectal cancer

Introduction

Colorectal cancer is the fourth commonest cancer worldwide. Around two-thirds of a million people will present with the disease each year. It affects men and women almost equally and tends to be more common in 'developed' countries and is particularly common in the US, Europe, and Australia.

Ethnic and racial differences, as well as migrant studies, suggest that environmental factors (probably diet) play a major role in the aetiology of the disease. Several distinct, inherited, predisposition syndromes have been described such as familial adenomatous polyposis (FAP) and hereditary non-polyposis colon cancer (HNPCC), but these account for a minority of cases (<8%).

The left side of the colon was more commonly affected, but over the last two decades there has been a steady increase in the incidence of cancer in the proximal colon.

Colorectal cancers are almost always adenocarcinomas. The tumour often starts as a polypoidal mass and then tends to infiltrate into and through the bowel wall. The loco-regional lymph nodes tend to be involved before the development of disseminated disease. This behaviour is the basis for all the staging systems for colorectal cancer. In rectal cancer specifically there is also a propensity for the tumour to infiltrate laterally into the perirectal fat and lymph nodes.

Colorectal cancer—surgery

Introduction

Surgery is the mainstay of curative therapy for colorectal cancer. There is considerable controversy about who should perform this surgery—general or colorectal surgeons. Currently there is no clear answer, but surgeons working regularly in the pelvis may get better results in rectal cancer.

Curative resection requires the excision of the primary tumour and its lymphatic drainage with an enveloping margin of normal tissue.

Pre-operative preparation

The precise **site** and local **extent** of the tumour should be known before laparotomy; knowledge of distant spread is helpful. Full colonoscopy or proctosigmoidoscopy and air-contrast barium enema (in the absence of obstruction or perforation) is required. The liver is imaged with CT and/or ultrasound examination; CT and endo-anal ultrasound imaging of the pelvis may offer additional information of the depth of invasion of rectal cancers.

Additional decisions are required before surgery for rectal cancer:

- Should transanal local excision be considered?
- If radical surgery is contemplated, should/can the sphincters be spared?
- If a stoma is planned the stoma care team must meet with the patient and plan the site of the stoma with attention to belt lines and skin creases.
- In choosing the operative approach, especially in rectal cancer, functional consequences are of prime importance—will the patient be able to cope with a colostomy or the different bowel habit associated with altered anatomy consequent on avoiding a colostomy?

Peri-operative antibiotics and thrombo-embolic prophylaxis are mandatory.

Principles in primary resection

The local anatomy of the disease and signs of distant spread are sought, perhaps using intra-operative ultrasound liver scan. The extent of resection is defined and the appropriate segment mobilized, including the arteries and veins associated with its lymphatic drainage, dividing these at their origins. The bowel segment and its lymphatic field are excised intact. If an anastomosis is planned, it is fashioned without tension, ensuring a good lumen and secure apposition. Minimally invasive colon cancer surgery is still unproven.

Rectal cancer

The rectum is mobilized circumferentially by sharp dissection in the plane outside the mesorectal fascial envelope, either to 3 cm below the tumour if part of the rectum is being preserved, or to the pelvic floor if a coloanal anastomosis or abdomino-perineal resection (APER) are planned.

If performing an anastomosis with anal observation, the meso-rectum is divided and after cross-stapling the bowel, the specimen is removed and an anastomosis made, either hand-sutured or by transanal circular stapling. If an APER is planned, an oval incision is made around the anus; the ischiorectal fat and pelvic floor muscles are incised to allow the specimen to be delivered intact through the perineum. Total excision of the mesorectum is considered essential.

Local excision

Around 5% of rectal cancers may be removed by non-radical transanal surgery. This is particularly appropriate in small, low, well-differentiated cancers on the posterior wall, especially if the patient is not an ideal candidate for major abdominal surgery.

Via a Parks' anal retractor, a disc of rectal wall is marked with a 1 cm margin around the tumour. Diathermy is used to cut through the full thickness of the rectal wall, taking a sliver of extra-rectal fat. The specimen should be pinned on cork to orientate it for the pathologist. The rectal defect may be closed if possible. If the pathologist reports incomplete excision, spread through the rectal wall, or poorly differentiated carcinoma, radical surgery may be required to obtain local extirpation of tumour, if the patient is fit.

Some lesions not reachable by the Parks' approach may be locally removable by transanal endoscopic microsurgery (TEM), using a special 4 cm rigid endoscope with binocular vision.

Surgery of recurrent cancer

Local recurrence occurs most commonly in rectal cancer, usually outside the bowel lumen. If investigations suggest that a recurrence is isolated and potentially resectable, further surgery should be considered. Clearance may involve removal of residual rectum and other pelvic organs, including the bladder and/or uterus.

Metastasis confined to one lobe of the liver or less than four in both lobes may warrant resection, as there is up to a 30% chance of cure.

Adjuvant chemotherapy of colorectal cancer

Rationale

Nearly half the patients undergoing apparently curative resection of bowel cancer are destined to relapse and eventually die with either locally recurrent or distant metastatic disease. This is due to the presence of residual micro-metastases invisible at the time of surgery. The aim of adjuvant chemotherapy is to eradicate these micro-metastases and thereby prevent future relapse.

Current available chemotherapy does not completely eradicate bulky, advanced metastatic bowel cancer. It does however eradicate micro-metastases in a proportion of patients. In view of the high incidence of colorectal cancer, even a small percentage benefit with adjuvant chemotherapy may have a significant impact in terms of prevention of death and morbidity.

Indications

Adjuvant chemotherapy is an exercise in risk reduction. Questions to be considered after a potentially curative operation:

- What is the probability of micro-metastases?
- Will adjuvant therapy prevent/delay relapse?
- What are the side-effects?
- Multidisciplinary team is essential.

The risk that the patient has micro-metastases is estimated, after surgery, by examining the pathological features of the primary cancer; best-established is the histological stage (Dukes' or Astler—Coller). Dukes' A cancers, ie those which have not breached the muscle layers of the bowel wall, carry only a 10% chance of relapse, and adjuvant therapy is not considered worthwhile. Dukes' C cancers, which have spread to the nearby lymph nodes, carry a much higher risk (around 50%). There is good evidence that this risk is reduced by adjuvant chemotherapy, which is now offered routinely in most centres unless there is a strong contraindication.

Dukes' B cancers, which have breached the muscle layers but not spread to lymph nodes, carry an intermediate risk of around 30%. The evidence for adjuvant chemotherapy is less clear-cut in these patients, and other factors including other pathological features, the patient's age, fitness, and attitudes come into the equation. Further trials to assess benefits in these groups are under way.

Molecular markers in the primary tumour may potentially predict invasiveness or determine sensitivity to chemotherapy; sensitive PCR-based tests are being developed to detect micro-metastases in blood, bone marrow, or other tissues.

Rectal cancer, which accounts for nearly 40% of bowel cancers, presents some special considerations. A relative lack of a barrier to lateral spread and increased technical difficulty of surgery in the pelvis combine to make local recurrence a particular problem. Radiotherapy, targeted to the pelvis either before or after surgery, reduces local recurrence rates. Adjuvant therapy for rectal cancer may therefore include both radiotherapy and chemotherapy aimed, respectively, at local and systemic micro-metastases. The evidence for the contribution of chemotherapy in these combined programmes is less clear than for chemotherapy alone in colon cancer.

Treatment

The current 'international standard' adjuvant chemotherapy regimen for colon carcinoma is 5-fluorouracil (5FU) given in combination with folinic acid, by bolus intravenous injection. Two commonly used schedules involve treatment for five consecutive days, repeated every four weeks, or treatment on one day each week, in both cases continued for six months. 5FU interferes with nucleotide synthesis, and hence the synthesis of DNA in dividing cells. It also has effects on RNA. The addition of folinic acid enhances the DNA-directed effects of 5FU and prolongs its duration of action.

5FU given by these standard schedules appear to reduce the relative risk of death by around a quarter. For a patient with Dukes' C colon cancer the absolute gain may be more than 10%, but for a patient with an earlier-stage cancer, who is already at low risk following surgery, the absolute gain from adjuvant therapy may be much smaller.

5FU is also a radiosensitiser. For patients with rectal cancer, pre- or postoperative pelvic radiotherapy is sometimes given concurrently with chemotherapy to harness this effect. This may be followed by a more prolonged course of standard adjuvant chemotherapy aimed at distant micrometastases.

Side-effects

Both the wanted and the unwanted effects of 5FU are critically dependent upon the dose and schedules used, and vary considerably from patient to patient. The side-effect profile should, for most patients, be quite easily tolerable and consistent with continuing normal activity, including work. Treatment is feasible even in the elderly.

Side-effects:

- Hair loss and vomiting
- Oral mucositis

- Diarrhoea
- Tiredness

Rare side-effects of 5FU include:

- Red, painful palms and soles
- Photosensitivity of face
- Irritation to eyes and nose
- Myleosuppression
- Cardiotoxicity (angina, infarction, or arrhythmias)
- Cerebellar syndrome (ataxia, slurred speech, and nystagmus)

Some patients may also experience unwanted psychological or social effects of adjuvant chemotherapy:

- Prolongation of the 'patient' status
- Feelings of anxiety or depression
- Loss of earnings
- Strains on family relationships

Newer treatments

It is known from research in patients with advanced colorectal cancer that there are more effective methods of giving 5FU, involving higher doses delivered by continuous or intermittent intravenous infusions. Ongoing randomized trials are evaluating whether these are worthwhile as adjuvant therapy.

5FU itself is not reliably absorbed if given by mouth, but a number of new oral preparations involving pro-drugs of 5FU and/or inhibitors of 5FU catabolism are being evaluated. Other research approaches involve regional delivery of 5FU to the tissues most at risk of containing micrometastases, via the peritoneal cavity or the hepatic portal vein.

New cytotoxic agents are continually under investigation, the most promising of which are:

- Irinotecan (a drug which works by interfering with the nuclear enzyme topoisomerase-I)
- Oxaliplatin (which forms covalently bonded adducts with DNA)

Chemotherapy for advanced colorectal cancer

Advanced colorectal cancer is that which is metastatic or locally advanced such that surgical resection is not likely to be curative. This may be at initial presentation (25% of new cases) or develop during follow-up of previously treated patients (50% of 'curatively' resected). It has a poor prognosis with five-year survival <5%.

Indications for chemotherapy

Any patient with good performance status. Patients who are eligible for surgery for isolated metastasis (e.g. liver, lung) should be excluded. Resection of such metastasis may be curative in a small subset of patients.

Timing of chemotherapy

A single randomized study has demonstrated that chemotherapy given early imparts a small but significant survival advantage when compared to delaying treatment until symptoms arise.

First-line chemotherapy

5-Fluorouracil (5-FU)

First introduced in 1957, 5-FU is still the most widely used single agent. It acts, following conversion to active metabolites, as a false substrate for thymidylate synthase, preventing DNA synthesis. Several trials suggest a response rate of 10–20%. No increase in overall survival is seen when analyzing all patients treated. A number of small randomized trials, comparing chemotherapy to best supportive care, suggest that there may be an average survival benefit of around six months in favour of chemotherapy.

Modulation

Understanding the complex pathways by which 5-FU acts has allowed the development of biochemical modulation techniques. Leucovorin enhances 5-FU toxicity by stabilizing the interaction of thymidylate synthase and active 5-FU metabolites. Several studies, when meta-analysed, have shown a doubling of response rate with the addition of leucovorin to 5-FU compared to 5-FU alone (23% vs. 11%). No difference in response rate has been seen when comparing high-dose to low-dose leucovorin.

Table 18.1 Commonly used regimens in first-line treatment of advanced colorectal cancer

Regimen	Mode	5-FU	Leucovorin	Duration	Interval
Mayo	Bolus	425 mg/m^2	20 mg/m^2	Daily for 5 days	4–5 weeks
DeGramont	Bolus/infusion	400 mg/m^2 Bolus, 8 g/m^2, 46 hrs	200 mg/m2	2 days	2 weeks
Lokich	Continuous infusion	300 mg/m^2 per day	–	8–12 weeks	–
Tomudex	Bolus	3 mg/m^2	–	15 mins	3 weeks

Table 18.2 Toxicities of commonly used regimens in first-line treatment of advanced colorectal cancer

	Mayo	DeGramont	Lokich	Tomudex
Nausea/vomiting	+	+	+	+
Diarrhoea	+++	+	+	
Mucositis	+++	+	+	+
Myelosuppression	++	+	+	+
Alopecia	±	−	−	−
Hand/food syndrome	−	−	++	−

Modes of administration

The optimum schedule of 5-FU ± leucovorin administration has yet to be elucidated.

Intravenous bolus 5-FU, usually given with leucovorin, is currently most commonly used (e.g. Mayo). Such regimes have the advantage of being outpatient-based. Bolus/infusion regimes (e.g. DeGramont) have been shown to increase response rates and improve treatment tolerability. Continuous infusion 5-FU regimes, delivered by portable pumps, have the theoretical advantage of increasing the likelihood of cancer cells being exposed to 5-FU during cell cycle and show improved response rates and good tolerability compared to bolus 5-FU. They suffer from the disadvantage of venous thrombosis and intravenous line occlusion.

Raltitrexed ('Tomudex')

Raltitrexed is a potent inhibitor of thymidylate synthase. It can be used as an alternative to 5-FU-based regimes for first-line treatment. It does not require co-administration of a biochemical modulator. Response rates appear to be similar to those seen with 5-FU/leucovorin. It has the advantage of being administered as an intravenous bolus every three weeks and causes less neutropenia and mucositis.

Regional chemotherapy

Intra-hepatic 5-FU, following surgical placement of a hepatic artery catheter, may be considered for patients with unresectable liver metastases. Response rates of 40–60% have been reported, although survival benefits are marginal.

Second-line chemotherapy

Irinotecan, CPT-1

Further chemotherapy depends on patient wishes and performance status. For patients previously treated with 5-FU-based chemotherapy, there is currently no standard treatment regime. Irinotecan is a novel topoisomerase I inhibitor.

Several non-randomized studies have demonstrated activity in colorectal cancer. A recent randomized controlled trial, comparing irinotecan with best supportive care in patients with 5-FU-refactory disease, has shown a significant increase in one-year survival (36% vs. 14%) and a significantly improved quality of life favouring irinotecan. A further study, comparing irinotecan with infusional 5-FU, has demonstrated a 40% improvement in one-year survival in the irinotecan-treated group.

Novel cytotoxic agents

Oxaliplatin　This platinum derivative is not effective as a single agent against colorectal cancer. However, oxaliplatin combined with 5-FU/leucovorin can increase response rate and progression-free survival (but not overall survival) when compared with 5-FU/leucovorin alone.

Oral 5-FU analogues　Because of marked variability in bioavailability, 5-FU cannot be given orally. Capecitabine is an oral agent, which is activated by a series of enzymes, resulting in 5-FU release preferentially at the site of tumour. Preliminary data suggest activity against colorectal cancer, with fewer side-effects than intravenous 5-FU.

Future directions　Results of clinical trials using several new agents, including novel thymidylate synthase inhibitors (e.g. uracil/tegafur, UFT) and novel biochemical modulators (e.g. trimetrexate, 5-ethynyluracil) are awaited.

Radiotherapy in colorectal cancer

Radiotherapy in colonic cancer is limited to the palliative situation in most circumstances. It is used for painful bone metastases, skin secondaries, and occasionally for tumours with local infiltration into surrounding organs. The mobile nature of the colon makes it impossible to deliver multiple fractions of treatment to anatomically defined regions of the colon.

Conversely, the rectum is immobile and fixed within the pelvis and therefore a suitable target for radiotherapy. Radiotherapy has been used in both the pre-operative and post-operative setting in this disease.

In the pre-operative situation there are a group of patients (10–15%) who present with large fixed or tethered tumours that are non-resectable. Only half of this group will have distant metastases at presentation. The conversion rate to resectability is 35–75%, with a dose of 50–60 Gy given over a five-week period. This group is also often offered combined chemo-irradiation, though the precise benefits (or otherwise) of this approach are not yet known. The successful use of radiotherapy in this situation has helped promote it, even in those with initially resectable cancers.

- Local recurrence of rectal cancer in up to half of patients
- 13 trials—comparing surgery alone with surgery plus radiotherapy
- Data conflicting—local recurrence less
- Survival unchanged
- Post-operative radiotherapy for 4 weeks—less recurrence
  —no difference in survival

Further reading

Cancer Guidance Sub-Group of the Clinical Outcomes Group. (1997) *Improving outcomes in colon cancer: the research evidence*. NHS Executive, Department of Health, London.

Bleiburg, H. *et al.* (1997) *Management of colorectal cancer*. Martin Dunitz, London.

MRC Rectal Cancer Working Party. (1996) Randomised trial of surgery alone versus surgery followed by radiotherapy for mobile cancer of the rectum. *Lancet* **348**, 1610–14.

O'Connell, M., Martenson, J.A., Wieand, H.S., *et al.* (1994) Improving adjuvant therapy for rectal cancer by combining protracted infusion fluorouracil with radiation therapy after curative surgery. *NEJM* **331**, 502–7.

Punt, C.J. (1998) New drugs in the treatment of colorectal carcinoma. *Cancer* **83**(4); 679–89.

Swedish Rectal Cancer Trial. (1997) Improved survival with pre-operative radiotherapy in resectable rectal cancer. *NEJM* **336**, 980–7.

Introduction

Anal cancer accounts for only 3–5% of all large bowel malignancies. Most anal tumours arise from the epidermal elements of the anal canal lining (squamous cell—85% of anal tumours), though some arise from the glandular mucosa of the uppermost part of the anal canal or from the anal ducts and glands (adenocarcinomas—10% of anal tumours). Malignant melanoma of the anus is very rare (<5% of anal tumours) and carries a poor prognosis.

Traditionally, the anal region is divided into the anal canal and the anal margin or verge. The boundaries of these areas differ from one group of authors to another, making interpretation of studies difficult.

Anal squamous cell carcinoma

There is wide geographical variation in the incidence of anal cancers around the world. Areas of high incidence include Recife in Brazil and the Philippines. Interestingly, those areas with a high incidence of anal cancer also tend to have a high incidence of cervical, vulval, and penile tumours.

Epidemiological evidence has suggested that anal cancer may be associated with anal sexual activity. Male homosexual activity and HIV infection are strongly associated with the incidence of anal squamous carcinoma. Most specifically, human papillomavirus has been shown to be an important aetiological factor in anal, cervical, vulval, and penile squamous tumours.

- Ano-genital papillomavirus lesion
  —condylomata
  —intra-epithelial neoplasia
  —invasive carcinoma
- Colposcopy useful
- High-grade and intra-epithelial lesions (AIN 111)
  —pigmented or white
  —flat or raised
  —if ulcerated, may be invasive
- Biopsy is essential

Pathology

Included within the category of epidermoid tumours are:

- Squamous cell
- Basaloid (or cloacogenic) carcinomas
- Mucoepidermoid cancers

Anal canal cancer spreads locally. The anal sphincters and the recto-vaginal septum, perineal body, and the vagina (in more advanced cases) are common sites of spread. Lymph node spread occurs initially to the perirectal group of nodes and thereafter to inguinal, haemorrhoidal, and lateral pelvic lymph nodes. Approximately 10% of patients will present with inguinal lymph node involvement, but this rises to approximately 30% when the primary tumour is greater than 5 cm in diameter. Synchronously involved nodes carry a poorer prognosis than metachronous nodal involvement.

Blood-borne spread tends to occur late and is usually associated with advanced local disease. The most common sites of metastases are the liver, lung, and bones.

Clinical presentation and staging

• Symptoms of epidermoid anal cancer
  —pain
  —bleeding
  —itch
  —discharge
  —mass
• Later
  —faecal incontinence
  —ano-vaginal fistula

Cancer of the anal margin often has the appearance of a malignant ulcer, with a raised, everted, indurated edge. Lesions within the canal may not be visible, although they may spread to the anal verge. Digital examination of the anal canal is usually painful and the canal often feels indurated and distorted. It is often difficult to distinguish an anal cancer from a low rectal tumour.

Approximately one-third of patients with anal carcinoma have enlarged inguinal lymph nodes on presentation, but less than half this number have metastatic nodes. Often the nodes are secondarily infected or reactive. Biopsy or fine-needle aspiration is therefore necessary to confirm involvement of the groin nodes if radical block dissection is contemplated.

The most widely used staging system is that of the UICC (Union International Contré Cancer).

Investigations

Examination under anaesthesia is the mainstay in the diagnosis and investigation of this tumour. Ultrasound scanning, CT, and magnetic resonance scanning may provide additional information.

Treatment

Until 10 years ago the standard treatment for anal canal tumours was abdominoperineal resection, while anal margin growths were viewed as equivalent to skin tumours elsewhere and treated by local excision. Over the past few years, radiotherapy and/or chemotherapy have become increasingly popular and in many cases are the treatment of choice.

Compared to anal margin cancer, anal canal cancer is more likely to be locally advanced and to be associated with subsequent metastases, perhaps explaining the general preference for radical surgery. Around 20% are incurable surgically at presentation. Most recurrence occurs loco-regionally.

Non-surgical treatment (chemo-irradiation) for anal cancer has become increasingly popular after pioneering work in the US by Norman Nigro. The drugs used are usually 5FU and mitomycin C.

This particular combination of chemotherapy was developed empirically as a pre-operative regimen aimed at improving the results of radical surgery[1]. The radiotherapy consists of 30 Gy of external-beam irradiation over a period of three weeks.

Chemo-irradiation was shown to be superior to radiotherapy alone in a recent British trial[2].

Small lesions at the anal margin may still best be treated by local excision alone, obviating the need for protracted courses of non-surgical therapy.

An important role for the surgeon is in treatment after failure of primary non-surgical therapy, either early or late. The appearance of the primary site can be misleading after radiotherapy. A proportion of patients develop complications such as radio-necrosis, fistula, or incontinence, following radical radiation or combined therapy.

Rarer tumours

Adenocarcinoma

Adenocarcinoma in the anal canal is usually a very low rectal cancer that has spread downwards to involve the canal, but true adenocarcinoma of the anal canal does occur, probably arising from the anal glands that arise around the dentate line and pass radially outwards into the sphincter muscles. This is a very rare tumour; although it is radio-sensitive, it is still usually treated by radical surgery.

Malignant melanoma

This tumour is excessively rare, accounting for just 1% of anal canal malignant tumours. The lesion may mimic a thrombosed external pile due to its colour, though amelanotic tumours also occur. It has an even worse prognosis than at other sites. As the chances of cure are minimal, radical surgery as primary treatment has been all but abandoned.

Practical points

- Rectal bleeding and anal pain are common—a high degree of suspicion is required to diagnose anal cancer correctly.
- Multifocal anal and genital disease may co-exist—be sure to examine the anal and genital areas.
- Examination under anaesthetic is essential for adequate staging and also permits a generous biopsy.
- Biopsy or needle aspiration of enlarged inguinal lymph nodes is essential prior to treatment.
- Local excision may be appropriate for small anal margin cancers.
- Chemo-irradiation is the treatment of choice for most anal squamous carcinomas.

1. Nigro, N.D., Vaitkevicius, V.K., Considine, B. (1974) Combined therapy for cancer of the anal canal. *Diseases of the colon and rectum* **27**, 763–6.
2. Arnott, S.J., Cunningham, D., Gamacher, J., *et al.* (1996) Epidermoid anal cancer: Results from the UKCCCR randomized trial of radiotherapy alone versus radiotherapy, 5-fluorouracil and mitomycin. *Lancet* **348**, 1049–54.

Chapter 20
Upper gastrointestinal cancer

Oesophageal cancer

Incidence and aetiology

In the UK, approximately 4000 people die each year from oesophageal cancer (0.7% of cancer deaths). It is at least twice as common in males than females, except for tumours arising in the post-cricoid area, for which there is a female preponderance. The incidence increases with age eight-fold between 45–54 and 65–74 years.

In most published series, squamous cell carcinoma is the most common histological type, but adenocarcinoma is increasing in incidence, especially in younger, white men. This trend is evident in the US where 50% of cases are now adenocarcinoma.

Historically, alcohol and smoking have been major risk factors in the West—heavy smokers and drinkers have a 100-fold increased risk. Other associated conditions include:

- Barrett's oesophagus (up to 1 in 2 risk if high-grade dysplasia is present)
- Tylosis palmaris (90% probability of developing oesophageal cancer)
- Chronic iron-deficiency states
- Chemical or radiation exposure
- Achalasia

Obesity may increase oesphageal reflux and incidence of Barrett's oesophagus and offers one possible explanation for the increase in incidence of adenocarcinoma.

Diagnosis and staging

The onset of dyspepsia or dysphagia in a person over 50 years of age requires investigation with upper GI endoscopy and biopsy. When the diagnosis is made, adequate staging is essential to decide on the appropriate treatment. A combination of the TNM and AJCC systems is commonly used:

T1   Tumour involves mucosa or submucosa
T2   Tumour invades the muscularis propria
T3   Tumour invades the adventitia
T4   Tumour invades adjacent organs
Stage 1   T1 N0
Stage II   T2–3 N0, T1–2 N1
Stage III T3 N1, T4 N0–1
Stage IV   M1 disease

A barium swallow/meal will delineate the length of the tumour. CT scan indicates the apposition of the tumour to major structures (aorta and carina) in addition to giving information about nodal involvement and distant metastatic disease. Endoscopic ultrasound (EUS) allows evaluation of the depth of oesophageal wall penetration in up to 85% of cases, provided that stenosis does not prevent full assessment. Regional nodes are more accurately evaluated with EUS than with CT scan. Bronchoscopy may be necessary to inspect the carina and the bronchial tree. Laparoscopy may also be valuable, especially in low oesophageal tumours, to exclude peritoneal metastases.

Treatment

Following adequate staging, case selection is important in the treatment of oesophageal cancer. A multidisciplinary approach involving surgeon, gastroenterologist, radiologist, oncologist, and dietitian is strongly advised for optimum patient management.

Resectable tumours

Surgical resection is the treatment of choice for Stage I and II disease; for more advanced localized tumours there is no definite evidence that surgery is superior to radiotherapy or chemo-irradiation. Most surgeons believe that there is no role for palliative oesophagectomy. Various techniques are used to resect the oesophagus and, most commonly, the stomach is used to re-establish continuity of the GI tract. Operative mortality is around 10%.

Fit patients with Stage I and II tumours treated with resection alone have expected five-year survival rates of 68–85%. Even with T1 tumours, 30% of patients have nodal metastases and the evidence from patterns of relapse and autopsy studies is that oesophageal cancer is often a systemic, not localized disease. Stage III disease patients treated by resection have a five-year survival rate of only 15–28% and it is for these patients that other treatment strategies such as pre-operative chemo-irradiation are being investigated.

Despite the chemosensitivity of advanced disease, adjuvant chemotherapy has not been shown to confer a survival advantage and is difficult to deliver after major oesophageal surgery. Post-resection irradiation improves the loco-regional control in patients with positive resection margins, but not if there is nodal involvement. The dose is limited to 50 Gy in 25 daily fractions (usually delivered with an anterior and two posterior oblique fields) in patients who have undergone a gastric pull-up or intestinal interposition procedure.

The principles underlying pre-operative (neo-adjuvant) chemotherapy are that in addition to downstaging the primary tumour, micro-metastases are treated before the post-operative, stimulatory surge of growth factors. Drugs effective in oesophageal cancer include:

- 5-fluorouracil (5FU)
- Cisplatin
- Mitomycin

- Paclitaxel
- Methotrexate

Bleomycin was used in early studies but pulmonary toxicity has led to its replacement. The most commonly used combination is continuous infusion of 5FU and cisplatin.

Despite reported response rates with chemotherapy of up to 60%, no randomized trial has shown a survival advantage for pre-operative chemotherapy for oesophageal cancer. However, most studies have randomized fewer than 200 patients.

Pre-operative radiotherapy has been studied but no reliable data are available to suggest increase in resectability improvement in local control or survival. A recent overview suggests that combined pre-operative chemoradiotherapy holds some promise in this disease.[1]

Pre-operative chemo-irradiation may be delivered with the combined modalities applied concurrently or sequentially. Inevitably, combination therapy causes increased normal tissue damage, in particular oesophagitis and pneumonitis, and as a result both chemotherapy and radiotherapy doses may be compromised. Some studies have included only squamous tumours and in these there has been no significant improvement in survival. An Irish study included 113 patients with adenocarcinoma and at three years the survival rates were 32% for combined therapy compared with 6% for surgery alone.

It is not certain whether treatment should be determined according to histological type, and stratification for histology within large randomized trials is essential for resolution of this issue. Pathological complete response rates of up to 70% have been reported in phase II studies of chemo-irradiation and the necessity for oesophageal resection after combined therapy questioned.

Many patients with oesophageal cancer will have serious co-morbid conditions due to age or lifestyle. In elderly or unfit patients (e.g. poor respiratory reserve) with apparently resectable tumours, oesophago-gastrectomy may be poorly tolerated and insertion of an oesophageal stent—usually metal—is often the most appropriate palliative measure. With proper technique, the risk of perforation is less than 5%. The stent should extend 3 cm beyond each end of the tumour. At least one randomized trial has demonstrated superiority of palliation with stenting rather than laser therapy.

Unresectable tumours

The majority of oesophageal tumours are diagnosed at an advanced stage when resection is not possible. Combined chemo-irradiation is more effective than radiotherapy alone in locally advanced oesophageal cancer and cure is not impossible, although rare. In one of the larger randomized trials, Herskovic reported an increase in 5-year survival from 0 to 27% (median survival 9.3 months v. 14.1 months) in 123 patients randomized to receive either cisplatin and 5FU with

50 Gy RT or 64 Gy RT alone. These encouraging results in advanced tumours indicate that randomized trials of combined modern chemo-irradiation (where optimal doses of each modality are delivered) versus surgery alone are warranted in earlier stage disease.

In patients with metastatic disease, those of ECOG performance status <2 should be considered for chemotherapy. The median survival for Stage IV disease remains around eight months. Palliation of dysphagia, usually through stenting, is often necessary before chemotherapy starts, although effective chemotherapy may return swallowing to normal after one course of treatment. Intraluminal radiotherapy (brachytherapy), laser treatment, and intratumoural alcohol injection are alternative palliative measures for control of local symptoms only.

References

1. Gen, J.I., Crellin, A.M., Glynne-Jones, R. (2001) Preoperative (neoadjavant) chemoradiotherapy in oesophageal cancer. *British Journal of Surgery* **88**, 338–56.

Gastric cancer

Aetiology

- Helicobacter pylori—3–6-fold increase in risk
  —causes atrophic gastritis, decrease in acid secretion, bacteria overgrowth, increase in nitrites
- Barrett's oesophagus—associated with increase in gastro-oesophageal cancer
- Blood group A
- Pernicious anaemia (3-fold increase)
- Lower social class

Epidemiology

Globally, stomach cancer is the second commonest cancer with an estimated 775 000 new cases per annum. In the UK, there were 11 851 new cases in 1990, being the sixth commonest cancer in men and the seventh in women (male:female ratio 3:2).

The diagnosis is rare prior to the sixth decade with the incidence rising steeply thereafter. Wide variations in incidence are observed, from rates of >90 per 100 000 in Japan to <10 per 100 000 for Caucasians in the US, Africa, and India. China and Eastern Europe have relatively high rates—28–50 per 100 000, whilst Western European rates are 15–20 per 100 000.

In most countries the incidence of stomach cancer is declining. However, despite this decline, several countries, including the UK, have detected an increase in cancers of the oesophageal gastric junction (OGJ).

In Japan, screening for gastric cancer is routinely performed with a double-contrast barium meal and gastroscopy. This increases the proportion of resectable early gastric cancers by 30–40%. In Western Europe and the US, screening of asymptomatic patients is not practicable because of the lower incidence of the disease. A British study in which patients over 40 years presenting with dyspepsia underwent gastroscopy detected tumours in 2%.

Pathology

90% of stomach tumours are adenocarcinomas, that are further divided into 'intestinal' and 'diffuse' types. The remainder are mainly lymphomas (up to 8%) and leiomyosaromas (1–3%). Intestinal type gastric cancers are ulcerative and occur more often in the distal stomach than diffuse types, including linitis plastica, which occur throughout the stomach. Gastric cancers are evaluated according to the TNM staging system. This system stages tumours according to:

- Depth of invasion of the primary tumour
- Degree of lymph node involvement
- The absence (M0) or presence (M1) of distant metastases

Endoscopy with biopsy is the optimal means of diagnosis of gastric cancer. CT scanning detects spread to regional lymph nodes and distant metastases. Endoluminal ultrasound is superior to CT in determining the depth of invasion of the primary tumour and presence of local adenopathy. Laparoscopy should be used in patients being considered for curative surgery to confirm operability and exclude peritoneal metastases.

Surgery

The best results are achieved in patients with T1N0 or T1N1 tumours; 70% of such patients are alive at five years. However, under 5% present with T1 tumours. Penetration of the serosa by the tumour predicts a risk of recurrence of 80–85%.

The type of operation will depend on the site of the tumour; oesophagogastrectomy may be required for cancers of the OGJ and proximal stomach, total gastrectomy for mid-stomach tumours, and partial gastrectomy may be adequate treatment for tumours in the distal stomach.

A further consideration is the extent of lymphadenectomy undertaken. In Japan, patients routinely undergo extensive lymphadenectomy, whereas in Western countries most patients have more limited lymph node resection. MRC and Dutch studies have compared R1 dissection (lymph nodes within 3 cm of the tumour) to R2 dissection (more extensive lymphadenectomy). In both studies postoperative mortality was significantly higher with R2 resection and no survival advantage has been observed. Consequently, R2 resection should not be used as standard treatment at present; long-term survival data are awaited from these studies.

Chemotherapy and radiotherapy

Adjuvant

- Post-operative adjuvant radiotherapy—no survival effect
- Meta-analysis of 11 trials, 2096 patients—no benefit from adjuvant chemotherapy
- More recent trials encouraging—patient should go into trial if eligible
- Mitomycin C (MMC), tegafur-encouraging results
- Current MRC trial of peri-operative chemotherapy (ECF)

Palliative

Many patients will be suitable for palliative chemotherapy, with radio-therapy being reserved for the control of pain from bone metastases. Four randomized studies comparing chemotherapy with best supportive care have been reported, three of which demonstrate benefit with palliative chemotherapy.

Many cytotoxic agents demonstrate single-agent activity in gastric cancer. Few randomized studies compare single agents with combination chemotherapy. One study comparing single-agent 5-fluorouracil (5-FU) to 5-FU combined with cisplatin and to FAM (5-FU, adriamycin, MMC) demonstrated significantly improved response rates and progression-free survival with cisplatin/5-FU. However, overall survival was similar in the three groups. This study suggests that response and survival benefits may be achieved with the use of effective combinations compared to single-agent treatment.

While FAM, with response rates of 22–40% in patients with gastric cancer, was once the most used regimen in gastric cancer, this has now been surpassed by other combinations. In a randomized trial, FAMTX (5-FU, adriamyicn, and methotrexate) demonstrated superior response rates and survival when compared to FAM. The ECF regimen (epirubicin, cisplatin, protracted venous infusion 5-FU) was developed at the Royal Marsden Hospital. The rationale for the three drugs was based on single-agent activity and the synergy between 5-FU and cisplatin in experimental models. An anthracycline was included because of the enhanced cytotoxicity afforded in combination with the other two drugs. 5-FU was given as a protracted infusion because of its improved therapeutic index compared to bolus 5-FU. A multi-centre randomized comparison to FAMTX demonstrated superior response rates, failure-free survival, and overall survival with ECF. In addition, global quality of life was improved with ECF at 24 weeks.

New drugs being evaluated in gastric cancer include irinotecan (a topoisomerase I inhibitior) and docetaxol, both of which have response rates of 20%. In addition, orally bioavailable fluoropyrimidines such as UFT and capecitabine are being evaluated in combination therapy in place of intravenous 5-FU.

High-dose chemotherapy

In a Phase II study of 235 patients treated with ECF, 10% survival at four years was observed. One way to attempt to increase the proportion of long-term survivors is to use high-dose chemotherapy as consolidation in patients achieving a partial or complete remission. A previous study observed an 89% partial remission rate with high-dose etoposide and cisplatin. The lack of complete response was probably due to the fact that patients were not cyto-reduced with conventional chemotherapy prior to high-dose therapy. A randomized study is underway in patients who achieve complete or partial remission at 12 weeks, with randomization to high-dose carboplatin/etoposide with peripheral stem cell transplant or to continuation of initial treatment.

Palliative therapies

Patients with dysphagia from inoperable tumours of the OGJ and cardia may benefit from the insertion of rigid or expandable metal stents. Bleeding from intraluminal tumours can be reduced by ablation of the tumour with endoscopic laser treatment. There remains a role for palliative surgery to bypass gastric outlet obstruction.

Small intestine and carcinoid tumours

Introduction

Small bowel tumours, both benign and malignant, are exceedingly unusual, and constitute less than 10% of all gastrointestinal tumours; and approximately 65% of all small bowel tumours are malignant. More than 35 pathological variants have been described. Most common are adenocarcinomas that constitute 40% of all malignant small bowel tumours. Carcinoid tumours represent 30% of all small bowel malignancies. Other forms of tumours are lymphomas, sarcomas, as well as benign tumours such as leiomyomas, angiomas and lipomas.

The incidence of small bowel tumours is 0.4–1.0/100 000 population with a slight male predominance. The prevalence increases with age and is rare below 30 years of age, peaking between 50–60 years. Occasionally, small bowel tumours are related to the Peutz–Jegher' syndrome or von Recklinghausen's neurofibromatosis. Metastases from melanoma may be found in the small bowel.

Aetiology

Despite the fact that the small bowel constitutes about 75% of the length of the gastrointestinal tract, small bowel tumours account for only 1–3% of all gastrointestinal malignancies. Rapid transit of its liquid contents might be one explanation. Increased incidence is noticed in immunocompromised patients e.g. AIDS, chronic immunosuppressant therapy.

Frequent consumption of red meat or smoked foods has been associated with a two- to three-fold increased risk of small bowel tumours. There is also a correlation between dietary fat intake and risk of small bowel carcinoma. Crohn's disease is associated with an increased risk of small bowel malignancies.

Pathology

Tumours can derive from all cell types of origin in the small intestine. The same staging system as for colorectal tumours is usually used.

In general, initial symptoms of small bowel tumours are rather vague and a diagnostic delay of 8–12 months is common. Tumour markers are useful for carcinoids, particularly chromogranin A and 5-HIAA. Markers such as CEA, CA-19-9, CA-50 are too non-specific for diagnosing small bowel tumours. Any patient who has a primary small bowel malignancy should be monitored for the development of a second malignant tumour, frequently in the colon.

Adenocarcinoma

- Commonest in proximal small bowel (80%)
- presents with abdominal pain and jaundice (obstruction)
- Anaemia—occult bleeding
- Diagnosis—barium studies
  Endoscopy

Carcinoid tumours

90% arise in the ileum and appendix and although they are often silent, abdominal pain is a common symptom. Small bowel obstruction can result from intense desmoplastic reaction around the primary tumour. The syndrome of chronic mesenteric ischaemia has been described, related to elastic vascular sclerosis. Less than 20% present with the carcinoid syndrome which includes:

- Flushing
- Diarrhoea
- Bronchial constriction
- Right-sided valvular heart disease

A majority of these patients are found to have liver metastases and have elevated urinary 5-HIAA levels and plasma chromogranin A and tachykinins (neurokinin A and substance-P). Approximately 30% of small bowel carcinoids are multiple. Pre-operative diagnostic tests are both biochemical and radiological. Urinary 5-HIAA and chromogranin A are assayed, the latter is particularly useful in earlier stage disease.

The primary tumours and metastases can be seen by somatostatin receptor scintigraphy (Octreoscan); 80% of these tumours express somatostatin receptor subtype 2 that binds this somatostatin analogue. This investigation should be supplemented with CT or MRI scan for detection of lymph node and liver metastases. Sometimes a small bowel contrast enema can be informative in patients with intermittent obstructive symptoms.

Lymphoma

Primary small bowel lymphoma constitutes about 1% of all gastrointestinal malignancies. There are five clinical distinct subtypes of primary small intestinal lymphoma:

- Adult Western type
- Paediatric type
- Immunoproliferative small intestinal disease
- Mediterranean type, enteropathy-associated T-cell lymphoma
- Hodgkin's lymphoma

Most small bowel lymphomas show intermediate or high histological grade. The diagnosis of small intestinal lymphoma is often made only at laparotomy. Radiological findings that might suggest this diagnosis include diffuse segment-thickened distal small bowel on a follow-through barium examination. CT can sometimes better demonstrate this finding. However, the radiological appearances are easily confused with other segmental diseases of the distal small intestine such as Crohn's disease.

Sarcoma

These tumours are exceedingly rare and most are of smooth muscle origin (leiomyoma/sarcoma). Recently, tumours derived from the autonomic nervous system have also been described. The clinical presentation is either bleeding or obstruction.

Treatment

Surgery

Surgical resection is the most important therapy for all small bowel tumours. All benign tumours, such as leiomyomas, small bowel adenomas, angiomas, and lipomas, can be cured by adequate segmental resections with clear serosal margins. The same holds true for the malignant tumours, although surgery should include lymph node resection.

Pancreaticoduodenectomy may be required in patients with tumours arising in the proximal and second portion of the duodenum. Carcinoid tumours confined to the distal ileum require resection that sometimes includes part of the caecum. In patients with Peutz–Jeghers' syndrome and multiple polyps only limited resection should be performed and most of the tumours can be removed by endoscopic polypectomy.

Resection of involved bowel is recommended for lymphomas, except the Mediterranean type, that often involves the entire small bowel and responds to systemic therapy.

Chemotherapy

Chemotherapy for most malignant small bowel tumours is based around 5-fluorouracil (5FU). 5FU can be applied either alone or in combination with leucovorin and/or α-interferon. Sarcomas are treated, as at other sites, with doxorubicin-based regimens. Similarly, lymphomas are commonly treated with regimens such as CHOP.

Carcinoid tumours, although malignant, should not be treated with cytotoxics in most cases. Streptozotocin and 5-FU or doxorubicin give modest (10–20%) response rates of short duration. Most patients with low-grade carcinoid tumours can be treated with α-interferon alone or in combination with somatostatin analogues.

Five-year survival in patients with malignant adenocarcinoma of the small intestine is only 20–30%. For carcinoid tumours with local disease, five-year survival is 75–95%; with regional lymph node involvement, 40–60%; and with liver metastases and the carcinoid syndrome, 20–30%. 'Aggressive' surgery combined with biotherapy (α-interferon plus somatostatin analogue) has recently afforded a five-year survival rate of 60% in patients with liver metastases and the carcinoid syndrome. For lymphomas of the small bowel the majority of deaths occur within two years of diagnosis, with five-year survival of 20–30%. Combination therapy with resection and chemotherapy has been reported to give five-year survival of 60%. The survival rate for patients with small bowel sarcoma is about 20%.

Radiotherapy

Radiotherapy is of limited value in most small bowel malignant tumours, not least because of the difficulty of localizing disease in a mobile organ and because of the low tolerance of the small bowel for ionizing radiation. However, tumour-targeted radiotherapy can be applied to carcinoid tumours, using either Indium[111]-DTPA-octreotide or MIBG. Response rates of 30–50% have been reported, but these are still considered investigational treatments.

Cytokine therapy

α-interferon can be used both for adenocarcinomas and carcinoids of the small bowel, either alone or in combination with 5-FU. Biochemical response rates of 40–50% are reported in malignant carcinoids, although only 10–15% show measurable reduction in tumour bulk. α-interferon can be combined with somatostatin analogues in carcinoid tumour patients.

Somatostatin analogue treatment

Somatostatin analogues are particularly useful for ameliorating clinical symptoms such as diarrhoea and flushing related to carcinoid tumours. They also demonstrate some anti-tumour effects with about 10% of patients showing significant tumour reduction and 30–40%, stabilization of the disease. High-dose therapy (>3 mg/day) has been shown to induce apoptosis in carcinoid tumours.

Their parenteral administration is simplified with the recently marketed long-acting formulations (10–30 mg intramuscular injection monthly).

Future treatment

Novel approaches will be based on tumour biology, taking into consideration the proliferation capacity, expression of adhesion molecules, and angiogenic factors. The carcinoid tumour determination of somatostatin receptor subtypes will be of importance as subtype-specific analogues are developed. New tumour-targeted radioactive treatments are also in development.

Cancer of the liver

Epidemiology

Primary liver cancer or hepatocellular carcinoma (HCC) is uncommon in the Western world but is prevalent in areas where hepatitis B is endemic. In the UK, HCC is most commonly associated with cirrhosis secondary to alcohol-induced liver injury or haemochromatosis. The majority of cases present under the age of 50 years and males are affected more frequently than females. In the UK, chronic hepatitis B does account for a small proportion of cases but hepatitis C infection is becoming an increasing cause. Tumours may also be found incidentally at the time of post-mortem examination in patients with cirrhosis.

Symptoms

Symptoms are often a late feature of the disease and can be divided into those arising from the mechanical effects of tumour growth, para-neoplastic symptoms, and deterioration of liver function. Right upper-quadrant abdominal pain is the most common symptom of HCC. Symptoms associated with advanced disease include:

* Weight loss
* Anorexia
* Abdominal distension
* Fever
* Intra-peritoneal haemorrhage

In cirrhotic patients, HCC may present as a rapid deterioration in hepatic function. Jaundice is uncommon unless liver function is severely impaired or the tumour has impinged upon a major intra-hepatic bile duct. Clinical examination may reveal stigmata of chronic liver disease, and hepatomegaly is usual; 30–60% have ascites.

Para-neoplastic effects include:

* Hypoglycaemia
* Erythrocytosis
* Hypercalcaemia
* Hypercholesterolaemia

Diagnosis

The diagnosis of HCC is usually made on the basis of the history associated with radiological findings of a mass lesion within the liver. The differential diagnosis includes:

- Secondary metastatic cancer
- Focal nodular hyperplasia
- Haemangioma
- Macronodular cirrhosis

Biopsy should be deferred in any patient in whom the potential for surgical resection exists because of the risk of tumour seeding outwith the liver. However, if coagulation is satisfactory, fine-needle aspiration is safe.

Pathology

Macroscopically, HCC may appear as a large solitary tumour or as a multicentric tumour with satellite lesions evident around a central tumour. True multifocal tumours can also occur. The tumours may appear as yellowish-white nodules and may be punctuated with areas of haemorrhage or necrosis.

Microscopically differentiated tumours contain large cells identifiable as being hepatocytic in origin, with clear cytoplasm, and often have a similar appearance to renal cell carcinoma. Undifferentiated or anaplastic tumours have a variable appearance with multiple mitoses and differing cell shape and size depending on type.

Investigations

- CT scan
- Laparoscopy
- Laparoscopic ultrasound
- Angiography
- Lipiodol and CT scanning—picks up multifocal tumours
- CXR + CT chest to exclude metastases
- α fetoprotein—useful for diagnosis and monitoring recurrence
- Liver function tests—to assess functional reserve

Therapeutic options

Surgical resection

Surgery offers the only hope of cure of HCC. However, resection is not possible in many patients. The most common reasons for irresectibility are bilobar or multifocal disease and liver failure associated with cirrhosis. Non-cirrhotic patients can tolerate extensive hepatic resection through compensatory hypertrophy of the unaffected liver, but in cirrhotic patients even limited segmental resection can induce liver failure. Multicentric tumours are most common in patients with cirrhosis and resection of the primary tumour may leave other, undetected deposits; higher recurrence rates following resection are observed in cirrhotic compared with non-cirrhotic patients.

Liver transplantation is appropriate for some cirrhotic patients with HCC <3 cm and is preferred to resection in the treatment of HCC arising from hepatitis C because of the high likelihood of further tumour development in these patients.

Systemic chemotherapy

For irresectable tumours systemic chemotherapy has been used. A variety of cytotoxic drugs including doxorubicin, mitozantrone, methotrexate and cisplatinum have been used as single agents or in combination with 5-fluorouracil. Response rates are however poor.

Tumour devascularization techniques

Surgical ligation of the hepatic artery and insertion of a hepatic artery catheter have been used to deprive the tumour of oxygenated blood and to provide a route for the direct administration of cytotoxic chemotherapy. Such techniques have been superceded by the use of chemo-embolization via radiologically placed catheters in the hepatic artery. This technique is less invasive and, using chemotherapy such as adriamycin combined with lipiodol uptake by the tumour, is demonstrable on CT scan. Repeat embolization is performed at 2–3 month intervals and tumour regression with associated regeneration of normal liver may render some tumours resectable.

Chemo-embolization or hepatic artery ligation can be complicated by acute hepatic decompensation and liver failure, although this is uncommon with appropriate patient selection.

Interstitial therapy

Instillation of absolute alcohol has been used during operation to avert haemorrhage following spontaneous rupture of a tumour, and alcohol can be injected percutaneously in patients under ultrasound guidance if resection is not being considered. Cryotherapy and laser ablation of tumours have been proposed but are not generally established therapies.

Palliation

Pain due to stretching of the liver capsule may respond to tumour regression following chemo-embolization or systemic chemotherapy. In recalcitrant cases, dexamethasone may provide symptomatic relief and reduce opiate analgesic requirements. Associated features of liver disease including peripheral oedema, ascites, and encephalopathy may require treatment.

Prognosis

Accurate prognosis is difficult to estimate due to the rarity of HCC in the UK, but overall survival is poor, with <10% of patients alive at three years. Surgical resection provides five-year survival rates of up to 50% for non-cirrhotic patients with clear resection margins.

Cancer of the biliary tract

Introduction

Microscopically, tumours of the biliary tract are adenocarcinomas of the papillary, nodular, or sclerosing type. Papillary tumours develop more commonly in the gall bladder or in the distal bile duct; sclerosing and nodular tumours, in the proximal bile duct. Adenocarcinomas without specific features are the most common. Papillary tumours represent 10% of cases and have a better prognosis, contrary to mucus-secreting tumours (5%) with a worse outcome.

Tumours of the bile ducts

In the Western world, the annual incidence is approximately 1.5/100 000. The most important predisposing factor is sclerosing cholangitis, with tumours developing in 9–20% of the patients (often heralded by a recent worsening of symptoms or an increase in the tumour markers CEA or CA19–9). Other predisposing diseases are chronic infection with *Clonorchis sinensis*, intra-hepatic stones, and bile stasis (such as in congenital choledochal cysts).

Anatomical classification and mode of spread

Tumours of the bile duct can develop within the head of the pancreas (lower third tumours), in the hepatoduodenal ligament (middle third tumours), or at the level of the hepatic hilum, defined by the portal bifurcation, where the ducts converge into the right and left hepatic duct and into the main hepatic duct. Hilar cholangio-carcinomas (Klatskin's tumours) account for more than half in most series.

Cholangiocarcinomas, especially of the sclerosing and nodular type, infiltrate along the walls of the ducts and the perineural tissue before obstructing the lumen. Metastases to the lymph nodes are seen in 13–30% of patients undergoing surgery. Direct duodenal invasion and peritoneal carcinomatosis occur late.

Clinical presentation

- Painless jaundice (occasionally intermittent)
- Palpable gall bladder (Courvoisier's sign)
- Weight loss
- Fatigue
- Itch

Diagnosis

- Blood tests—obstructive jaundice
  —if cholangitis (transaminases × 5)
  —tumour markers CA19–9, ACE elevated
  —coagulation abnormality (Vitamin K deficiency)
- Ultrasound—level of obstruction
  —excludes stones
  —may see nodes or hepatic secondaries
  —doppler to assess vessels
  —endoscopic ultrasound good for tumour of lower one third
- CT scan—excludes cancer of head of pancreas
  —assesses liver
- Angiography—useful 'road map' for surgeon
- MRI cholangiography—good biliary tree map
- ERCP
- Percutaneous cholangiography

Treatment

Cholangiocarcinomas should be resected if there are no distant metastases and no irreparable involvement of the hepatic artery and portal vein. Lower third tumours can be treated by a standard pancreatico-duodenectomy and middle third tumours by resection of the bile duct. It is advisable to perform a full lymph-node dissection, including the retro-pancreatic and para-aortic stations, as cure has been reported even with hilar nodal metastases.

The results of surgery are good, with microscopically curative resections possible in over 75% of the patients, and five-year survival of approximately 50% in the best series.

In cases of unresectable tumours, cholestatic jaundice requires surgical, endoscopic, or percutaneous palliation. Cholangiocarcinomas often grow slowly, and in young patients surgical bypass is preferred. A gastroenterostomy can also be performed to prevent duodenal obstruction. Endoscopic stenting is less invasive but the failure rate is high and the prostheses often need to be replaced (polyethylene tubes) or unblocked (Wallstent). The percutaneous transhepatic route is generally superior because of better access to negotiate the obstruction.

The results of trials comparing the different modalities are inconclusive. Percutaneous transhepatic stenting is definitely preferred in cases of recurrence after surgery. Although cholangiocarcinomas are not generally considered chemosensitive or radiosensitive, responses to chemotherapy with cisplatin and 5-fluorouracil and folinic acid have been observed, occasionally allowing resection of apparently unresectable tumours. Newer agents such as gemcitabine and irinotecan are under investigation.

Tumours of the gall bladder

In Western countries, the annual incidence is 1–1.5/100 000, with women affected twice as often as men because of their increased predisposition to gallstones, the most important aetiological factor. The risk of gall bladder cancer is 1%, 20 years after diagnosis of cholelithiasis. Endemic peaks are observed in some populations of Chile and in some native American tribes with a very high prevalence of gallstones. Gall bladder polyps may degenerate and, if larger than 10 mm, should be removed by laparoscopic cholecystectomy.

Mode of spread and clinical presentation

The tumour infiltrates the muscular wall of the gall bladder and the neighbouring liver tissue in segments 4 and 5, and spreads to regional lymph nodes and to the liver. Distant metastases occur late.

Two modes of presentation are common. During cholecystectomy for gallstones (approximately 1% of cholecystectomies) either a small, non-penetrating mass is found on examination of the resected specimen or an obvious mass is seen penetrating the gall bladder wall. Alternatively, patients present with obstructive jaundice, abdominal pain, and a mass in the right upper quadrant—either the tumour itself or lymph node metastases.

Diagnosis

- Liver function tests may be abnormal
- CEA, CA19–9 may be increased
- Ultrasound—may reveal tumour
                —invasion of ducts
                —nodes
                —liver secondaries
- CT scan
- Angiogram—vessel invasion

Treatment

Incidental tumours diagnosed after a laparoscopic cholecystectomy need no further action unless the gall bladder was ruptured, in which case the trocar sites should be excised because abdominal wall metastases may occur. Tumours of more advanced stages should be treated with radical surgery (resection of segments 4 and 5, bile duct, and lymphadenectomy). Post-operative chemotherapy with cisplatin is of no proven benefit. Radiotherapy is used in cases of incomplete resection. For unresectable tumours, surgical or radiological biliary drainage is performed according to the same principles as for the palliative treatment of cholangiocarcinoma.

Outcome

The five-year survival rate for Stage I tumours is 90% and for Stage II tumours is 80%. The results of surgery for more advanced disease have improved in centres performing very extensive resections, where a five-year survival rate of 40% for Stage III tumours has been obtained.

Pancreatic cancer

Aetiology

The cause of this disease is largely unknown. Smoking accounts for about 30% of the risk. Diets high in saturated fats may be important, but not the previously controversial factors such as alcohol and caffeine intake. Sporadic chronic pancreatitis is associated with a 5% lifetime risk. In hereditary pancreatitis there is an elevated 40–70-fold risk of pancreatic cancer. There is also increased risk in various familial cancer syndromes, for example:

- Peutz–Jeghers' syndrome
- von Hippel–Lindau disease
- Lynch II families
- Familial atypical multiple-mole melanoma (FAMMM)
- Breast and breast–ovarian cancer families
- Familial pancreatic cancer

Epidemiology

There is relatively high incidence in North America, northern Europe, and Australasia. The age-standardized incidence is 8–11 per 100 000 women, and 10–12.5 per 100 000 men. The male:female incidence ratio of 2:1 decreases with age. 40% of cases present before the age of 75 years. The mean age of presentation is 67 years for men and 63 years for women. Pancreatic cancer is the seventh commonest cause of cancer death in the UK (7000 deaths per annum).

Pathology

The majority of exocrine tumours are ductal adenocarcinomas (90%) and 1–2% are acinar; the remainder are of diverse histology. 75% arise in the head of the organ, 15% in the body, and 10% in the tail. Genetic abnormalities found in pancreatic cancer include the K-*ras* oncogene (90–100%) and mutations in p53 (60%), p16 (80%), and SMAD4 (50%) tumour suppressor genes.

Spread is mainly to retroperitoneal tissue, the liver, and the peritoneum, with distant metastases to the lung, liver, and the bone.

The most significant prognostic indicators are tumour size, grade, stage, and resection margin status. Staging is according to TNM classification.

Presentation

Classical symptoms are painless jaundice, weight loss, and back pain (70–90%). Anorexia is present in 60%. It may present with:

- Pruritus
- Diabetes mellitus
- Acute pancreatitis
- Ascites
- Cholangitis
- Deep-vein thrombosis

Signs of pancreatic cancer are:

- Jaundice (85%)
- Cachexia (70%)
- Hepatomegaly (60%)
- Palpable gall bladder (Courvoisier's sign—40%)

Epigastric masses, ascites, and abdominal tenderness are common. Rare signs include:

- Trousseau's syndrome (migratory thrombophlebitis)
- Troisier's sign (left supraclavicular lymph-node enlargement)
- Splenic-vein thrombosis
- Gastric fundal varices

Investigations

- Tumour markers CA19–9, CA125—poor sensitivity
- Ultrasound—75% accuracy
- Endoluminal ultrasound—90% accuracy
- CT, MRI—identify liver metastases >1 cm
- ERCP—positive cytology in 60%
- Laparoscopy—unexpected peritoneal deposits
- Laparoscopic ultrasound
- Fine-needle aspiration—percutaneous

Treatment options

For all patients the aim is to relieve jaundice, duodenal obstruction, weight loss, and pain. The majority of patients will present with advanced disease, and a third present with disease so advanced only pain relief and symptomatic palliative care is possible.

Oral pancreatic enzyme supplements may be required for pancreatic exocrine insufficiency. Non-surgical relief of jaundice is indicated for patients with unresectable disease and those unfit for resection of localized disease. Prior to any procedure attention is required to ensure adequate urine output and correction of coagulopathy, anaemia, and hypoproteinaemia. Antibiotic prophylaxis is mandatory.

Endoscopic stents have relative low morbidity rates and metallic stents are preferred for patients with expected longer survival. Percutaneous transhepatic stenting has a higher complication rate. Surgical biliary bypass is indicated for younger patients with a low tumour burden; 10–15% of these will develop duodenal obstruction, so prophylactic duodenal bypass may be indicated.

Following these palliative manoeuvres the median survival rate is dismal—between 3 and 6 months; the overall five-year survival rate is 0.5%.

Surgery

Resection is the only treatment that offers the possibility of cure, but its feasibility will depend on individual criteria such as tumour size and invasion, medical fitness of the patient, and the surgical expertise available. Resection is possible in 10–15% of cases—most commonly, Kausch–Whipple's procedure with or without pylorus preservation.

Post-operative complications include bronchopneumonia, pancreatic fistulae, sepsis, abscess, and haemorrhage—but the mortality rate is less than 10% in specialist centres.

Although surgery is curative for the minority, resection can result in good palliation. The median survival time after surgery is 10–18 months, with a five-year survival rate of 10–24%. The sites of tumour recurrence are:

+ Loco-regional (60–80%)
+ Hepatic (40–80%)
+ Peritoneal (27–62%)
+ Distant (6–20%)

The majority occur within two years following surgery.

Chemotherapy

There is no standard chemotherapy for pancreatic cancer. One randomized controlled study has shown that the nucleoside analogue, gemcitabine, marginally improved survival compared to a simple 5-fluorouracil (5FU) regimen—median survival, 5.7 months vs. 4.6 months. Adjuvant therapy using 5-FU, doxorubicin, and mitomycin C doubled median survival in a randomized controlled trial (11 months vs. 23 months) but did not improve long-term survival.

Radiotherapy

Patients with good performance status and localized resectable tumour may be considered for radiotherapy, with or without chemotherapy. Moertel showed that 5FU increased median survival after radiotherapy (35–40 Gy) by 4 months (10.4 months vs 6.3 months). With 3D-CT planning of external-beam radiotherapy it is possible to deliver 50.4 Gy in 28 daily fractions to pancreatic tumours without exceeding tolerance for the adjacent stomach, bowel, or kidneys.

Both external-beam radiotherapy (EBRT) and intra-operative radiotherapy (IORT) have been used in the adjuvant settings. The EORTC and ESPAC-1 randomized controlled trials have shown no benefit from adjuvant chemoradiotherapy.

Future treatments

The ESPAC trial has shown evidence of a benefit for adjuvant chemotherapy and justifies further randomized trials.[1] The possible value of gemcitabine needs repeating in other randomized controlled trials.

Other drugs under examination in advanced disease are:

- Thymidylate synthase inhibitors (e.g. tomudex)
- Topoisomerase I inhibitors (topotecan, irinotecan)
- Taxanes
- Angiogenesis inhibitors

Reference

1. Neoptolemos, J.P., Dunn, J.A., Stocken, D.D. *et al.* (2001) Adjuvant chemoradiotherapy in resectable pancreatic cancer: a randomized controlled trial. *Lancet* **358**, 1576–85.

Controversies in management

The proposed superiority of radical extended pancreaticoduoden-ectomy has been advocated to increase patient survival. However, a small randomized trial comparing radical and standard pancreatico-duodenectomy showed no significant difference in survival between the two groups. The use of chemotherapy in advanced cancer and as adjuvant therapy still needs to be confirmed in large randomized con-trolled trials.

Further reading

1. Berlin, J.D., Rothenberg, M. (2001) Chemotherapy for resectable and advanced pancreatic cancer. *Oncology* **15**, 1241–590.
2. Bonenkamp, J.J. *et al.* (1999) Evaluation of extended lymph node dissection in the randomized D–D2 Dutch Gastric Cancer Trial. *New England Journal of Medicine* **340**, 908–14.
3. (1997) Improving outcomes in colorectal cancer: the research evidence. Wetherby UK: NHS Executive Department of Health.
4. Nerenstone, S.R., Ihde, D.C., Friedman, M.A. (1988) Clinical trials in primary hepatocellular carcinoma: current status and future directions. *Cancer Treatment Reviews* **15**, 1–31.

Chapter 21
Endocrine cancers

Thyroid cancer

Thyroid cancer has a UK incidence of 1:100 000 and a median age at presentation of 47 years, and is three times more frequent in females (amongst whom there is a young adult rise in incidence). It usually presents as a painless lump in the neck. Classification is on a histological basis:1. differentiated (papillary or follicular); 2. anaplastic; 3. lymphoma; 4. medullary.

Differentiated thyroid cancer

Management is similar for all cases and commences with radical thyroidectomy preserving parathyroid and recurrent laryngeal nerve function. Low risk patients (those with small intrathyroidal papillary or micro-angioinvasive/minimally invasive follicular tumours) are sometimes managed by thyroid lobectomy but most clinicians prefer the radical approach for all patients. Radioiodine therapy (40–80 mCi = 1500–3000 MBq) to ablate the thyroid remnant follows the operation. This rids the body of all iodine avid normal thyroid, obviating the risk of future second tumours (papillary) and rendering the subsequent screening programme (both thyroglobulin and radioiodine) more sensitive and specific for detecting relapse. External beam radiotherapy is delivered to the neck where the tumour was locally invasive at operation (giving a dose of 5000 cGy in 5 weeks via a well executed, CT planned, three field MV photon plan in a shelled patient, the volume being parallel to a straight cervical spine).

If the patient presents with metastatic disease, or at relapse after partial thyroidectomy, radical thyroidectomy and ablation is still required because optimal management is based on the ability of most differentiated cancers to concentrate radioiodine (I^{131})—albeit usually less avidly than the parent gland. A carefully conducted radioiodine programme can prolong life substantially in many of these patients and achieve complete and durable response in a significant number—small bulk relapse and high iodine avidity being better response predictors.

Following radical thyroidectomy and radioiodine ablation of the stump, the patient has serial clinical examinations with at least two whole body radioiodine whole body profile scans in the next 1½ years (each performed after 3 months off thyroxine, 8 days off liothyronine and the tracer dose being given when the TSH is known to be above 30 Uu/L or after 200 μg of TRH iv—hereafter referred to as 'optimal conditions for radioiodine'). Serum thyroglobulin is measured at each clinical consultation and this important serum marker is more sensitive for relapse under the optimal conditions just described, although worthwhile when the patient is on thyroid replacement. If two iodine scans over the first 1.5 years are negative, and the clinical examination and thyroglobulin are negative, then iodine scanning is only used in suspected relapse (and even then many would go straight to an iodine therapy dose with a whole body scan on the 'tail-end' of the dose, because of the possibility of a tracer dose scan missing low avidity, but therapeutically relevant, uptake).

Papillary cancer tends to relapse first in neck nodes (and then mediastinal nodes) before the lungs and then bones. The treatment of neck nodal disease is surgical resection (preceded by an iodine profile scan under optimal conditions) followed by radiodine therapy where appropriate. Pre-operative imaging to define the extent of the nodal disease should be with MRI and not CT, because of the iodine load with CT contrast agents.

Metastatic disease further afield is treated by serial doses of radioiodine (150 mCi = 5500 MBq), using the whole body scans after each dose and the serial thyroglobulin estimation to guide progress, as well as other imaging. Iodine therapy is continued at 4–6 monthly intervals until maximal remission, so long as the FBC and creatinine are satisfactory; care is needed after a cumulative dose of 1 Ci.

In patients who do not relapse, physical examination (with careful attention to the neck and CXR) and blood checks to ensure TSH suppression and minimal serum thyroglobulin readings (<2 μg/L) constitute follow-up, the periodicity of which decreases with the passage of time; remember that this disease can relapse up to 15 years from diagnosis.

Anaplastic carcinoma

Again presenting as a lump in the neck, the treatment is altogether more palliative as these tumours are rarely a radical surgical proposition and do not take up iodine. Radiotherapy to the neck is the standard treatment, with palliative chemotherapy a not very promising systemic alternative (as indeed it is not in differentiated cancers).

Lymphoma

Lymphomas tend to occur in elderly women, frequently against a background of prolonged autoimmune thyroid disease. They are high grade immunoblastic non-Hodgkin's tumours and are treated with a combination of combination chemotherapy and wide field radiotherapy to the neck. Prognosis is guarded.

Medullary carcinoma

Medullary carcinoma of the thyroid arises from the parafollicular C cells (the cell of origin of calcitonin), and may be sporadic or familial. If the latter, it may or may not be part of the MEN syndrome, and the diagnosing clinician should take a family history and screen for phaeochromocytoma. Surgical clearance of apparently localized disease to the neck is the only curative hope and is the first therapeutic step. For recurrent disease (for which the serum calcitonin serves as a good marker), occasional avidity of uptake to meta-iodo-benzyl-guanadine (MIBG) makes radioiodinated MIBG therapy a possibly useful therapeutic modality. Otherwise there is no useful therapy except for palliative radiotherapy where appropriate; we have had little to no success with palliative chemotherapy.

Adrenal cancer

The adrenal gland is composed of a cortex and a medulla and the tumours that arise in these two regions are aetiologically and functionally different, reflecting their cells of origin.

Aetiology

The aetiology of adrenocortical carcinomas is generally unknown. There are rare reports of familial incidence. About 10% of adrenal medullary tumours are familial, although in future more may be identified as hereditary. These are usually associated with multiple endocrine neoplasia (MEN) syndrome II and, occasionally, von Hippel–Lindau disease. The RET proto-oncogene was the first to be associated with MEN IIA and familial medullary thyroid cancer and, subsequently, MEN IIB. The ability to identify this oncogene is of considerable importance in prophylaxis of the disease (discussed later). In over 80% of cases exons 10 and 11 are affected, which is useful for screening purposes.

Epidemiology

Both medullary and cortical tumours are rare. The incidence is about 1.0 per 10^6 population for cortical tumours and lower for phaeochromocytomas, at 0.6 per 10^6 population.

Pathology

Both benign and malignant tumours are seen in the adrenal gland and, in the hereditary variants, hyperplasia and pre-malignant changes may be evident. The differentiation between benign and malignant tumours is usually only made by their clinical behaviour—the presence of local invasion or metastases indicates a malignant tumour.

Only about 10% of adrenal medullary tumours are malignant. The hereditary tumours often occur in younger age groups, are more likely to be bilateral, and tend to be more benign in their behaviour. Adreno-medullary tumours are usually phaeochromocytomas, so-called because of their golden or tan-coloured appearance. About 10% of phaeochromocytomas are extra-adrenal and arise anywhere in the sympathetic chain. Rarely, neuroblastomas may present in late adolescence or adulthood.

Immunocytochemistry is important in establishing the diagnosis.

Adrenocortical carcinomas are usually adenocarcinomas and malignancy is confirmed by the presence of metastatic spread. These tumours extend locally to nodes and the liver but have a high frequency of distant spread when malignant.

Presentation

Adreno-medullary tumours (phaeochromocytomas) tend to present at a younger age when associated with the MEN syndrome, whereas sporadic tumours tend to occur in older patients. Classical symptoms include paroxysmal headaches, palpitations, tremors, and sweating attacks. A few may be diagnosed incidentally and a rare, but occasional case may be diagnosed after a maternal death in an unrecognized MEN family. Intermittent, severe hypertension is a rare but classical presentation.

Patients often have a long history and these tumours can be difficult to diagnose. Many doctors will never see a patient with this condition, but a low threshold for investigation is appropriate.

Adrenocortical tumours have a more varied presentation. About 40% are functioning; the rest are non-functional and only present with pressure symptoms such as pain in the abdomen or flank. They may also present with metastases. Others secrete steroids including oestrogens, testosterone, aldosterone, or even combinations and, depending upon the predominant steroid produced, the symptoms will vary.

Diagnosis

* Clinical signs—Cushing's syndrome
                —virilization
                —feminization
                —neuromata, 'café au lait' spots
* Family history
* Haemoglobin, electrolytes, urea, liver function tests
* Urinary VMA, catecholamines

Table 21.1 Endocrine syndromes associated with adrenocortical tumours

Syndrome	Steroid
Cushing's syndrome (ACTH-independent)	Cortisol
Conn's syndrome/primary hyperaldosteronism	Aldosterone
Virilization syndrome	Androgen secretion
Feminization syndrome	Oestrogen secretion
Precocious puberty syndrome/adrenogenital syndrome	Sex hormones
Non-functioning	None

- Plasma catecholamines
- Chromogranin assays
- Blood, urinary cortisols
- Blood oestrogen, testosterone
- Chest X-ray, ultrasound, CT, MRI abdomen
- Ultrasound thyroid (MEN)
- ^{123}I-MIBG, octreoscan—adrenal tumour
- Selenocholesterol imaging—cortical tumour

Treatment

The mainstay of treatment in all these tumours is surgical resection. This is the only treatment likely to achieve cure. Before considering surgery it is necessary to carry out staging investigations, as already described, to exclude the presence of metastases. It may still be appropriate to resect the primary tumour in the presence of metastases if it is slow-growing or where there are a small number of metastases, in order to achieve local control. The surgical resection of phaeochromocytomas requires a skilled multidisciplinary team approach. As a rule, surgery for adrenocortical tumours is less hazardous, but patients with electrolyte disturbances require careful preparation prior to surgery. Following surgery, persistent biochemical disturbance indicates residual disease. This is best handled by a multidisciplinary experienced team.

The identification of the gene causing MEN has led to the screening of affected families and prophylactic surgery in children. When performed in specialist units this carries minimal morbidity. Thyroid surgery for MCT is carried out at 5–7 years of age.

For phaeochromocytomas with residual or unresectable disease, anti-hypertensive medication may be required to control the blood pressure. If the tumour takes up the radionuclide MIBG, a therapeutic dose of up to 10 000 MBq of ^{131}I-MIBG may be administered and repeated at 3–6 monthly intervals. A number of tumours will not take up MIBG and consideration should be given to chemotherapy. These tumours were traditionally considered to be chemo-resistant, but a combination of DTIC, vincristine, and cyclophosphamide shows activity. Other regimens which include cisplatin and etoposide have shown promise.

For unresectable or metastatic adrenocortical tumours, Mitotane (opDDD) is the first-line treatment. This drug may be associated with unpleasant symptoms and the dosage is usually built up slowly, to a maximum of 10–12 g daily. Control of the disease is transient and after 6–12 months there is evidence of biochemical progression or symptoms return. Metyrapone, aminoglutethamide, and ketoconazole are second-line medical therapies.

Chemotherapy is of limited benefit. There are no randomized clinical trials, but the most active drugs appear to be cisplatin and etoposide. There are anecdotal reports of long-term remission. The role of external radiotherapy is limited to the treatment of symptomatic metastases, usually in bone.

Neuroblastoma

Neuroblastoma is the commonest extracranial solid tumour in childhood—approximately 6% of all childhood cancers. Tumours arise in sympathetic nervous tissue (adrenal 30%, abdomen 30%, thorax 15%). The peak age incidence is 1–3 years of age.

Localized intra-thoracic neuroblastoma may present with cough, pain, or Horner's syndrome or be detected on a chest X-ray (taken for an unrelated symptom). With abdominal disease there may be pain, abdominal distension, or general malaise. Bone or bone marrow metastases usually result in the child developing non-specific limb, joint, or back pain, which may be misdiagnosed as arthritis or irritable hip. There may be persistent unexplained fever. Pancytopenia from bone marrow involvement causes anaemia, petechiae, or infection. Periorbital ecchymoses indicate disseminated neuroblastoma.

Staging investigations

- Abdominal ultrasound
- CT, MRI abdomen
- CT, MRI spine
- CT, MRI chest
- Urinary catecholamines
- Serum neurone-specific enolase (NSE) elevated
- Serum LDH—if very high, poor prognosis
- Techetium or I^{123}MIBG scan

Pathology

Morphology ranges from a very undifferentiated, small, round cell tumour that may be difficult to distinguish from rhabdomyosarcoma, PNET, and NHL, to a highly differentiated ganglioneuroblastoma. The Shimada classification combines age with an evaluation of tumour cell necrosis (karyorrhexis) and the extent of stromal component. Amplification of *n-myc* oncogene, deletions on chromosome 1, gains on chromosome 17, and diploid or tetraploid tumours all indicate a poor prognosis.

Treatment

Stages 1 and 2

In the absence of *n-myc* amplification the cure rate for these tumours is extremely high, irrespective of completeness of excision. Surgery is usually performed at the thoracic site, although the indications for this are somewhat controversial, as the procedure may be associated with sequelae such as Horner's syndrome. A 'wait and watch' policy may be appropriate following non-invasive tumour biopsy to demonstrate favourable biology.

Stage 3

In the past this stage was routinely treated with intensive chemotherapy, but it is now clear that the non *n-myc* amplified tumours behave in a similar fashion to Stage 2 disease and a more conservative approach may be applied. If possible, surgical clearance should be attempted but if this is not feasible then non-intensive chemotherapy, such as OPEC/OJEC, followed by delayed surgery is appropriate. In the face of incomplete resection, local radiotherapy is not indicated. Recently, a 'wait and watch' policy has been advocated as for stage 2 disease.

There remains controversy about the importance of attempting to achieve complete clearance at the primary site, as this is often difficult and necessitates several hours of complex surgery. The main problem is infiltration of the tumour around IVC and aorta, or infiltration of the adjacent liver.

MIBG positivity, post-operatively, indicates likely residual primary tumour, and local radiotherapy is indicated. An alternative is the use of I^{131} MIBG-targeted radiotherapy. High-dose melphalan with peripheral blood stem rescue is standard in some protocols but this approach remains to be clearly proven. One randomized study indicates a significant prolongation of progression-free survival. Alternative high-dose intensity strategies, such as administering treatment every 10 days or escalating the dose of cyclophosphamide, are currently under evaluation.

Stage 4

This unusual stage occurs in infants less than one year of age and requires a careful balance between a very conservative 'wait and watch' policy and appropriate intervention with chemotherapy or radiotherapy. In the majority, disease will resolve spontaneously, but where there is significant respiratory decompensation, low-dose irradiation to the liver or low-dose chemotherapy using vincristine or combinations of cyclophosphamide, doxorubicin, or carboplatin/etoposide are indicated.

Screening of neuroblastoma

Attempts have been made to detect neuroblastoma within the first year of life by screening for raised urinary catecholamines. Almost invariably the tumours detected by screening are localized and of favourable biology and there is a significant incidence of spontaneously resolving

Table 21.2 International staging system for neuroblastoma

Stage 1	Localized tumour with complete gross excision, with or without microscopic residual disease; representative ipsilateral and contralateral lymph nodes negative for tumour microscopically (nodes attached to and removed with the primary tumour may be positive).
Stage 2a	Localized tumour with incomplete gross excision; representative ipsilateral and non-adherent lymph nodes negative for tumour microscopically.
Stage 2b	Localized tumour with complete or incomplete gross excision; with ipsilateral non-adherent lymph nodes positive for tumour. Enlarged contralateral lymph nodes must be negative microscopically.
Stage 3	Unresectable unilateral tumour infiltrating across the midline with or without regional lymph node involvement; or localized unilateral tumour with contralateral regional lymph node involvement; or midline tumour with bilateral extension by infiltration (unresectable) or by lymph node involvement.
Stage 4	Any primary tumour with dissemination to distant lymph nodes, bone, bone marrow, liver skin, and/or other organs (except as defined in Stage 4S).
Stage 4S	Localized primary tumour (as defined for Stage 1, 2a, or 2b) with dissemination limited to skin, liver, and/or bone marrow (limited to infants less than one year old).

neuroblastoma at this age. Screened patients have double the expected incidence of the disease. There is no evidence that the detection of tumours by this method, for this age group, reduces the incidence of unfavourable biology or metastatic tumours during the following 2–3 years. Screening at a later age is under consideration.

Further reading

Mazzaferri, E.L. and Samaan, N.A. (1993) *Endocrine tumors.* Blackwell, Oxford.

Sheaves, R., Jenkins, P. and Wass, J. (1997) *Clinical endocrine oncology.*
   Blackwell, Oxford.

Chapter 22
Genitourinary cancers

Renal cancer

Epidemiology and aetiology

Renal cancers are more common in men (1.9% of male cancers) than in women (1.2%) and increase in frequency with increasing age, being most common in the sixth, and eighth decades. There has been a slow increase in the incidence over the past 10 years. Approximately 65% of patients die of their disease.

The most important aetiological factor is smoking. A higher incidence of renal carcinoma has also been reported in urban dwellers, workers in the petroleum industry, and in the obese. Chronic renal dialysis is a risk factor, as is analgesic abuse.

Over 98% of adult renal cancers are sporadic, but an inherited predisposition occurs in the von Hippel-Lindau familial cancer syndrome (1/36 000 births) and in the rarer hereditary papillary renal carcinoma syndrome.

Pathology

Adenocarcinomas make up the vast majority (85%) of renal cancers. They were previously known as 'Hypernephroma' or 'Grawitz tumours' and demonstrate several histological types:

* Clear cell
* Papillary
* Spindle cell or sarcomatoid

Transitional cell carcinomas can arise within the urothelium of the renal pelvis and represent the majority of the remaining tumours.

Presentation and natural history –

The presenting symptoms are:

* Haematuria (50%)
* Loin pain (50%)
* Palpable mass (40%)
* Anaemia (40%)
* Weight loss (35%)
* Pyrexia (20%)
* Hypertension (37%)
* Hypercalcaemia (6%)
* Polycythaemia (<5%)

Renal tumours may invade locally causing pain and occasionally lymphoedema, or may metastasize to the lungs, lymph nodes, bone, and brain.

Investigations

- CT scan, chest and abdomen
- Chest x-ray
- Brain CT and bone scan if indicated by symptoms
- Routine blood and coagulation studies
- Tumour markers are unhelpful

Staging

The Robson staging system is commonly used.

Surgery

Resection of all the tumour is the only potentially curative modality and should be offered to patients without metastases who are fit for surgery. In patients with limited metastatic disease who are fit, nephrectomy may be indicated to control local symptoms. There are documented cases of regression of metastases following nephrectomy. However, this is extremely rare and nephrectomy cannot be justified on this basis in patients who are frail or have extensive metastatic disease. Partial nephrectomy is occasionally performed for localized tumours or in patients without a second kidney.

Surgery for metastases is occasionally indicated for isolated metastases that occur after a long disease-free interval or, rarely, at presentation in young, fit patients. Although supported by anecdotal evidence, randomized data are lacking.

Although surgery is the cornerstone of management of localized disease, some patients are unfit for nephrectomy. Tumour embolization (infarction) may provide some symptom control but can itself

Table 22.1 The Robson staging system

Stage	Description	% of cases	5-year survival
I	Confined to the kidney	20–40%	50–60%
II	Extends into peri-renal fat but confined to Gerota's fascia	4–20%	27–60%
III	Involvement of renal vein or IVC or lymph node involvement	10–42%	20–50%
IV	Involvement of adjacent organs or metastatic disease	11-49%	0–18%

cause considerable morbidity. Adjuvant therapy has not been proven to offer a survival benefit. Cytotoxic chemotherapies, endocrine therapy, radiotherapy, and interferon have been tested. There is current interest in testing more complex biological therapies in this setting, but no positive studies have yet been reported.

Spontaneous remissions

One of the most pervasive of 'oncological folklore' is the expectation of spontaneous remissions in renal cancer. Although these certainly occur, the true rate is less than 1%, and they tend to occur following resection of the primary tumour or after an episode associated with immune activation, such as following severe sepsis. Such regressions are not usually durable.

Management of advanced disease

The management of patients with advanced and/or metastatic disease is palliative. There is now good evidence that a very small subset of patients who have complete responses to biological therapy may enjoy long-term, disease-free survival.

Treatment

Radiotherapy

Irradiation is indicated for painful or obstructing lesions, but responses are seen in only 50% of patients. Higher palliative doses may be appropriate to give durable control of isolated non-resectable metastases after nephrectomy.

Endocrine therapy

Progestins are widely used on the basis of the identification of progesterone receptors in some renal tumours and evidence of activity in animal models. The objective response rate for systemic progestagen therapy is less than 10% and probably only 1–2% by modern response criteria. However, the anabolic effects of progesterone are often valuable in patients with advanced disease, who may feel better on treatment.

Chemotherapy

Cytotoxic drugs are of little value in renal carcinoma. The chemoresistance may, in part, be due to the very high expression of a multidrug resistance phenotype in both normal and malignant renal tissue. Response rates for single agents are generally under 15% and for combination regimens no more than 25%. Vinca alkaloids have been the most commonly prescribed drugs but there are no gains in survival after chemotherapy.

Biological therapy

Biological therapy has been extensively tested in renal cancer, partly because of its chemo-resistance, but mainly because of the presumption that immunological mechanisms underly the occasional spontaneous regression of metastases. In addition, the very late relapses seen in some patients and the increased incidence of renal cancers in immunosuppressed patients suggest that some intrinsic immunological surveillance can operate in patients with renal cancer.

Interleukin-2 (IL-2) is the most widely tested biological agents and induces responses in 10–25% of patients with advanced disease. Those patients with a complete radiological response have a significant survival benefit, with durable remissions in a few.

The original studies of IL-2 employed high-dose intravenous IL-2, either alone or in combination with lymphokine-activated killer cells (LAK). These regimens are associated with considerable morbidity, in particular capillary leak syndrome, and some mortality.

Less toxic subcutaneous (SC) IL-2 regimens are probably equally effective and can be combined with interferon-α (IFN) and/or cytotoxics, although comparative studies are lacking to confirm a benefit for combination regimens. As a single agent, SC IFN also provides a response rate of approximately 15% and use of this agent has a proven survival advantage over endocrine therapy in an important MRC trial.

Prognostic factors that predict better response and survival time after biological therapy include:

• Long time for diagnosis to relapse
• Nephrectomy
• Good performance status
• Pulmonary metastases as the sole site of disease

Transitional cell carcinoma

These tumours arise in the renal collecting system and may be associated with TCC in the ureter and bladder. Their biology, management, and prognosis is similar to that of TCC of the bladder.

Wilms' tumour

Introduction

Wilms' tumour (WT) is an embryonal neoplasm arising in the kidney. Classical 'triphasic' WT has stromal, blastemal, and epithelial elements. the bone-metastasizing renal tumour (clear cell sarcoma) and malignant rhabdoid tumour are pathologically and genetically distinct entities, with their own clinical courses.

WT represents about 8% of all childhood neoplasia. The peak age for diagnosis is 3–4 years of age. It is very rare after the age of 10 years, but is occasionally diagnosed in adults.

There are a number of conditions known to predispose to the development of WT:

- Genitourinary abnormalities
- Hemihypertrophy
- Aniridia
- Beckwith–Wiedeman syndrome
- Denys–Drash syndrome
- Perlmann syndrome
- Simpson–Golabi–Behmel syndrome

This group of patients represents only a small proportion of the total number seen however.

Clinical features

- Abdominal mass—smooth, rounded, or lobulated mass arising in the loin
- Pain
- Haematuria
- Hypertension

Investigations

- Abdominal ultrasound to confirm organ of origin, determine extent of any spread within the abdomen, confirm patency of the inferior vena cava
- Chest X-ray to detect pulmonary metastases
- Full blood count to detect anaemia resulting from haemorrhage into the tumour
- Prothrombin and partial thromboplastin times—some patients may acquire von Willebrand disease

- Urea, creatinine, and urinalysis to detect any gross abnormalities of renal function
- Urinary catecholamines to exclude neuroblastoma
- CT scan of chest and abdomen

It is important to know that the contralateral kidney is functioning adequately before surgery and IVU, DMSA scan, or excretion of contrast at the end of a CT scan of the chest/abdomen is useful in this role.

Pathology

Two broad groups of tumours may be recognized by their histological appearances:

Favourable histology—by far the larger group
- Classical triphasic histology—epithelial, blastemal, and stromal elements are all present.
- Rhabdomyoblastic differentiation, such that the cells resemble fetal rhabdomyoblasts.
- Monomorphic epithelial variant.

Unfavourable histology
- Anaplasia is an unfavourable, often patchy occasionally observed in triphasic tumours. The major unfavourable histological types are probably distinct tumours, rather than true variants of Wilms' tumour.
- Bone-metastasizing renal tumour of childhood.
- Malignant rhabdoid tumour.

Treatment

There is overwhelming evidence that Wilms' tumour ought to be treated only in paediatric oncology centres and there is no place for the casual therapist. Surgeons, radiotherapists, paediatricians, or nephrologists not working in a centre with paediatric oncological expertise who find themselves unexpectedly dealing with a child with Wilms' tumour should make an urgent referral to an appropriate unit.

Surgery

Surgical extirpation is, and almost certainly will remain the fundamental treatment for Wilms' tumour. There is debate about the timing of surgical intervention, the place of percutaneous needle biopsy, and the use of pre-operative chemotherapy. US practice remains steadfastly in favour of immediate surgery followed by adjuvant therapy dictated by the surgical stage. In contrast, the SIOP group in Europe has conducted a series of trials based on the use of pre-operative therapy, and while it remains to be proven that the latter approach is superior, there is increasing recognition that pre-operative treatment may be of benefit in some circumstances.

In an attempt to resolve the issues posed by the findings from these two groups, the UKCCSG is currently conducting a prospective randomized trial comparing immediate surgery with six weeks of chemotherapy and delayed surgery.

Adjuvant therapy

The use of chemotherapy and radiotherapy as adjuvants to surgery is now an essential part of WT treatment. Major advances in treatment have come as a result of multicentre co-operative trials run by the US National Wilms' Tumour Study (NWTS) Group, the International Society of Paediatric Oncology (SIOP), and the UK Children's Cancer

Table 22.2 Main findings in NWTS 1, 2, and 3

NWTS 1	
Group I	Patients under two years of age do not all need radiotherapy.
Group II/III	AMD plus VCR is better than either alone.
Group IV	Pre-operative vincristine is of no benefit.
Other findings	Unfavourable histology and lymph-node involvement are adverse features.
NWTS 2	
Stage I	No patients benefit from radiotherapy regardless of age. 6 months of VCR and AMD is as good as 15 months.
Stages II, III, and IV	Addition of doxo to VCR and AMD improves survival.
Other findings	Stages II and III have the same survival. Local spillage and invasion of the renal vein do not affect outcome.
NWTS 3	
Stage I	10 weeks therapy with VCR/AMD is as effective as 6 months.
Stage II	Intensive VCR/AMD is as effective as three drugs. Addition of radiotherapy does not affect survival.
Stage III	Intensive VCR/AMD is as effective as three drugs. 10 Gy flank irradiation is as effective as 20 Gy.
Other findings	Addition of cyclophosphamide to VCR/AMD/doxo does not improve survival.

Key: VCR = vincristine; AMD = actinomycin D; doxo = doxorubicin

Table 22.3 Outcome for patients in NWTS III

Stage	2-year relapse-free survival (%)	2-year overall survival (%)	Treatment
I	92	97	10 weeks vincristine + actinomycin D
II/III	87	91	15 months vincristine + actinomycin D + doxorubicin
III	78	86	10 Gy + vincristine + actinomycin D +/- doxorubicin
IV + UH	72	81	

UH = Unfavourable histology

Table 22.4 Outcome for patients in UKW1

Stage	3-yr event-free survival (%)	3-yr overall survival (%)	6-yr event-free survival (%)	6-yr overall survival (%)
I	90	96	89	96
II	85	94	85	93
III	82	83	82	83
IV	58	65	50	65

Study Group (UKCCSG). An essential part of all therapy protocols is the 'stage' of the tumour. The NWTS staging system is:

- **Stage I**   Tumour within renal capsule and fully resected.
- **Stage II**   Tumour outside renal capsule but fully resected; biopsy; ruptured; confined to the flank.
- **Stage III** Tumour outside capsule and incompletely resected; lymph-node involvement at the hilum or paraortic chain.
- **Stage IV**   Haematogenous metastases e.g. to lungs, liver, bone, or brain.
- **Stage V**   Bilateral renal tumours.

Cancer of the bladder and ureter

Aetiology

The occupational risk of developing bladder cancer for workers in the dye industry was established more than 90 years ago. The association was supported when 2-napthylamine was shown to cause bladder cancer in animals and related carcinogens were associated with increased risk for those working in the aniline dye and the rubber industries. Now, the range of known human bladder carcinogens identifies risks associated not only within these industries mentioned but also for those working in:

+ Gas works
+ Rodent care
+ Laboratory work
+ Sewage work
+ Textile printing
+ Manufacture of firelighters.

Squamous cancers of the bladder are associated with chronic bladder infection by *Schistosoma haematobium*.

Cigarette smoking is known to increase, 2–6-fold, the risk of developing bladder cancer.

Epidemiology

The incidence increases with age with rates of 90 per 10^5 population in American men aged 60–69 years and 26 per 10^5 for women of the same age. These incidences almost double in the age range 70–79 years.

Pathology

The majority of urothelial tumours presenting in the UK are transitional cell carcinomas. Pure squamous carcinomas and adenocarcinomas represent 5% of tumours, though metaplasia can occur in a primary transitional tumour. There is a link between adenocarcinoma of the bladder and presentation of the tumour in the bladder dome, often associated with persisting urachal remnant. This type of tumour also occurs in the context of a congenital malformation exstrophy. Primary squamous cancers are the commonest subtype with bladder schistosomiasis.

Transitional carcinomas have a number of characteristic chromosomal abnormalities including, in particular, loss of chromosome 9. Other common abnormalities include a mutation of the p53 gene that appears more often in advanced cancers and has been associated with an increased risk of treatment failure.

Transitional cancers are characterized by definition of both grade and local T stage. There is a strong association between well-differentiated tumours and early stage. Most recent reports are based on the UICC TNM staging classification (1987):

- T1 tumours are confined to the urothelium.
- T2 tumours invade superficial muscle.
- T3 tumours extend to deep muscle and through the bladder wall.
- T4 tumours extend into adjacent organs.

Even when the tumour is localized the T stage is highly relevant to prognosis, with five-year survival rates of 75% for T1 tumours, 40–50% for T2 tumours, 20–30% for T3 tumours, and 10% or less for T4 tumours. Recently, this classification has been revised in UICC TNM staging (1997).

Typical metastatic sites include:

- Pelvic and para-aortic lymph nodes
- Lung fields
- Liver
- Bone

Bone metastasis is recognized increasingly as more patients have systemic control of disease with combination chemotherapy.

Presentation

The commonest presentation is with macroscopic haematuria, though some patients also have frequency of micturition, dysuria, or symptoms of metastases.

Haematuria should be confirmed by urine analysis and investigated by analysis of the cytology of voided urine and by cystoscopy. An IVU can demonstrate the possibility of disease involving the ureter and the diagnosis is established by resection of the primary tumour at cystoscopy. During the same procedure, bimanual examination is performed and this, together with the biopsy findings with associated evidence of depth of tumour invasion, enable the T stage of the tumour to be established. Nodal and metastatic staging is achieved with a CT scan of the thorax and abdomen. MRI is an excellent alternative for investigating the local extension of disease and the possibility of pelvic lymphadenopathy.

The staging demonstrated following radical cystectomy may in many cases be different from that established from pure clinical investigation; this is important for comparison of different treatment series.

Treatment options

- Superficial tumours (Ta, T1)
  —resection
  —superficial recurrence is common (60%)
  —poorly differentiated, worse prognosis

- Frequent recurrences/high-risk tumours
  —intravesical chemotherapy: mitomycin C; doxorubicin
  —intravesical immunotherapy: BCG
    monitored by cystoscopy
    reduces recurrences; no long-term effect on survival
- Muscle-invasive, local tumour
  —radical radiotherapy
  —radical cystectomy
  —occasionally radiotherapy followed by salvage cystectomy
- Metastatic disease
  —palliative chemotherapy
  —usually relapse again after 2 years

Surgical principles

The usual procedure is cystoprostatectomy in male patients or anterior bladder exenteration in female patients, with dissection of local lymph nodes. Bladder resection is associated with urinary diversion—most commonly, a non-refluxing ileal conduit and urinary bag. Complications include loss of sexual potency in the male and loss of the vagina in the female. It is important for patients to have advice from a specialized stoma therapist before surgery.

In specialist centres, excellent results can be achieved in selected patients treated by radical cystectomy with continent diversion based on urinary tract reconstruction by ileocystostoplasty. This can produce urinary continence and, in experienced centres, the surgical complication rates are less than 10% and operative mortality less than 2%.

Radical radiotherapy based on CT scan has led to increased precision and more accurate dosimetry. Usually, the entire bladder is treated to encompass the risk of subclinical disease at other sites in the urothelium. The technique uses either three or four fields and the common fractionation regimens include treatment to a dose of 64 Gy in 32 fractions over $6\frac{1}{2}$ weeks or 55 Gy in 20 fractions over 4 weeks. Most patients suffer some side-effects during radiotherapy, such as increased frequency of micturition, dysuria, and, occasionally, strangury requiring analgesics. There may also be proctitis associated with diarrhoea. Chronic side-effects of this type are uncommon.

Chemotherapy

Combination chemotherapy has an established role in the palliation of patients with incurable bladder cancer. M-VAC comprises:

- Methotrexate
- Vinblastine
- Adriamycin
- Cisplatin

CMV comprises:

• Cisplatin

• Methotrexate

• Vinblastine

These regimens can be toxic, especially for an elderly patient with poor general health and impaired renal function associated with the primary tumour, and achieve a response with palliation of symptoms in approximately 50–60% of patients. However, complete responses are uncommon (approximately 20%) and prolonged complete response is rare (less than 10% of patients).

Chemotherapy is being investigated as an adjuvant therapy in localized disease either prior to, or following, definitive local treatment with surgery or radiotherapy. As yet, the role of chemotherapy in this context is controversial since trials have failed to show clinically significant impact on survival.

Future treatments

New drugs under investigation for the management of bladder cancer include the taxanes, gemcitabine and ifosphamide. There is continued investigation of the role of these agents as a complement to definitive local therapies for patients with local muscle-invasive cancers.

Controversies in management

Superficial, poorly differentiated cancers

Conventionally, these are managed by transurethral resection. However, the relatively poor prognosis of these tumours has led to investigation of adjuvant treatments with cytotoxic chemotherapy intravesically, BCG, or external-beam radiotherapy to the bladder. Results of these studies are awaited.

Localized muscle invasive cancer

Internationally, the commonest pattern of management is radical cystectomy. Prospective trials comparing cystectomy with radical radiotherapy have not show a significant survival difference and the use of radiotherapy in order to seek tumour control with organ conservation is preferred by some clinicians and patients. Improved tumour characterization and other methods of establishing appropriate local treatment should enable better selection of patients for organ conservation with a low risk of local tumour recurrence.

Adjuvant chemotherapy in local disease

Trials reported so far have failed to demonstrate a clinically significant benefit to early adjuvant chemotherapy and more intensive regimens are currently being explored. Promising results have been reported recently with chemo-irradiation.

Prostate cancer

Introduction

Cancer of the prostate gland is one of the most controversial malignancies. Its pathogenesis is clearly androgen-dependent, and men who are castrated or are hypopituitary before 40 years rarely develop this tumour. Age is the most important risk factor and it is estimated that 70% of men over 80 years have histological evidence of cancer in the prostate; 5% of cases are due to inheritance of a susceptibility gene such as *BRCA1*. Other clinical observations such as the increased incidence in African–Americans are unexplained.

During the last 20 years the incidence and the number of deaths from prostate cancer in the US and Europe has inexorably risen. Since the development of assays to measure serum prostate-specific antigen (PSA) to diagnose prostatic disease, the condition has been increasingly diagnosed at an earlier stage. In 1974, in the UK, more than 50% of patients presented with metastatic disease. Twenty years later, more than 50% of patients are diagnosed as a result of PSA testing without any symptoms of prostatic disease.

The use of PSA has proved to be an ambiguous advance. In the US, in 1995, with widespread use of PSA testing in asymptomatic men, nearly 400 000 patients were diagnosed suffering from prostate cancer; in the same year approximately 38 000 patients died of prostate cancer. In Europe, 85 000 patients were diagnosed and around 20 000 died of prostate cancer. These figures suggest that too many cases were diagnosed in the US and treated without clear evidence that they would have died of the disease, or that European patients were diagnosed too late for curative treatment with a consequent higher death rate. In either case the net result is that more patients are presenting with early stage disease and suitable treatment strategies are required to cure those that can be cured and palliate optimally those that cannot.

Assessment of disease

- PSA measurement
  —routine screening not recommended in UK
  —measure in all patients with outflow symptoms
  —PSA > 4 ng/ml: clinical suspicion, requires transrectal ultrasound and needle biopsy
  —PSA > 50 ng/ml: often distant metastases
- Pathological grading: Gleasons' score predicts behaviour
- Isotope bone scan, CT, MRI in selected patients

Table 22.5 TNM staging of prostate cancer

T0	No evidence of tumour
T1a	Tumour, incidental finding at TURP (<5% chippings)
T1b	Tumour, incidental finding at TURP (>5% chippings)
T1c	Impalpable tumour identified by raised PSA
T2a	Tumour involves half of a lobe or less
T2b	Tumour involves more than a half of a lobe but not both lobes
T2c	Tumour involves both lobes
T3a	Unilateral extracapsular extension
T3b	Bilateral extracapsular extension Tumour involves seminal vesicles
T4	Tumour invades bladder neck, rectum, pelvic side-wall

Treatment of localized prostate cancer

A localized prostate cancer of 1 cm diameter will metastasize within 8 years in over half the patients, regardless of their age. Furthermore, patients who present with metastatic disease with >10 metastases in the skeleton and symptoms from metastases will, in spite of optimal palliative therapy, die within three years. Between these ends of the spectrum, patients' therapy should be tailored to the individual needs of the patient and his cancer.

Organ-confined disease

* Age less than 70 years
* Co-morbidity not significant
* Consider radical local therapy
  —prostatectomy
  —radiotherapy
* No trials
* Staging lymph node dissection, may be done laparoscopically
* Surgery may be better long-term for local control but effect on survival is uncertain
* High dose of conformal radiotherapy or brachytherapy may be as good
* Complications
  —radical prostatectomy: 50% impotence; 8–15% long-term incontinence
  —radical radiotherapy: 40% impotence; rectal stricture/bladder irritation but no incontinence
* Patients over 70 years
  —'wait and see' policy

Locally extensive disease

- Localized T3, T4 disease not cured by radical surgery or radiotherapy
- Good results with neo-adjuvant anti-androgen therapy—if followed by radiotherapy, better results than radiotherapy alone

Node-positive disease

- USA—radical prostatectomy followed by surgical castration
- Europe—hormone therapy and radiotherapy
  —early hormone therapy prolongs survival in Mo cases

The treatment of metastatic disease

Once the tumour has spread beyond the local lymph nodes and particularly if bony metastases are present, the chances of the patient dying of prostatic is 75%, regardless of age. Nonetheless, useful palliation of the disease can be readily achieved by hormonal therapy.

A number of treatments may be used to exert much the same biological effect, namely the cessation of androgen-driven growth of the cancer. The following will produce symptomatic response in about 70% of men with bone metastases, with a median response duration of 12–18 months:

- Surgical castration
- Oestrogens (no longer used because of cardiovascular toxicity)
- Steroidal anti-androgens such as cyproterone acetate (best avoided for long-term use because of occasional hepatotoxicity)
- Non-steroidal anti-androgens (flutamide, bicalutamide)
- Medical castration with LHRH agonists

More than 20% of patients will continue to respond for up to five years. The price for this is the toxicity of long-term castration, including:

- Loss of libido and potency
- Hot flushes
- Alteration of body form
- Loss of energy
- Inability to concentrate
- Osteoporosis

Although initial reports on the combination of medical castration and anti-androgen therapy (Maximal Androgen Blockade or MAB) suggested a benefit over monotherapy, recent meta-analysis has shown that monotherapy and combined treatment are equivalent in efficacy. At least 30% of patients who relapse following androgen antagonist primary therapy will respond to subsequent medical or surgical castration. In addition, some patients respond to withdrawal of anti-androgens. However, the responses to second-and third-line endo-crine therapy are incomplete and short-lived, and ultimately patients return with hormone refractory metastatic disease. The results of chemotherapy in this disease are poor, although responses to anthra-cyclines and the related mitoxantrone have been reported.

Radiation therapy offers useful palliation of advanced disease both in bone and soft tissue. In addition, radioactive strontium given by IV injection (150 MBq) has proved effective in relieving bone pain and delaying the progression of symptomatic bone disease.

Screening for prostate cancer

Introduction

Prostate cancer is the second most common cause of cancer death in the UK and causes over 9500 deaths each year. The incidence of prostate cancer appears to be rising. It is difficult to know whether this reflects a real increase, an increase in case finding, or the fact that men are living longer and failing to die from other causes. Intuitively, it would seem obvious that early detection of prostate cancer would lead to earlier treatment and an increased cure rate.

In the US, where treatment has been historically more aggressive than in the UK, death rates from prostate cancer have gone down (despite increasing incidence). Surgical pundits attribute this to earlier surgery. This is not entirely supported by data.

Screening can be defined as a performance of tests in apparently well men, to detect those with unrecognized prostate cancer. The ultimate aim of screening is to reduce morbidity and mortality from a disease by its detection and treatment before symptoms appear.

Procedure

Screening for prostate cancer involves the examination of asymptomatic men, firstly by digital rectal examination (DRE) and a blood test of prostatic-specific antigen (PSA). Those men with a suspicious DRE or raised PSA are then investigated by ultrasound transrectally (TRUS) and/or biopsy, either randomly of the prostate or of suspicious areas.

Those who have the disease can then be staged and offered treatment, such as radical prostatectomy or radical radiotherapy, or monitored until they develop symptoms.

National screening

Screening for prostate cancer has operated in Germany since 1978 and rectal examination is included in insurance annual check-ups in Belgium. In France, work-site PSA screening has been launched by Occupational Health Services for men aged 50–65. However, no consensus exists on the validity of such screening. The US National Cancer Institute stated there is insufficient evidence to establish that a decrease in mortality from prostate cancer occurs with screening by DRE, TRUS, or serum markers; yet the American Urological Association and the American Cancer Society have published guidelines advocating annual DRE and PSA testing for men over the age of

50. Although formal screening is not taking place widely, there is certainly marked case finding in many parts of the world.

There have been a number of small screening studies, but many rely on volunteers willing to respond to invitations for screening and this introduces selection bias.

The cancers that are confined to the prostate can be slow-growing and may be biologically insignificant as far as the patient is concerned, and yet 70% of tumours detected through screening are organ-confined and could potentially be eradicated by radical prostatectomy. This eradication is measured by undetectable PSA levels for up to 10 years after surgery.

Slowly growing or latent tumours may be more likely to be detected by screening but might have a longer pre-clinical course. The rate of detection of these tumours would increase if the screening was applied over a number of years.

Other factors that must be addressed before the introduction of screening include the morbidity of screening—the unnecessary anxiety it induces, especially for a high proportion of men found to have a falsely positive initial result. Finally, and probably most importantly, there is lack of true evidence regarding the effective treatment for early prostate cancer.

There is a debate as to the desirability of including DRE at the initial screen. Although its use will increase the number of cancers detected, there is some evidence that DRE may miss life-threatening tumours. Although in two GP studies in the UK, DRE and PSA were acceptable to members of the general male population, in larger pilot studies in Belgium and the Netherlands acceptance rates were as low as 35–40% when both tests were used. Acceptance rates in UK males of screening for other diseases by blood tests are of a higher order, up to 60%.

The combination of serum PSA and DRE screening results in a higher overall cancer detection rate than each used in isolation—4–6%. This means, however, that 20% of the screened population will require biopsy. If PSA is used alone, three patients must undergo biopsy to find one case of prostate cancer. In PSA-based screening, over 97% of cancers detected on initial evaluation are clinically localized to the prostate.

The case for screening would therefore appear to be strong, except for one major flaw: there have been no randomized controlled trials with sufficient power to detect any improvements in mortality from medical intervention. Two trials evaluating randomized treatment of prostate cancer after detection—the PIVOT study in the US and a smaller Scandanavian study—will soon report.

In those patients who have organ-confined prostate cancer, about 90% are free of PSA relapse at five years after radical prostatectomy, as are about 70% of men with only focal capsular penetration. Prior to

PSA testing, many patients were found to have positive lymph nodes, but the trend now is to operate on patients with lower PSAs and to focus on those who can theoretically be cured.

The absence of data to support prostatic screening does not mean such a benefit may not exist.

Testicular cancer

Introduction

The majority of testicular cancers are germ cell tumours. Germ cell tumours are relatively rare, being the fourteenth most common cancer in men overall. It is, however, the commonest cancer in young men (20–40 years) and its incidence has doubled over the last 30 years. The reason for this increase in incidence is not clear. The age group which the disease affects and the fact that the majority of patients are curable, even when the disease has metastasized, makes this a particularly important disease for oncologists. It is one of the few curable solid tumours once it has metastasized and there is an overall survival of about 90%.

Pathology

Germ cell tumours arise from the germinal epithelium and both seminomas and teratomas are thought to arise from pre-existing carcinomas *in situ*. In the UK, the British classification is still the most commonly used.

The natural history of seminoma and teratoma differs and these differences largely dictate the variation in management between the two. The majority of seminomas (75%) present with Stage I disease—that is with no evidence of metastases. Spread tends to be predictable, to the para-aortic lymph nodes in the first instance and, subsequently, to the supra-diaphragmatic lymph nodes and thereafter to other metastatic sites.

Table 22.6 Pathological classification of testicular cancers

British	WHO
Seminoma	*Seminoma*
Spermatocytic seminona	Spermatocytic serinoma
Teratoma	*Non-seminomatous germ cell tumour*
Teratoma differentiated (TD)	Mature teratoma
Malignant teratoma intermediate (MTI)	Embryonal carcinoma with teratoma (teratocarcinoma)
Malignant teratoma undifferentiated (MTU)	Yolk sac tumour, embryonal carcinoma
Malignant teratoma trophoblastic (MTT)	Yolk sac tumour; choriocarcinoma

Only about half of testicular teratomas present as Stage I disease and spread tends to be less predictable, with blood-borne metastases occurring earlier than with seminoma. In addition to this, teratomas produce markers in the form of the human chorioric gondotrophin (HCG) and/or alpha feta protein (AFP) in 75% of cases. Seminomas on the other hand have no reliable tumour marker to monitor disease, although the HCG may be raised in about 25% of cases. The lactate dehydrogenase (LDH) may be raised in both tumours and is useful for defining a prognostic group, but is not a reliable marker for monitoring response to treatment or subsequent relapse.

Presentation

+ Lump in/on testis
+ Metastases—back pain (para-aortic nodes)
                    —chest symptoms (lung secondaries)
+ Differential diagnosis—epididymo-orchiditis

Initial management of testicular germ cell tumours

This includes:

+ Ultrasound of both testicles
+ Chest X-ray
+ Blood levels of the testicular tumour markers (AFP, HCG, LDH)

Where the patient has obvious and widespread metastases, immediate referral for chemotherapy may be necessary, but in general the initial management will be inguinal orchidectomy. A biopsy of the contra-lateral testis should be considered where there is a high risk of carcinoma *in situ*. Such patients include those with a history of maldescent, a small testis (less than 12 ml), and patients less than 30 years. Further staging investigations will usually be performed post-operatively.

Staging investigations and prognostic grouping

Staging investigations will include, in all patients, a CT scan of the thorax, abdomen, and pelvis. In patients with a high HCG (greater than 10 000 international units per litre) or bulky mediastinal disease, a brain scan is advisable. Post-operative tumour markers should be serially checked, if raised, to assess whether or not they are falling according to a satisfactory half life (4–6 days for AFP, 24 hours for HCG). Other investigations such as a bone scan may be necessary if specifically indicated.

Until recently the Royal Marsden Hospital (RMH) staging has been used for both teratomas and seminomas. The IGCCC prognostic grouping is now more applicable, particularly for teratomas.

Sperm storage

Sperm count and storage should be considered at an early stage where patients are likely to require further therapy. It should be remembered

Table 22.7 RMH staging

1	No evidence of disease outside the testis
1M	As above but with persistently raised tumour markers
11	Infradiaphragmatic nodal involvement
11A	Maximum diameter <2 cm
11B	Maximum diameter 2–5 cm
11C	Maximum diameter 5–10 cm
11D(*)	Maximum diameter >10 cm
III	Supra-and infradiaphragmatic node involvement
	Abdominal nodes a, b, c, as above
	Mediastinal nodes M+
	Neck nodes N+
IV	Extralymphatic metastases
	Abdominal nodes a, b, c, as above
	Mediastinal or neck nodes as for Stage III
	Lungs:
	—L1<3 metastases
	—L2 multiple metastases <2 cm in diameter
	—L3 multiple metastases >2 cm in diameter
	Liver involvement H+
	Other sites specified

* The Stage IID category was formulated at the 1989 Seminoma Consensus Conference

that up to 50% of patients with testicular germ cell tumour may be subfertile at presentation.

Management

The management of seminoma and teratoma depends on the stage of disease and involves all three major modalities for the treatment of cancer—surgery, radiotherapy, and chemotherapy.

Management of carcinoma *in situ*

Carcinoma *in situ* will progress to invasive cancer, either seminoma or teratoma, with 50% producing invasive tumours five years from diagnosis. Once this diagnosis is made, treatment should be offered, although this may not need to be given immediately. Carcinoma *in situ* can be eradicated by low-dose radiotherapy to the testis (20 cGy in 10 fractions given over two weeks). The advantage of this treatment is that, in the majority of cases, it will not affect Leydig cell function, and long-term hormone therapy with its attendant problems should not be necessary.

Table 22.8 IGCCCC prognostic grouping

Teratoma (NSGCT)	Seminoma
Good prognosis with all of:	
Testis/retroperitoneal primary	Any primary site
No non-pulmonary visceral metastases	No non-pulmonary visceral metastases
AFP <1000 ng/ml	Normal AFP
HCG <5000 iu/ml	Any HCG
LDH 1.5 upper limit of normal	Any LDH
56% of teratomas: 5-year survival 92%	90% of seminomas: 5-year survival 86%
Intermediate progress with any of:	
Testis/retroperitoneal primary	Any primary site
No non-pulmonary visceral metastases	Non-pulmonary visceral metastases
AFP >1000 and <10 000 ng/ml	Normal AFP
HCG >5000 and <50 000 iu/ml	Any HCG
LDH >1.5 normal <10 normal	Any LDH
28% of teratomas: 5-year survival 80%	10% of seminomas: 5-year survival 73%
Poor prognosis with any of:	
Mediastinal primary	No patients in this group
Non-pulmonary visceral metastases	
AFP >10 000 ng/ml	
HCG >50 000 iu/ml	
LDH >10 normal	
16% of teratomas: 5-year survival 48%	

Management of Stage I seminoma

- 20% seminomas recur after orchidectomy
- 90% of relapse is in para-aortic nodes
- Radiotherapy to para-aortic/pelvic nodes reduces relapse to 4%
- Current trials for chemotherapy in Stage 1 seminoma
- Radiotherapy to para-aortic nodes in all stages (T10–S1)
- Risk factors for pelvic node involvement
  —previous inguino-scrotal surgery
  —maldescent
- If risk factor is present give pelvic node radiotherapy

- IVU to identify kidney position
  —limit radiation to kidney
  —horseshoe kidney is contraindication to radiotherapy
- Standard dose of radiotherapy is 30 Gy in 15 fractions over 3 weeks
- Side-effects of radiotherapy—nausea
                                          —tiredness

Stage 2a and 2b seminoma

- Radiotherapy—30 Gy in 15 fractions over 3 weeks

Stage 2c, 3, and 4 seminoma

- Chemotherapy
- Toxic in older patient
- Bleomycin pneumonitis common

Stage 1 teratoma

- Relapse rate after orchidectomy alone—25%
- Vascular or lymphatic invasion relapse rate—50%
- If vascular or lymphatic invasion—2 courses of BEP reduce relapse rate to 1%
- No vascular or lymphatic invasion—surveillance (90% cure rate)
- Surveillance is 'active'
  —monthly clinic visits for first year
  —3 CT scans first year
  —80% who relapse do so in first year

Stage 2, 3, and 4 teratoma

- Standard treatment for metastases—Bleomycin
                                                    —Etoposide
                                                    —Cisplatin
- Cure rates—good prognostic group (90%)
              —intermittent group (75%)
              —poor prognosis (50%)
- Role of high-dose chemotherapy, marrow or stem cell transplantation—not clear
- Chemotherapy side-effects common
  —nephropathy
  —neuropathy
  —ototoxiciy
  —myelosupression
  —Bleomycin pneumonitis (fatal in 10%)
- Results better in specialized centres
- Monitor response—scans, tumour markers

Post-chemotherapy surgery or residual masses

Where residual masses are present after chemotherapy for metastatic testicular teratoma, surgery should be performed to resect these. The majority of these will be in the retroperitoneum, and extensive and difficult surgery is often necessary for a complete resection. The residual masses may contain differentiated teratoma, fibrosis, or indeed viable tumour, and further chemotherapy may be indicated. Surgery should usually only be undertaken when markers have normalized.

Residual pulmonary masses should also be resected where possible. The problem of surgical technique and anaesthetic risk, particularly as most patients will have been exposed to Bleomycin, again demand that patients are seen and operated on in a centre experienced in this surgery.

Following primary management of metastatic disease, fairly intensive follow-up is necessary as in those patients who relapse, salvage therapy can be effective in about 25% of cases.

Non-germ cell testicular tumours.

These represent a very small proportion of testicular tumours. Stromal tumours such as those arising from Leydig cells are generally thought to be benign, but metastases have been reported in approximately 10% of cases. Unfortunately, pathological examination of the primary tumour does not give a good indication of the propensity to metastasize, making management difficult. It is reasonable to perform normal staging investigations and monitor such patients for about two years. Testicular lymphomas are the commonest testicular cancer in elderly men and should be treated along the same principles as lymphomas arising at other sites.

Psychological issues

There is undoubtedly a significant psychological morbidity associated with diagnosis and subsequent management of men with germ cell tumours. The loss of a testicle alone in many patients is considered mutilating, and a testicular prosthesis should be inserted when possible. The optimal support for these patients is not clear, but psychological help should be available.

Further reading

Atzpodien, J. *et al.* (1990) Home therapy with recombinant interleukin-2 and interferon α- 2b in advanced human malignancies. *Lancet* 353, 1509–12.

Cookson, M.S., Herr, H.W., Zhang, Z.F., *et al.* (1997) The treated natural history of high risk superficial bladder cancer: 15 year outcome. *J Urol* 158, 62–7.

MRC Renal Cancer Collaborators. (1999) Interferon-α and survival in metastatic renal carcinoma: early results of a randomized controlled trial. *Lancet* 353, 14–17.

Raghavan, D., Shipley, W.U., Garnick, M.B., Russell, P.J., and Richie, J.P. (1990) Biology and management of bladder cancer. *N Eng J Med* 322, 1129–38.

Scottish Intercollegiate Guidelines Network (2000). *Management of adult testicular germ cell tumours: a national clinical guideline.*

Chapter 23
Gynaecological cancer

Ovarian cancer

Introduction

Ovarian cancer is the fifth commonest cancer in women with nearly 6000 cases diagnosed and over 4000 women dying of the disease each year. The majority of cases occur over the age of 55 years with the peak in the 65–75 age group. Treatment consists of surgery, followed for most patients by chemotherapy which, for over 20 years, has consisted of platinum-based regimens.

Aetiology

The risk of ovarian cancer appears to relate to the number of ovulatory cycles in a woman's lifetime and multiple pregnancies. Use of the oral contraceptive pill seems to offer protection, infertility raises the risk. Less than 5% are clearly hereditary—associated with *BRCA1* or *BRCA2* or Lynch II families.

Pathology

More than 80% of ovarian malignancies are epithelial, the rest comprise germ cell and stromal tumours. Epithelial cancers are classified by their cell type (serous, mucinous, endometrioid, Brenner, mixed) and by their grade.

CA125

80% of women with advanced ovarian cancer have elevated serum CA125 and this marker is valuable in monitoring response to therapy and in the detection of early relapse. However, it is not specific for ovarian cancer and is elevated in association with other peritoneal pathologies.

Presentation and staging

The vast majority of women present with disease that has spread beyond the ovary to involve the peritoneum and other abdomino-pelvic organs. The most common symptoms are of abdominal discomfort and swelling; vaginal bleeding and gastrointestinal and urinary symptoms also occur.

The two main prognostic factors in ovarian cancer are stage and the amount of residual disease after surgery. Five-year survival rates according to stage are as follows:

- Stage I   75%
- Stage II   45%
- Stage III   20%

Table 23.1 Staging of ovarian cancer

Stage	Description
Ia	Tumour confined to one ovary
Ib	Tumour confined to both ovaries
Ic	Tumour Stage I but with capsule ruptured or malignant ascites
II	Tumour with pelvic extension
III	Tumour with peritoneal implants outwith the pelvis or involved small bowel; retroperitoneal or inguinal nodes
IV	Distant metastases

- Stage IV   Less than 5%

The majority of patients present with advanced disease (Stage II–IV) with a corresponding poor prognosis. The three-year survival rate for patients with advanced ovarian cancer but no residual disease after surgery is 75%, and for those with maximum residuum less than 1 cm, 50%. Patients who have greater than 2 cm disease after their initial surgery have a poor prognosis with only 20% of patients surviving three years. Median survival times for patients with suboptimally debulked disease (greater than 1–2 cm) range from 16 to 29 months and from 26 to 96 months for patients with optimally debulked disease.

Surgery

Patients must undergo full surgical staging—generally early ovarian cancer of good prognosis (Stage Ia–b, well differentiated) does not require adjuvant chemotherapy. A surgical staging procedure consists of:

- A midline incision
- Total abdominal hysterectomy
- Bilateral salpingo-oophorectomy
- Omentectomy
- Multiple peritoneal biopsies and washings
- Lymph node sampling of the para-aortic and pelvic regions
- Careful assessment of the subdiaphragmatic areas

There is uncertainty as to which patients with Stage I disease require adjuvant chemotherapy and there are three trials (MRC, EORTC, and Scandinavian) currently addressing this issue.

Radical surgery plays an important role in the treatment of ovarian cancer. In addition, a randomized trial has shown that for patients who cannot be optimally debulked at initial laparotomy, interval debulking surgery after three cycles of chemotherapy confers a significant survival benefit. It is reasonable to treat with chemotherapy and plan interval debulking surgery if clinical and imaging assessment show that optimal debulking will not be possible. A small proportion of patients of child-bearing age who wish to preserve fertility may be treated by conservative surgery, but these patients need careful selection and counselling.

First-line chemotherapy

Cisplatin was introduced in the 1970s and the main controversy during the 1980s was whether patients required single-agent or platinum-based combination therapy. A meta-analysis published in 1991 suggested a survival benefit for platinum-based combinations but single-agent carboplatin remained standard treatment in the UK. In 1996, the Gynaecologic Oncology Group published the results of a pivotal study (GOG 111) which demonstrated a significant survival advantage for cisplatin–paclitaxel over cisplatin–cyclophosphamide (the gold standard therapy in the US and most of Europe). Median survival was improved by over one year in this study and cisplatin–paclitaxel became standard therapy in the US. In 1998, the Intergroup published confirmatory data from a similar study.

Cisplatin–paclitaxel causes significant neuro-toxicity particularly with shorter infusions of paclitaxel (the Intergroup used a three-hour, GOG 24-hour infusion), although these do reduce the risk of neutropenia. Phase II data of carboplatin–paclitaxel demonstrate similar response rates to cisplatin–paclitaxel, with less toxicity. These regimens are now being compared directly in Phase III studies.

Treatment at relapse

Patients who relapse after first-line therapy are incurable. The majority of patients relapse within 12 months and the length of the treatment-free interval before relapse is an important factor in predicting response to second-line therapy. People with a treatment-free interval of greater than 12 months should be re-challenged with a platinum-containing regimen. Other indicators of response are the bulk of disease, previous response to treatment, and the number of disease sites.

A number of new agents including topotecan, liposomal doxorubicin, etoposide, gemcitabine, and altretamine have response rates of 15–25% in this setting.

Follow-up

Clinical dilemmas arise after first-line therapy—what follow-up protocol is appropriate and when should second-line therapy be instituted? All patients have serial CA125 estimations but as soon as the marker rises, much anxiety is caused and many patients expect treatment. There is no evidence that treating simply because of a rising CA125 is of benefit, and because second-line therapy is not very effective within 12 months of previous treatment, there is good reason to try and withhold chemotherapy until patients are either symptomatic or have measurably progressive disease on imaging or clinical examination. An MRC–EORTC study is addressing this important issue, randomizing patients with a rising CA 125 to immediate second-line therapy or delayed treatment.

New approaches

The overall response rate to platinum–paclitaxel therapy is 70–75% with 30–50% of patients achieving a complete clinical remission. The question has been raised whether some form of consolidation or maintenance therapy should be investigated. Possible approaches include:

- Intra-peritoneal chemotherapy
- High-dose systemic chemotherapy
- Biological response modifiers
- Metalloprotinease inhibitors
- Anti-angiogenic agents

Cancer of the uterine corpus

Introduction

By far the commonest cancer of the corpus is carcinoma of the endometrium, which accounts for over 80% of tumours; less common are the uterine sarcomas. Of the latter, some have a glandular element, the so-called Mixed Mesodermal Mullerian Tumours (MMMT) or carcinosarcomas, and some are fibrosarcomas.

In some respects endometrial cancer has been unjustly regarded as the 'Cinderella' of gynaecological cancers, as it often appears straightforward to manage. In fact, it requires as much attention to detail as other cancers and the death rate, stage for stage, is no different from cervical or ovarian cancer.

Endometrial adenocarcinoma

Epidemiology

Endometrial cancer occurs principally in post-menopausal women and the incidence rises with age. Its aetiology has not been determined but it occurs more commonly in women who take unopposed oestrogen as hormone replacement therapy, and also in women with breast cancer taking tamoxifen, which exerts oestrogenic agonist effects on the endometrium. It is also commoner in obese women in whom oestrogen is peripherally produced in fat. These data suggest not so much a hormone—dependent tumour but one in which oestrogenic effects influence cell growth or perhaps inhibit apoptosis. Because it commonly presents early with post-menopausal bleeding, advanced disease at presentation is uncommon compared with other gynaecological cancers.

Pathology

The natural history of endometrial adenocarcinoma is not well understood. Precursor lesions in the form of atypical hyperplasia are recognized but it is not known whether these changes always precede cancer development.

Endometrial adenocarcinoma exhibits a spectrum of differentiation from well-differentiated lesions with acinar or glandular morphology to poor differentiation with none. Lymph node metastases and prognosis are strongly associated with the degree of differentiation.

Adenosquamous lesions, clear cell, and serous papillary tumours all carry a worse prognosis. The other major prognostic factor is the depth of invasion of the myometrium and this is reflected in the FIGO staging classification.

Diagnosis

Table 23.2 Revised FIGO staging for endometrial cancer

Stage	Definition
Ia	Tumour limited to endometrium
Ib	Invasion to <1/2 myometrium
Ic	Invasion to >1/2 myometrium
IIa	Endocervical glandular involvement only
IIb	Cervical stromal invasion
IIIa	Tumour invades serosa and/or adnexa and/or positive peritoneal cytology
IIIb	Metastases to pelvic and/or para-aortic lymph nodes
IVa	Tumour invasion of bladder and/or bowel mucosa
IVb	Distant metastases including intra-abdominal and/or inguinal lymph nodes.

Treatment

The mainstay of treatment for Stage I disease is hysterectomy and bilateral salpingo-oophorectomy. This should be performed through a vertical incision and peritoneal washings should be taken at the start of the operation. The role of lymphadenectomy remains to be defined. In North America, lymphadenectomy is preferred to stage the disease and, if the nodes are free of disease, adjuvant radiotherapy is avoided. In the UK, the traditional approach has been to determine the level of risk of nodal metastasis by uterine pathology and, in high-risk cases, to prescribe adjuvant radiation. The MRC is conducting a randomized trial of lymphadenectomy in endometrial cancer.

If the cervix is known to be involved pre-operatively, a radical hysterectomy should be performed. Occasionally the patient will present with a frozen pelvis that requires a non-surgical approach. Some surgeons are advocating laparoscopic lymphadenectomy together with a laparoscopically-assisted vaginal hysterectomy but, as yet, this is an unproven procedure.

Radiotherapy   Radiotherapy has two roles in endometrial cancer. The usual indication is adjuvant therapy following hysterectomy but, less commonly it may be required as primary treatment for women unfit to undergo surgery, usually through a combination of co-morbidity and marked obesity. It may also be required for advanced disease where residual tumour remains following surgery or where the tumour was inoperable from the outset or for local recurrence.

Adjuvant radiotherapy is generally delivered with external-beam irradiation of a planned volume (usually four fields) to around 50 Gy over four weeks. Vault brachytherapy reduces the risk of vault recurrence in Stage II disease.

Although currently given to 40–50% of cases treated in the UK, the value of adjuvant radiotherapy is not certain. While early trials have demonstrated that loco-regional control is improved by irradiation, there is no evidence that radiotherapy improves survival, and it does carry a risk of radiation damage to bowel and bladder. The current MRC trial randomizes women with regards to adjuvant radiotherapy for high-risk disease, with the aim of answering this question.

Chemotherapy   Chemotherapy alone has relatively little to offer in endometrial carcinoma. Combinations such as cisplatin and doxorubicin have some activity but response rates are low. Progestagens, which have been widely prescribed in the past, have never been shown to be of significant benefit and should not be prescribed as adjuvant long-term therapy.

Prognosis

Overall, endometrial cancer has the best survival rate of the gynaecological cancers, with a 70–75% five-year survival. Low-risk Stage I disease carries a five-year survival in excess of 90%, but in high-risk Stage I disease this may drop to nearer 50%. In Stage II, III, and IV disease the five-year survival falls to 50%, 30%, and 10% respectively.

Sarcomas

The epidemiology of these tumours is less well-defined than endometrial carcinoma, although cases of mixed Mullerian tumour have been reported following tamoxifen therapy. The mixed Mullerian tumours (MMTs) are divided into homologous and heterologous.

Homologous MMTs are composed of tissues native to the uterus, whereas heterologous MMTs involve tissue from outside the uterus. The tumours vary also in the frequency of mitoses seen on pathology sections, and this predicts prognosis. Tumours with fewer than 5 mitoses per 10 high-power fields are regarded as low-grade and carry a good prognosis, whereas those with a mitotic rate of over 20 per 10 high-power fields often have a more aggressive course with a high risk of nodal and systemic metastasis. Even low-grade tumours can behave unpredictably and if there is any residual disease it tends to be very unresponsive to non-surgical treatment.

Fibrosarcomas may arise *de novo* or rarely are found in a fibroid uterus. These tumours also exhibit a spectrum of mitotic activity that determines prognosis.

Successful treatment depends very much on surgery for localized disease. Residual disease or tumours with nodal or distant metastases are usually incurable. Hysterectomy and bilateral salpingo-oophorectomy should be performed, together with pelvic and para-aortic lymphadenectomy to stage the disease. Residual disease can be treated with radiation. Adjuvant radiation may improve pelvic control but does not confer a survival benefit. Chemotherapy (e.g. doxorubicin and ifosfamide) can be prescribed for metastatic disease, especially outside the pelvis, but long-term survival is very poor under these circumstances.

The future

Endometrial cancer will probably continue to increase in incidence as more women live longer. Long-term tamoxifen treatment for breast cancer may merit endometrial screening to identify early change, but screening on a population basis is not currently regarded as an effective strategy.

Cancer of the cervix

Aetiology

- Sexual intercourse
- Human papillomavirus (HPV)
- HPV types 16, 18—USA and Europe
- Vaccination programme in development

Epidemiology

The epidemiology of this disease has been extensively studied and strong associations demonstrated with:

- Low social class
- Multiparity
- Cigarette smoking
- Early onset of sexual intercourse (before 17)
- Non-barrier forms of contraception

More recent studies have focused attention specifically on papillomavirus transmission and the increased susceptibility of the cervical epithelium of the sexually active teenage female.

This disease has dramatic variations in incidence around the world. In the developing countries of South-East Asia, Africa, and South America, it is the commonest female cancer. Limited regional studies in South America have revealed massive incidences up to 96/100 000 (against 14.5/100 000 in the UK and only 2/100 000 in Israel).

The UK saw significant incidence changes during the different decades of the twentieth century. High rates occurred in the cohorts of women who were aged 20–30 years during the First and Second World Wars when they entered their 50s and 60s. More recently, a rise in incidence occurred in the late 1970s and early 1980s in women aged 30–50 years. The UK incidence is now falling for the first time in a century. This is attributed to the success of the population-based screening programme, which was introduced following success in Finland and British Columbia.

Pathology

When the disease is confined to the cervix, patient management depends on the cytology and/or histology specimens. These can reveal a spectrum of changes in the epithelium of the cervix:

- Slight dysplastic changes to the cell architecture
- Viral cytoplasmic changes

- Intra-epithelial neoplasia (CIN 1, 2, or 3)
- Micro-invasive carcinoma
- Frank invasive carcinoma

A number of changes may be present in the same patient at one time. The changes are often maximal at the junction zone where the squamous epithelium of the ectocervix meets the cuboidal epithelium of the endocervix close to, or at, the external os. The changes can be a single focus, multiple foci, or confluent change extending up the endocervical canal.

These early changes may first be identified by examination of a smear of cells, collected by a special wooden (Ayers) spatula or a brush, from the vaginal surface of the cervix. The specimen is a sample of the cells that are being shed from the ectocervix along, sometimes, with cells that are being shed from the endocervix and the endometrium. They are examined on a slide after staining with Papanicolou stain and an impression of the health of the epithelium can be formed.

To accurately map changes in the cervical epithelium patients require colposcopy where the cervix is examined by binocular microscopy at ten times normal magnification. A skilled operator can discriminate between different grades of change identifiable histologically, map the abnormalities, and biopsy the most abnormal areas. If changes extend up the cervical canal the operator will proceed to a formal cone biopsy in which the abnormal ectocervix along with the endocervical canal up to the internal os of the cervix is removed in one piece and examined histologically.

Viral changes, dysplasia, CIN 1 and 2 are common in the sexually active adult female, particularly among those in their 20s when multiple partners and non-barrier contraception are involved. They can all revert to normal without treatment and are monitored by regular smears. CIN 3 changes are more commonly part of a process that can progress over months or years to invasive carcinoma. Invasive cancer can also develop *de novo*. Most patients have changes to the squamous cell population, some have pure adenomatous cell changes, and others have mixtures of the two cell types. Papillary or small cell carcinomas are seen occasionally.

The pathology report should indicate the cell type(s), the level it has reached relative to the basement membrane, the maximum depth of any invasion below the membrane, and the width of invasion. These last two points are particularly important when invasion is only a few millimetres as this determines whether the problem is micro-invasion (less than 5 mm in depth or 7 mm in width) or invasive carcinoma.

Staging

The FIGO staging system is based predominantly on the extent of the primary tumour. Metastatic spread is normally by the lymphatic system and tends to be sequential—to the parametrial nodes, the obturator

Table 23.3 FIGO staging system for cervical cancer

Stage	Definition
Ia	Micro-invasive disease (max depth 5 mm, max width 7 mm)
Ib	Clinical disease confined to the cervix
IIa	Disease involves upper 1/3 vagina but not parametrium
IIb	Disease involves parametrium but does not extend to pelvic wall
III	Disease involves lower 2/3 vagina and/or pelvic wall
IV	Involvement of bladder, rectum, or distant organs

group, the internal then common iliacs, and on through the para-aortics to the left neck. Systemic metastases are rare outside the chest.

Presentation

Patients with CIN and micro-invasive carcinoma have no symptoms. The diagnosis typically follows an abnormal cervical smear or colposcopic examination. Symptomatic patients should not be investigated by cervical smear alone. The earliest symptoms of invasive carcinoma are:

• Increased vaginal discharge
• Post-coital bleeding
• Inter-menstrual or post-menopausal bleeding

Increasing tumour bulk and pelvic infiltration leads to pressure on the bladder (frequency), rectum (altered bowel habit), or ureters (often asymptomatic until uraemia appears). Deep lateral pelvic pain can be due to direct extension of nodal disease. This can progress to lymphoedema, venous thrombosis of a lower limb, and even sciatic nerve palsy. Rarely in Western countries patients may present with a vesicovaginal or recto-vaginal fistula.

Investigation

Asymptomatic patients with CIN 1, 2, or 3 or micro-invasive carcinoma do not require any further investigation prior to treatment. Symptomatic patients should have an examination under anaesthetic to complete FIGO staging, cystoscopy or sigmoidoscopy if these organs appear to be involved, and an IVU in Stage 2–4. CT or MRI scanning of the pelvis and abdomen define more fully the size of the primary tumour and any lymphadenopathy.

Treatment

Surgery

• CIN 3 disease localized to ectocervix—colposcopy and loop diathermy, cryoprobe or laser

- CIN 3 disease extending into endocervical canal or micro-invasion—cone biopsy
- Complete excision still requires follow-up or if patient wants no more children—hysterectomy and surveillance for vaginal vault
- Invasive carcinoma (less than 4 cm, confined to cervix)—Wertheim's hysterectomy removes parametrium and pelvic nodes
- Radiotherapy if—incomplete excision of tumour
  —poor tumour differentiation
  —vascular invasion
  —node involvement
  —all other stages/medically unfit

Radiotherapy

- External-beam irradiation followed by intra-cavitary brachytherapy (ICT)
- 40–45 Gy—pelvis over 4 weeks
- Sterilizes pre-menopausal patients
- ICT gamma sources (^{137}Cs on ^{192}Ir) in uterus/upper vagina (GA)
  —left for minutes (high dose rate)
  —left for days (low dose rate)
- ICT—dose to central pelvic structures
  —80 Gy to 2 cm lateral and superior to external os
  —dose to bladder and rectum below 70 Gy
- Pelvic radiotherapy for advanced cancer
  —5% late morbidity (bowel and urinary tract)
  —bleeding
  —stricture
  —ulceration
  —fistula
  —vaginal shortening/dryness

Chemotherapy

Despite a considerable number of studies, chemotherapy has no established role in the radical treatment of any stage of this cancer. Patients with recurrent pelvic or systemic metastatic disease may benefit from palliative chemotherapy. The principal active agents are

- Cisplatin
- Mitomycin C
- Ifosfamide
- Methotrexate
- 5-fluorouracil
- Bleomycin

Combined therapy

Modern management of advanced cancer regularly involves the use of concurrent or sequential chemotherapy and radiotherapy.

Results

Survival at five years is typically—Stage 1a, 100%; Stage 1b, 70–90%; Stage 2, 50–70%; Stage 3, 25–60%; Stage 4, 10–20%. The wide ranges reflect the large variation in disease volume seen within the present staging system that is based on tissue involvement rather than volume of disease. Relapse after five years is unusual.

Vaginal and vulval cancer

Vaginal cancer

Primary vaginal cancer is uncommon, constituting only 1–2% of malignant female genital tract malignancies. Most vaginal maligacies are metastatic, from primaries in the cervix, vulva, endometrium, or trophoblast (choriocarcinoma). The most common histological types of primary cancer are squamous (80%) and adenocarcinoma (10%).

Aetiology

The cause of primary squamous carcinoma is uncertain. The recognized association with squamous intra-epithelial and invasive neoplasia at other anogential mucosal and cutaneous sites such as the cervix, vulva, and anus suggests a common aetiological agent. Oncogenic human papillomavirus (HPV) subtypes 16 and 18 and/or primary p53 polymorphisms are likely to be important in this tumour's biology.

Symptoms and signs

+ Symptoms—abnormal vaginal bleeding
            —vaginal discharge
            —bladder, rectal symptoms
+ Signs—vaginal examination: best method of detection
        —speculum examination
        —most lesions in upper 1/3 and are exophytic

Staging and investigations

The staging is clinical but may include results of invasive investigations such as cystoscopy, protoscopy, and appropriate radiography in order to detect local and distant spread. MRI is the preferred investigation for evaluating local spread, particularly if body or transvaginal coils are used. The negative predictive values of CT and MRI for regional nodal involvement remain unsatisfactory.

Treatment

Radical radiotherapy with a combination of pelvic external-beam and utero-vaginal intra-cavitary brachytherapy is the treatment of choice. The literature is unclear regarding optimum dosimetry and field design. Lower vaginal involvement should prompt consideration of either additional groin node dissection or irradiation. Para-aortic irradiation (extended field) is associated with high morbidity and is of uncertain value.

Overall five-year survival is 40%, and salvage after first relapse is uncommon. Bad prognostic features are primary adenocarcinoma, large tumour bulk, tumour site (lower vaginal lesions fare worse), and posterior vaginal wall involvement. One in five long-term survivors will suffer from serious radiotherapy-related complications.

If the uterus is intact, the tumour involves the upper posterior vagina, and there is small volume disease (highly selected Stage I disease), then a radical hysterectomy, partial vaginectomy, and bilateral pelvic lymphadenectomy may be performed.

Treatment of vaginal cancer should be limited to centres with expertise in gynaecologic oncology.

Vulval cancer

Primary invasive vulval cancer occurs as commonly as cervical cancer in women over 60 years. One in four tumours occur in women under the age of 65 years. The majority (85%) are squamous carcinoma. Other types include basal carcinoma (10%) and malignant melanoma (4%).

Aetiology

The known associations with oncogenic HPV DNA (types 16 and 18), p53 mutations, and pre-existing abnormal vulval skin conditions such as a thickened epidermis (squamous hyperplasia), lichen sclerosis, and intra-epithelial atypia, suggest a complex aetiology. Little prospective data exist to clarify the aetiology further. Women with these skin disorders should be kept under regular review by experienced clinicians and advised to report persistent symptoms or new skin changes that might herald malignant change.

Symptoms and signs

Many tumours are preceded by chronic vulval skin symptoms such as pruritus and irritation, which probably reflect pre-existing skin disorders. Patients complain of the sensation of a painful lump. Abnormal genital tract bleeding or haematuria may occur.

A simple, thorough examination of the external genitalia will identify the majority of tumours. Persistent erythematous areas that are raised or tender should be suspected as invasive disease and a confirmatory full thickness skin biopsy should be performed.

Staging and investigations

Staging requires a combination of surgical and histopathological investigations. The incidence of nodal metastases rises from less than 1% for tumours with less than 1 mm depth of invasion to over 10% for tumours over 3 mm in depth. The confirmation of groin lymph node status is therefore mandatory in all but early stage I disease. Non-invasive modalities such as ultrasound, CT, or MRI are of insufficient negative predictive value for regional (groin) node metastases. The routine dissection of groin nodes therefore remains important for most stages of this disease.

Treatment

- Surgical excision with clear margins and removal of groin nodes
- Care if tumour involves distal urethra, anal mucosa (preserve function)
- Extensive disease may require complex reconstruction
- Psychosexual dysfunction, body image problems frequent
- Chemo-irradiation for advanced disease: 5 FU and mitomycin C combined with radiotherapy—encouraging results
- 5-year survival—85% if node-negative
- Bad prognosis if—>3 regional nodes involved
  - —Stage III, IV disease
  - —large tumour bulk
  - —node metastases
  - —poor performance status
  - —tumour type (melanoma)
- Treatment in specialized centres

Trophoblastic tumours

Introduction

Gestational trophoblastic disease (GTD) includes a spectrum of disorders ranging from the pre-malignant complete hydatidiform mole (CHM) and partial hydatidiform mole (PHM), to the malignant invasive mole, gestational choriocarcinoma, and the highly malignant placental-site trophoblastic tumour (PSTT). Both CHM and PHM can develop into invasive moles. However, it is thought that only CHM may progress to the highly malignant choriocarcinoma and the rare PSTT.

Difficulty in diagnosis occurs most frequently with choriocarcinomas and PSTT, which can arise after any type of pregnancy and may not present until many years later with widespread metastases. GTD remains an important group of disorders for the clinician to recognize, because they are nearly always curable if appropriately managed and, in most cases, fertility can be preserved.

What is trophoblast?

Within a few days following conception a ball of cells is formed called the blastocyst and the outer layer of this ball differentiates into trophoblast. This consists of an inner layer of cytotrophoblast cells that migrate outwards and fuse to form large multinucleate syncytiotrophoblast cells. The latter produce the pregnancy-associated hormone, human chorionic gonadotrophin (HCG), and invade the myometrium, triggering the formation of new maternal blood vessels which are leaky and supply nutrition to the growing foetus. Trophoblast tissue frequently invades these blood vessels, both in normal and molar pregnancies, and circulates in the blood.

Hydatidiform moles

Epidemiology

* 1/1000 pregnancies in UK
* Two-fold frequency in South-East Asia
* More common after pregnancy when aged <16 years or >40 years

Pathology

* Ovum lacking maternal nucleus DNA fertilized by one or two sperm—duplicate its chromosomes
* Conceptus is androgenetic
* Proliferate to give abnormal trophoblastic tissue

- Partial mole—arises when two sperm fertilize an ovum that has retained nuclear DNA
    —triploid conceptus proliferation, to give abnormal trophoblast and variable foetal tissue
    —abnormal trophoblast forms hydropic villi which resemble grapes

Histology

- Dilated villi of hyperplastic syncytiotrophoblast and cytotrophoblast
- Later, cisterns form
- Large AV shunts form—facilitates spread

Presentation and staging

- Bleeding in early pregnancy
- Anaemia
- Toxaemia, hyperemesis, hyperthyroidism

About 15-20% of complete moles and 0.5% of partial moles will require chemotherapy. Staging of the disease involves ultrasound of the pelvis, serum HCG, and chest X-ray. In most instances the CXR will be normal but metastatic disease can present with:

- Cannonball secondaries
- Pleural effusions
- Wedge infarcts
- Oligaemic areas
- Cavitating lesions
- Miliary appearance

If there are chest lesions then a CT or preferably MRI brain scan is indicated prior to lumbar puncture for HCG analysis of the CSF (an HCG ratio of >1:60 (CSF: blood) indicates CNS involvement).

Diagnosis

- Ultrasound—large uterus for dates
    —CHM: snow-storm appearances, no foetal parts
    —PHM: abnormal placenta, foetal parts seen
- HCG level high
- DCIS in 2%
- Trophoblastic embolism

Treatment

- Gentle suction curettage
- Spontaneous abortion

* Hysterotomy, caesarean section increases the risks two-fold of chemotherapy required to eradicate persistent trophoblastic disease

The information from the staging investigations is used in the scoring system to determine the risk of developing drug resistance to methotrexate. Patients who score <5 will be cured with methotrexate alone in at least 75% of cases, while only 30% are cured who score 5–8. Nevertheless, the latter patients are also offered methotrexate therapy to start with since this treatment carries no risk of long-term sequelae. Methotrexate may cause bleeding through rapid involution of metastases. Patients scoring >9 receive 'high-risk' intravenous combination chemotherapy comprising etoposide, methotrexate, and actinomycin D (EMA), alternating weekly with cyclophosphamide and vincristine (CO). Treatment with either methotrexate or EMA/CO regimens continues until the HCG has been normal for six weeks.

Registration

Three specialist centres in the UK register and oversee therapy of this rare tumour: Dundee, Sheffield, Charing Cross (London).

Follow-up

* Regular HCG measurement
* Subsequent pregnancies increase risk of further molar pregnancy
* Rise in HCG means persistent gestational trophoblastic disease or invasive mole or choriocarcinoma has developed

If the HCG plateaus or starts to rise, this indicates that the patient has persisting molar disease or has developed an invasive mole (progression to choriocarcinoma and PSTT is rare). If a repeat ultrasound shows evidence of trophoblastic proliferation within the uterus, suction curettage may be performed. However, performing more than two D&Cs is not usually beneficial and will not prevent the subsequent need for chemotherapy. Uterine perforation is more likely if the HCG is >20 000 when a second D&C is contraindicated.

Other factors which increase the risk of needing subsequent chemotherapy include age >50 years and use of the oral contraceptive pill whilst HCG is still elevated. Accordingly, all patients are advised to use a barrier method of contraception following evacuation of a mole.

Choriocarcinoma

Epidemiology

* Follows any type of pregnancy
* Incidence 1/50 000
* 3% of CHM develop into choriocarcinoma
* No geographical trends

Pathology

• Highly malignant
• Soft, purple, haemorrhagic mass
• Histology—mimics early blastocyst
      —cores of mononuclear cytotrophoblast
      —rim of multinucleated syncytiotrophoblast
      —no chorionic villi
      —surrounding necrosis, bleeding
      —tumour in venous sinuses

Presentation

• Presents within one year of pregnancy
• Vaginal bleeding
• Abdominal pain
• Pelvic mass
• One third present with metastases to liver, brain, or lung

Management

In most instances the patient will be transferred to the specialist centre. In addition to the staging investigations previously outlined, patients may undergo further tests including:

• Measurement of other tumour markers
• Whole body CT/MRI
• PET scanning
• Anti-HCG antibody scanning

Where it can be safely achieved, excision biopsy of a metastasis should be considered. This not only enables histological confirmation of the diagnosis but also permits genetic analysis to prove the gestational nature of the tumour. If there are only maternal genes and no paternal genes present then the patient has a non-gestational tumour (an ovarian choriocarcinoma or, more rarely, an epithelial tumour that has differentiated into choriocarcinoma). Frequently, however, biopsy is not possible and the diagnosis is made on the clinical history and other investigation findings. The patients are then scored and treated as described for molar disease.

The indications for chemotherapy are:

• Evidence of metastases in brain, liver, or gastrointestinal tract; or radiological opacities >2 cm on chest X-ray.
• Histological evidence of choriocarcinoma.
• Heavy vaginal bleeding or evidence of gastrointestinal or intraperitoneal haemorrhage.
• Pulmonary, vulval, or vaginal metastases unless HCG falling.

Table 23.4 Scoring system for gestational trophoblastic tumours

Prognostic factor	Score*			
	0	**1**	**2**	**6**
Age (years)	<39	>39		
Antecedent pregnancy (AP)	Mole	Abortion or unknown	Term	
Interval (end of AP to chemo in months)	<4	4–7	7–12	>12
HCG iu/l	10^3—10^4	<10^3	10^4—10^5	>10^5
ABO blood group (female × male)		A × 0 0 × A O or A × unknown	B × A or 0 AB × A or 0	
No of metastases	Nil	1–4	4–8	>8
Site of metastases	Not detected Lungs Vagina	Spleen Kidney	GI tract	Brain Liver
Largest tumour mass	<3.0	3–5 cm	>5 cm	
Prior chemotherapy			Single drug	2 or more drugs

* The total score for a patient is obtained by adding the individual scores for each prognostic factor. Lower risk, 0–5; medium risk, 6–8; high risk, >9.

- Rising HCG after evacuation.
- Serum HCG = 20 000 iu/l more than 4 weeks after evacuation, because of the risk of uterine perforation.
- Raised HCG 6 months after evacuation even if still falling.

Any of these are indications to treat following the diagnosis of GTD.

Placental-site trophoblastic tumour (PSTT)

PSTT can develop following a term delivery, non-molar abortion, or CHM. There are currently about 100 recorded cases of PSTT in the literature and so estimates of its true incidence may well be inaccurate. Nevertheless, PSTT is thought to constitute about 1% of all trophoblastic tumours (choriocarcinoma, invasive mole, and PSTT).

PSTTs are slow-growing, malignant tumours composed mainly of cytotrophoblast with very little syncytiotrophoblast, so producing little HCG. However, they often stain strongly for human placental lactogen (HPL) which helps to distinguish this tumour from carcinomas, sarcomas, exaggerated placental-site reaction, and placental nodule. The raised HPL may cause hyperprolactinaemia that can result in amenorrhoea and/or galactorrhoea. In most cases spread occurs by local infiltration with distant metastases occurring late via the lymphatics and blood.

The behaviour of PSTT is thus quite different from other forms of GTD and it is relatively chemo-resistant. The best management is hysterectomy when the disease is localized to the uterus. When metastatic disease is present, patients can respond and be apparently cured by multi-agent chemotherapy either alone or in combination with surgery.

Patient follow-up and prognosis

On completion of their chemotherapy, patients are advised to avoid pregnancy for one year and remain on HCG follow-up for life to confirm that their disease is in remission. About 2% of low-risk and 4% of high-risk patients will relapse. All low-to middle-risk patients are salvaged with further chemotherapy (EMA/CO or alternative regimens) and the cure rate is almost 100% in this group. The high-risk group has 90% survival rate beyond 10 years. With the addition of platinum and other new agents salvage rates for patients relapsing following EMA/CO therapy can be in excess of 70%. Neither methotrexate nor EMA/CO therapy reduce fertility or cause abnormalities. Thus women treated for GTD can expect to have healthy children.

Further reading

1. Advanced Ovarian Cancer Triallist Group (1998) Chemotherapy in ovarian cancer: four systematic meta-analyses of individual patient data from 37 randomized trials. *British Journal of Cancer* **78**, 1479–87.
2. Rose, P.G., Bundy, B.N., Watkins, E.B. *et al.* (1999) Concurrent cisplatin-based chemotherapy and radiotherapy for locally advanced cervical cancer. *New England Journal of Medicine* **340**, 1144–53.

Chapter 24
Head and neck cancer

Cancer of the larynx

Introduction

The use of the operating microscope (microlaryngoscopy), rigid and fibre laryngoscopes, stroboscopy, CT, and MRI, and the improved histopathological diagnosis by immunohistochemistry, electron microscopy, cytometry, and morphometry have made major contributions in laryngeal pathological diagnosis.

Radiotherapy is, in many countries, the prime treatment for laryngeal carcinoma. Surgery has, however, been successfully refined, with various voice and airway conservation procedures. Rehabilitation of the laryngectomized patient has been easier with insertion of differing voice prostheses.

Squamous cell neoplasm

Tumours arising from the mucosa of the larynx make up the majority of tumours in the larynx. Juvenile laryngeal papillomas are virus-induced benign tumours that are most commonly located on the vocal cords and occasionally remain or arise in adults. They may be solitary or multiple. Malignant degeneration of non-irradiated juvenile laryngeal papillomas is extremely rare. Surgical excision with the aid of the operating microscope and the carbon dioxide laser is the treatment of choice. Interferon may be used in very selective troublesome cases.

Pre-malignant lesions

Classification should be based on grade of dysplasia, as this has a bearing on prognosis. Most of these lesions are diagnosed on the vocal cords with hoarseness as the symptom. These lesions should be endoscopically excised (conventional technique or laser) and the specimens should be carefully examined by an experienced pathologist working in close collaboration with the clinician. Radiotherapy may be used for frequently recurring or diffuse lesions. These patients should be carefully followed up as there is not only a risk of development of invasive carcinoma but also a high risk of other primary malignant neoplasms, especially within the upper aero-digestive tract and lungs.

Epidemiology and carcinogenesis

Laryngeal cancer makes up less than 2% of all carcinomas in males, with an annual incidence of 3–10 per 100 000. It is a predominantly male disease, with a higher incidence in urban than rural areas.

Smoking and alcohol are documented risk factors and act synergistically. Occupational risk factors may include asbestos and solvents. Human papilloma virus has also been suggested as a risk factor.

Symptoms

Hoarseness is the most common presenting symptom for primary glottic carcinoma (the most common laryngeal cancer in North America, England, and Scandinavia). Dysphagia, irritation, and coughing are characteristic of supraglottic carcinomas (which make up more than 50% of the laryngeal cancers in Mediterranean countries and South America). Subglottic carcinomas are rare (<5%) and cause dyspnoea and stridor as they grow circumferentially in the subglottis. They usually present late. Most laryngeal carcinomas are diagnosed between 40–80 years of age.

Diagnostic examinations

Indirect and direct laryngoscopy, including stroboscopy, complemented by CT or MRI and histopathological studies are requirements for correct diagnosis. Ultrasound-guided fine-needle aspiration cytology is the most accurate technique for assessment of neck masses.

Treatment

The main treatment modalities are radiotherapy and surgery with the aim to provide optimal cure with the best functional results. Induction chemotherapy may select patients with advanced carcinoma suitable for full-course radiotherapy to save the larynx. Patient factors such as general condition, lifestyle, previous treatment, and personal views are all important in the treatment decision.

Limited glottic carcinomas are treated with equal results by radiotherapy and surgery with external techniques or endoscopically using the CO_2 laser, which is increasingly employed. The voice may be better spared by radiotherapy, the cure rate being 70–90%.

Advanced glottic carcinomas (T3–T4) are treated by primary radiotherapy at many centres and surgery or induction chemotherapy are reserved for salvage of failures. Near total laryngectomy is an operation that saves the voice, but the patient is given a stoma for breathing

In advanced carcinomas the neck nodes are included in the treatment planning; the survival rate is 50–60%. Partial voice conservation laryngectomy techniques are employed in some centres as primary treatment for early supraglottic carcinomas. Endoscopic laser surgery is reported to give the same cure rate and less functional morbidity, at least in experienced hands. As 30–40% of the patients have nodal metastases, neck dissection is usually performed when surgery is the sole treatment. Primary radiotherapy gives nearly the same cure rate, but any recurrence means that a total laryngectomy is most often necessary. Local control rates with primary surgery and radiotherapy are 80–90%. Subglottic primary carcinomas are rare and the high risk of paratracheal and upper mediastinal nodal metastases must be taken into account.

Miscellaneous tumours

Verrucous carcinoma is a distinct variant of well differentiated squamous cell carcinoma (also named Ackerman's tumour) and is characterized by a verrucous appearance and pushing margins histopathologically, surrounded by a marked inflammatory cell response. Lymphatic spread is rare. Surgical treatment is usually advocated, but a good response to radiotherapy is also reported.

Spindle cell carcinoma is a rare, well-described tumour making up less than 1% of laryngeal malignant tumours. The term 'pseudo-sarcoma' has been used for some of these tumours as the spindle elements were once considered reactive. Immunohistochemical and electron microscopy suggest they are epithelial cells.

Rehabilitation and follow-up after total laryngectomy

The greatest handicap for the patients after a total laryngectomy is the loss of voice. 40% of patients acquire socially useful oesophageal speech. Some people use the artificial larynx. Fistula operations with insertion of speech valvulas are increasingly performed and well tolerated. Heat and moisture exchangers are commonly used to lower the risk of respiratory problems and can be positioned in front of the stoma.

Follow-up should be strict—90% of recurrences occur within three years. The high risk of multiple primary malignancies (12–20%) should be considered, making routine chest X-rays and broncho-scopies part of the follow-up programme. All patients should be advised to stop smoking.

Cancer of the oral cavity

Pathology

Squamous cancers of the oral cavity are associated with heavy consumption of both tobacco and alcohol. Other aetiological factors are:

- Diet (deficient in Vitamin A, fruit, and vegetables)
- Poor dental hygiene
- Syphilis

The other less common malignancies in the oral cavity include:

- Salivary tumours (adenoid cystic, mucoepidermoid, adenocarcinoma)
- Melanomas
- Plasmacytomas
- Sarcomas

Squamous cancers in the mouth present with a mucosal irregularity which progresses either into an ulcerated destructive lesion or a more exophytic growth. These can be highly aggressive tumours, invading and destroying adjacent local tissues including the bone of the mandible, and disseminating to regional lymph nodes in the neck and submandibular region.

The region is divided anatomically but tumours commonly involve more than one region:

- Alveolar ridge/retromolar trigone (10%)
- Floor of mouth (15%)
- Tongue (60%)
- Hard palate (5%)
- Buccal mucosa (10%)

Staging

The assessment of the patient requires examination under anaesthetic to assess the extent of disease and biopsy of the lesion. The primary and regional nodes are also usefully assessed by MRI scan. The malignant nature of lymphadenopathy should be confirmed by FNA cytology. CXR should be performed as much to exclude a coincidental lung primary as for infrequent lung metastases.

Treatment

- Multidisciplinary approach is essential
  —maxillofacial, plastics, dental

—radiation oncologist

—dietician

—speech therapist

• Surgery for early tumours

• Primary radiotherapy and reserve surgery for salvage

• Neck dissection for positive nodes

• Large lesions require osteomyocutaneous flap reconstruction

• If locally advanced—combination of surgery and radiotherapy

Radiation therapy is planned taking account not only of all clinical and radiological evidence of the tumour but also the likely sites of occult nodal disease. Doses of 50–65 Gy are delivered to the tumour volume, depending on the extent of residual tumour. At least part of this dose can be delivered by interstitial therapy, often using iridium wire. Inevitably radical irradiation of the oral cavity causes mucositis and a dry mouth, that may persist depending on the amount of salivary tissue spared from irradiation. Chronic ulceration of the mucosa and osteonecrosis are risks, particularly with locally advanced tumours involving the mandible.

As with head and neck squamous cancers at other sites, chemotherapy (cisplatin, 5-fluorouarcil, methotrexate, bleomycin) is active in advanced disease, but there is no proven benefit for chemotherapy given as either adjuvant or neo-adjuvant therapy.

Carcinoma of the nasopharynx

Anatomy

The nasopharynx is the part of the upper respiratory tract situated between the nasal and oropharyngeal cavities. The roof is the base of the skull and arch of the atlas with the first two cervical vertebrae forming the posterior wall. The anterior border is the posterior choanae and the floor is the upper surface of the palate.

Epidemiology

There is a wide variation of incidence of nasopharyngeal carcinoma (NPC) throughout the world.

The highest incidence is in South China and a large part of South-East Asia (Hong Kong, Singapore, Malaysia, Vietnam, and North Thailand) with an average incidence of 20–30/100 000 per year. The incidence amongst males aged 45–55 in South China is 120/100 000. There is an intermediate incidence amongst Maghrebian Arabs (from Ageria, Tunisia, Morocco, Libya, and Sudan) of 1.5–9/100 000 per annum. The only group in North America or Europe with a high incidence of NPC are Eskimos, with a prevalence similar to that of the Cantonese. Otherwise, this is a rare cancer with a typical incidence of 0.2–0.5/100 000 (West Midlands of England).

Aetiology

* Epstein–Barr virus (EBV)
* Genetic susceptibility—major histocompatability complex profile, H_2, BW46, B17 antigens
* Dietary-salty fish—contain nitrosamines
* Chinese herbal medicine contains esters—tumour promoters, reactivate EBV infection
* Lack of dietary vitamin C
* EBV infection—reactivated 18–60 months before detectable tumour
* EBV copies inside malignant cells

Pathology

The WHO divided NPC into three types:
* Type 1: keratinizing squamous carcinoma
* Type 2: non-keratinizing carcinoma (transitional cell carcinoma)
* Type 3: undifferentiated (lymph-epithelioma)

Squamous cancers are associated with a higher propensity for local persistence after treatment and a poorer prognosis. Undifferentiated tumours are the most common entity and, unlike most head and neck cancers, frequently spread to distant sites, initially via the lymphatic system.

Presentation and methods of spread

Unilateral deafness, secondary to Eustachian tube blockage, is the most common local symptom, followed by epistaxis. Nasal obstruction is common when the tumour is advanced. NPC spreads into the parapharyngeal space laterally, anteriorly to the orbit and paranasal sinuses, inferiorly to the oropharynx, and superiorly through the base of the skull. Any of the cranial nerves can be involved by the tumour. In practice, the Vth nerve is involved most frequently owing to tumour in or around the foramen ovale. Tumour in the cavernous sinus can lead to diplopia secondary to compression of the IV, III, or VI nerves. The posterior cranial nerves (IX to XII) can be involved by direct parapharyngeal spread or compression by retropharyngeal lymph nodes.

Cervical lymph node spread is common and is a frequent presentation. Bilateral or unilateral upper deep cervical nodes just below the mastoid are frequently involved. Caudal spread of nodal disease correlates with distant spread and this is the basis of the Ho staging scheme. Distant spread to bone (often with sclerotic metastases), the liver, and lung is common in advanced stage disease.

CT scanning of the base of the skull, nasopharynx and neck, thorax, and liver is an essential part of pre-treatment assessment. About a quarter of patients with low cervical or supraclavicular nodes have a positive isotope bone scan.

In the Far East, the Ho staging system is used instead of the UICC scheme. It is argued that it is often impossible to decide whether the tumour is confined to only one subsite and the UICC T staging does not correlate well with prognosis. The nodal staging system is particularly inappropriate as the tumour originates in the midline and bilateral spread is common. Nodal size or the degree of fixation are not important prognostic variables, but the level of nodal spread is related to the probability of distant spread.

Treatment

NPC is generally both radio- and chemosensitive. Radiotherapy is the mainstay of treatment. The role of surgery is restricted to staging and the elective dissection of neck nodes that have not regressed three months after radiotherapy.

Radiotherapy planning is complicated in this disease. The primary tumour should be irradiated with a wide margin including the base of the skull. The neck is invariably irradiated owing to the high frequency

Table 24.1 Ho staging scheme (1989)

T1	Tumour confined to nasopharynx
$T2_n$	Nasal involvement without parapharyngeal space involvement or T3 features
$T2_o$	Oropharyngeal involvement without T3 features
$T2_p$	Parapharyngeal involvement without T3 features
$T3_q$	Parapharyngeal involvement with T3 features
$T3_a$	Bone involvement below base of skull including floor of sphenoid sinus
$T3_b$	Involvement of base of skull
$T3_c$	Cranial nerve involvement
$T3_d$	Involvement of orbit, laryngopharynx, or infratemporal fossa
N0	No cervical lymph nodes palpable
N1	Nodes wholly above the skin crease extending laterally and backwards from just below the thyroid notch
N2	Nodes palpable between the skin crease and supraclavicular fossa
N3	Nodes palpable in the supraclavicular fossa or skin involvement

The groups can be condensed to five stages:

Stage I	T1 N0
Stage II	T2 and/or N1
Stage III	T3 and/or N2
Stage IV	N3 involvement irrespective of T stage
Stage V	Haematologous spread or nodal involvement below clavicles

Table 24.2 UICC staging (1992)

T1	Tumour limited to one subsite in the nasopharynx
T2	Tumour involving more than one subsite
T3	Tumour invades nasal cavity and/or nasopharynx
T4	Tumour invades skull and/or cranial nerves
N0	No regional lymph nodes
N1	Single ipsilateral node <3 cm
$N2_a$	Single ipsilateral node >3 cm
$N2_b$	Multiple ipsilateral nodes >3 cm but <6 cm
$N2_c$	Bilateral or contralateral nodes all <6 cm
N3	Any node >6 cm

of overt and occult neck metastases. However, the radiation dose to the brain, eyes, and spinal cord must be kept within tolerance. In order to reduce acute reactions as much normal mucosa as possible must be excluded from the irradiated volume. In general, doses of 65–70 Gy are given to the primary site in 6.5–7 weeks. Involved areas of the neck are treated to 60 Gy with boosts of 70 Gy with electrons if necessary. Parapharyngeal masses are also boosted. Brachytherapy may be used to increase the dose to the primary site.

Local or regional recurrence developing two or more years after radiotherapy can be successfully treated by a second radical course of radiotherapy with a reported five-year survival of 25–35% but with considerably increased morbidity.

Chemotherapy

* Chemo-responsive tumour
* 20% complete response
* 70% overall response rate in advanced disease
* 5FU, cisplatin, bleomycin
* May be advantage for chemotherapy before radiotherapy, especially in Stage IV

Results

The 10-year actuarial survival for 5037 patients treated in Hong Kong between 1976 and 1985 was 43%. Typical three-year survival figures, by stage, in Hong Kong are:

* I   (81%)
* II   (63%)
* III (54%)
* IV   (36%)

Future developments

The following are under investigation:
* Development of an EBV vaccine
* Conformal radiotherapy to reduce dosage to normal tissue
* Accelerated hyperfractionated radiotherapy
* Combined radiation and chemotherapy

Nasal cavity and paranasal sinuses

Aetiology

Unlike the rest of the upper aerodigestive tract, smoking plays little if any role in malignant tumour development. However, for certain histology occupational factors are important. Adenocarcinoma of the ethmoids may develop from exposure to hard wood dust, whereas soft wood dust may lead to the development of squamous cell carcinoma. The relative risk of a wood worker developing adenocarcinoma is 70 times normal; adenocarcinoma has also been associated with the manufacture of chrome pigment, isopropyl alcohol, textiles, clothing, leather, and shoes.

Epidemiology

Sinonasal malignancy is rare, constituting approximately 3% of head and neck cancer. Global figures suggest an incidence of <1/100 000 people per year in most countries, though occupational factors produce regional differences. The male to female ratio is approximately 2:1 overall and, while the tumour may occur at any age, the majority present between 50–70 years.

Pathology

The sinonasal region offers a great histological diversity of tumours. Of these, squamous cell carcinoma remains the commonest. Late presentation may make it difficult to define the exact site of origin. Generally, the maxillary sinus is regarded as the usual site, though lesions frequently arise in the lateral wall of the nasal cavity and ethmoids. The primary malignant tumours of the frontal and sphenoid sinuses are extremely rare.

The nasal cavity and sinuses are intimately related to the orbit and skull base (anterior and middle cranial fossae)—areas into which the tumours may spread early and covertly. In addition, anterior spread into the soft tissues of the face, posterior involvement of the pterygoid region and nasopharynx, and inferior spread to the oral cavity may all be encountered, generally along the routes of least resistance. Distant lymphatic and haematogenous spread are rare in the early stages of the disease and patients more often die of local disease before secondary spread is apparent.

Table 24.3 Sinonasal malignancy

Epithelial	Malignancy
Epidermoid/squamous	Carcinoma (spindle cell, verrucous, transitional)
Non-epidermoid	Adenoid cycstic carcinoma
	Adenocarcinoma
	Mucoepidermoid carcinoma
	Acinic cell carcinoma
	Metastases
Neuroectodermal	Malignant melanoma
	Olfactory neuroblastoma
Mesenchymal	
Vascular	Angiosarcoma
	Kaposi's carcoma
	Haemangiopericytoma
Muscular	Leiomyosarcoma
	Rhabdomyosarcoma
Cartilaginous	Chondrosarcoma (mesenchymal)
Osseous	Osteogenic sarcoma
Lymphoreticular	Burkitt's lymphoma
	Non-Hodgkin's lymphoma
	Extra-medullary plasmacytoma
	Midline destructive lesions
Miscellaneous	Fibrosarcoma
	Liposarcoma
	Malignant fibrous histiocytoma
	Ewing's sarcoma
	Alveolar soft part sarcoma

Presentation

From the maxilla the tumour may spread into the nasal cavity producing nasal obstruction and discharge (often serosanguinous). Anterior spread along the infra-orbital canal may produce pain and paresthesia. Orbital involvement produces displacement of the globe with:

• Proptosis
• Diplopia
• Epiphora
• Chemosis
• Visual loss

Inferior involvement of the dental roots may lead to loosening of the teeth and/or a malignant oro-antral fistula or a mass in the hard palate. Posterior extension into the pterygoid and infra-temporal fossa produces pain and trismus.

Spread from the ethmoid sinuses will involve the nasal cavity, contralateral ethmoid, and orbit with symptoms as described. Superior extension into the anterior cranial fossa is generally asymptomatic. The middle cranial fossa may be involved by direct spread from the anterior cranial fossa or orbital apex, whence a cavernous sinus syndrome may arise. Nasal cavity lesions, in addition to nasal symptoms, may spread posteriorly to obstruct the Eustachian tube producing a unilateral serous otitis media or anteriorly to erode and displace the nasal bones in the region of the glabella.

Surgical principles

The majority of tumours present late with involvement of important adjacent structures. Even histologically 'benign' tumours may be associated with significant morbidity and/or mortality at this site. The principle of oncological resection may be compromised by the proximity of vital structures. This, combined with the histological diversity in this area, necessitates specialist management.

Diagnosis and assessment of extent of disease relies upon expert imaging and histology. Ideally, CT scanning (direct coronal and axial cuts with intravenous contrast enhancement) combined with MRI should be undertaken. In addition, a chest X-ray and CT of the thorax, abdomen, and bone studies may be appropriate if occult primary or systemic metastases are suspected.

Biopsy should ideally be performed under general anaesthesia to obtain representative tissue. Tissue should also be removed via an endonasal endoscopic approach. Surgery alone, or in combination with radiotherapy, is required in the majority of cases. Surgical options include craniofacial resection, maxillectomy, or occasionally total rhinectomy, with or without orbital exenteration. Prosthetic rehabilitation should be undertaken immediately when the palate is sacrificed.

Radiotherapy

Radiotherapy may be given before or after surgery where appropriate. Care must be taken to shield the brain stem and orbit wherever possible. Megavoltage photons are optimally used, in a dose of 60–66 Gy in 30–33 fractions given over 6–6.5 weeks. The neck nodes do not require prophylactic treatment. Radiotherapy alone may be appropriate for patients unfit for radical surgery, but local control rates are inferior to combined treatment.

Chemotherapy

Although a number of agents (cisplatin, 5FU, methotrexate, bleomycin) have significant activity in recurrent or metastatic disease, with response rates reported of 30–70%, responses are often short-lived and the median survival in this setting is six months. Although response rates of 90% have been achieved with neo-adjuvant chemotherapy, no proven survival benefit has yet been shown. Concurrent chemo-irradiation is under investigation.

Eye and orbit

Although primary intra-ocular and orbital tumours are rare, malignant involvement of the eye is not unusual. Skin tumours often arise on the upper face and ocular involvement by metastatic disease may not be appreciated or may be ignored due to spread to more critical organs.

External eye—skin, lids, lacrimal glands

Basal cell carcinoma

Basal cell carcinomas occur frequently on the face and particularly around the eye. They have a predilection for the lower lid margin and adjacent inner canthus. It is unusual for the upper eyelid to be involved. Surgical excision, with either local transposition or graft repair, is often appropriate. However, in more extensive lesions or where surgery is contraindicated, radiotherapy can be given.

Radiotherapy can be used as primary treatment, following excision when the surgical margins are positive or where a recurrence has occurred. Superficial X-rays (100–150 kV) are appropriate (e.g. 45 Gy in 10 daily fractions). It is easy to protect the eye using an internal eye shield and lead cut-outs. Margins around the lesion should be 5 mm, but increased if electrons are used rather than orthovoltage X-rays.

If the nasolacrimal duct is involved by the tumour, epiphora will occur due to duct stenosis. Cannulation or stenting of the duct may be necessary later. However, carefully planned and fractionated radiotherapy should not, of itself cause duct stenosis.

Non-Hodgkin's lymphoma

Lymphoma may involve the upper and lower lids/conjunctiva, major lacrimal gland, or orbit. Most commonly it appears as a pink fleshy lesion on the conjunctiva. Occasionally it presents with bilateral involvement but with no other evidence of more widespread disease. It is important to carry out staging procedures including CT scan through the orbits.

Low-grade lymphoma with localized disease is treated with local radiotherapy; high-grade lymphoma with localized disease, with chemotherapy followed by local radiotherapy. Other stages are treated with chemotherapy. Radiotherapy technique and dose depend on the location, stage, and grade of the disease.

Squamous and adenocarcinoma

Squamous carcinoma arising from the skin, lids, or, very rarely, conjunctiva contribute approximately 5% of tumours of the external eye.

They can be treated with radiotherapy as already discussed, although more generous margins should be given. Squamous carcinoma can affect the eye by direct spread from adjacent sites such as the maxillary antrum and paranasal sinuses. Sebaceous and lacrimal gland tumours are rare and not particularly radio-sensitive. Primary treatment should be surgery.

Intra-ocular tumours

Melanoma

Melanoma can affect the uveal tract; its most frequent location is the choroid. Often the patient presents having attended the optician for a routine visit and a pigmented lesion has been noted. The patient may present with visual loss. Biopsies should not be performed. Diagnosis should be made by an ophthalmologist with experience in this field. Management should ideally be carried out in a combined ophthalmic–oncology clinic.

Treatment may be observation, radioactive eye plaque (ruthenium or iodine), local resection, charged particles (proton beam), or enucleation. A small lesion may represent a naevus so it is important to document growth. This is carried out by three-monthly examinations with indirect ophthalmoscopy and serial photographs. An increase in size of 1 mm is significant.

Treatment with Ruthenium 106 radioactive eye plaques causes less morbidity than iodine 125 plaques but can only treat tumours up to a maximum depth of 5 mm. Iodine plaques omit low-energy gamma-rays, so that tumours up to 8 mm depth can be treated. A dose of 80–100 Gy is given to the apex of the tumour, or 500 Gy to the base. Local resection and proton-beam irradiation are used for larger tumours.

Results after local resection have been shown to be better if a radioactive eye plaque is inserted at the end of the operation to irradiate the tumour bed. Proton-beam irradiation showed great promise but the treatment is expensive, time-consuming, and can be only used for very selected cases. The prognosis depends on the location of the tumour, tumour dimensions, and histology. Tumours with spindle B-cell elements do better than mixed epithelioid and spindle B tumours.

Retinoblastoma

This is a rare intra-ocular tumour arising in young children, usually in the first two years of their life. In a large number of cases the disease is hereditary and often bilateral. As with melanoma, the diagnosis is made by clinical appearance of the lesions. Therefore patients should be managed in combined clinics by ophthalmologists experienced in management of retinoblastoma. Biopsy should not be performed.

Diagnosis may be made by routine screening in those with a family history, by parents noticing their child had a squint or difficulty in visual fixation, or by a white reflex that is indicative of a large intra-ocular tumour.

Treatment

* Small tumours not adjacent to the macula or optic disc—photo-coagulation
* Small/moderate tumours—radioactive plaques (iodine, ruthenium plaques–40 Gy)
* Large or multiple tumours—external radiotherapy
* May need to radiate whole eye (40 Gy, 20 fractions over 4 weeks), try to maintain vision
* Occasionally enucleation is required
* Tumour is also chemosensitive—platinum
                                  —etoposide
                                  —vincristine
                                  —doxorubicin
                                  —cyclophosphamide
* Chemotherapy is useful if tumour has a bad prognosis or in neo-adjuvant setting
* Prognosis—90% survival; 80% of patients can have eye preserved

Optic nerve tumours

Optic nerve tumours are rare and usually their treatment is surgery. When excision is not possible high-dose radiotherapy can be given, usually using paired wedge fields and giving doses of the order of 55 Gy conventionally fractionated.

Rhabdomyosarcoma

This is a rare tumour but its most frequent location is the orbit.

Metastatic disease

Metastatic disease involving the eye is usually associated with choroidal metastases. The commonest tumours implicated are lung and breast. Presentation is usually with visual loss and sometimes pain. This is an oncological emergency. Treatment with radiotherapy should usually be with a lateral field to the orbit giving 20 Gy in five fractions over a week. The field may be angled five degrees posteriorly to avoid the contralateral lens. However, the prognosis is usually poor and cataract is not an issue.

Widespread bone metastases may affect the eye. This can lead to ocular pain, diplopia, and exophthalmos. When this occurs it is usually due to a breast primary, but does also occur with lung and prostate cancers. Systemic treatment is often appropriate, although local radiotherapy may be helpful.

Salivary gland tumours

Salivary gland tumours present initially as a painless lump within the substance of a salivary gland, as opposed to an enlargement of the whole gland. This is usually obvious with parotid gland tumours, but the outline of the submandibular salivary gland is more difficult to define and the differentiation between an enlarged gland and a lump in the gland is often impossible.

Pleomorphic adenoma (mixed parotid tumour)

This benign epithelial tumour is the most common tumour of the parotid gland. It may present at any age, normally as a painless, slowly growing, firm lump with a smooth surface with no deep tissue fixation. Rarely, the tumour may be soft and feel cystic. Distant metastases are very rare but local recurrence following enucleation is common. This is because the slowly expanding tumour compresses surrounding salivary tissue, forming a pseudo-capsule through which the tumour may penetrate. Occasionally this benign tumour can undergo malignant transformation.

Other benign tumours

Much less common benign tumours arising in the salivary gland include:

• Monomorphic adenoma

• Adenolymphoma

• Sebaceous lymphadenoma

• Oncocytoma

• Myoepithelioma

• Vascular tumours

The majority are clinical indistinguishable from pleomorphic adenoma, and their true nature is revealed only after pathological examination of a removed tumour.

Acinic cell and mucoepidermoid tumours

Whereas most of these tumours are microscopically low-grade, some are high-grade and more aggressive with local invasion and a tendency to metastasize to lymph nodes and through the bloodstream. Most present as a painless mass and a potentially malignant tumour is revealed only on microscopic examination after surgical removal. With wide removal, as recommended for the pleomorphic adenoma, the majority of well-differentiated tumours of this type will be cured.

Carcinomas

These may be immediately apparent clinically because of their more aggressive behaviour. Adenoid cystic carcinoma sometimes presents as a very slowly growing, painless mass of many years' duration. Epidermoid carcinoma occurs usually in adults but in the rare case in children the disease can be highly malignant.

Adenocarcinoma and undifferentiated carcinoma are usually aggressive. There is a particular tendency for salivary gland carcinomas, especially of the mucoepidermoid type, to infiltrate and spread along the perineural spaces. Eventually, all the characteristics of malignancy, including adherence to and infiltration of surrounding structures such as skin, muscle, and bone, develop. With parotid gland cancer, facial nerve malfunction is common. Submandibular gland cancers are more difficult to recognize pre-operatively.

Lymphoid tissue occurs within the parotid and submandibular glands where it may be involved with secondary carcinomatous spread, for example from the lung and breast. This also explains the occurrence of lymphoma, apparently within the salivary glands. Most commonly, however, there are other adjacent lymph nodes involved and biopsy confirms the diagnosis.

Management of clinically benign lumps

At least 50% of submandibular lumps prove to be malignant and the only logical treatment is therefore submandibular excision if suspicious. In the parotid, about 50% prove to be benign pleomorphic adenomas, but potentially malignant tumours may present with identical clinical features.

Investigations must provide reliable information on the relationship of a lump to the facial nerve and its branches, and of the histological diagnosis. Sialography is often performed but provides no such useful information. Ultrasound examination of salivary lumps is also misleading because both benign adenomas and carcinomas may have cystic areas. CT, in combination with tissue-density assessment studies, may be informative, but cannot provide an accurate diagnosis. However, CT or MRI scanning do help determine the extent of deep invasion.

Pre-operative histological diagnosis could refine management, but biopsy by incision or with a Tru-cut needle carries risks of tumour seeding. Fine-needle aspiration (FNA) cytology is probably risk-free but is not always helpful. Some 90% of FNA specimens are adequate and of these, the precise histological nature of a tumour cannot be determined in 10%. Thus FNA will provide a reliable diagnosis in about 80% of cases.

Parotidectomy

The aim of this operation is to remove the parotid lump with as wide a margin of normal tissue as possible while preserving the facial nerve.

Because tumour infiltration of the facial nerve may require a total parotidectomy, with sacrifice of the facial nerve trunk, patients must be warned of this possible outcome beforehand.

When a clinically unremarkable lump is removed by formal parotidectomy with a wide margin of normal tissue and is shown to be malignant, no further treatment is necessary with muco-epidermoid or acinic cell tumours. If histology reveals adenoid cystic or carcinoma, or if the margin of normal tissue is inadequate, then post-operative radiotherapy is advisable because of the known risks of perineural invasion and spread.

Management of clinically malignant lumps

The characteristic features of fixation to adjacent structures, facial nerve malfunction, and enlarged lymph glands are usually indications of malignancy. In this situation the diagnosis may be safely established by incisional biopsy. If malignancy is confirmed, the subsequent wide surgery will remove the biopsy wound and there will be no risk of tumour seeding.

Following microscopic confirmation, a CT or MRI scan will help to determine the local extent of the tumour. Treatment must be planned in conjunction with radiotherapy, faciomaxillary, and plastic surgery colleagues. Adjuvant radiotherapy is most commonly delivered post-operatively, but also as a split course, giving two-thirds of the treatment before and one-third after the operation.

Pre-operative radiotherapy has two advantages: a large tumour mass may shrink considerably, simplifying removal; and sometime an in-operable tumour will be rendered operable. However, surgery after radiotherapy is technically demanding.

Radiotherapy

Pleomorphic adenomas are essentially benign tumours. However, the rate of local recurrence after local enucleation has led to the use of post-operative radiotherapy by some; there is no proof that this is beneficial. A lapse of 10 years or more is seen in about half of all those patients who relapse. Better treatment is the removal of the lump with an adequate wide margin of normal tissue.

When a mucoepidermoid or acinic cell tumour is removed, there is no place for radiotherapy unless there is concern about the margin of normal tissue.

In malignant salivary gland tumours, post-operative radiotherapy reduces the incidence of local recurrence. With clinically malignant tumours arising in the parotid gland, post-operative radiotherapy is indicated when:

- The tumour is high-grade
- The surgical margins are close
- Resection has been performed for recurrent disease

• There is invasion of extra-parotid tissue
• There is regional node involvement
• There is gross residual post-operative disease

Orthodox radiotherapy techniques use 6–10 MV photons, often with a wedged pair of fields, to give a dose of 55–65 Gy over 6–7 weeks. The tumour volume will include the courses of adjacent cranial nerves up to the skull base, to control any perineural spread (which is particularly common with adenoid cystic carcinoma). Dryness of the mouth is usual but recovers if the opposite salivary glands are avoided. Trismus is common following treatment.

Pre-operative radiotherapy may be advantageous in the management of large tumours, particularly those considered to be inoperable. The situation should be reviewed after 45–50 Gy, when tumour shrinkage may have already made surgery possible. Split-course post-operative radiotherapy is given as soon as possible after healing—a further 20–25 Gy in 2–3 weeks.

Electron therapy has potential advantages in the treatment of parotid tumours. More recently other forms of particulate irradiation have been used, in particular neutrons. In a multi-centre randomized study of patients with locally advanced parotid gland cancer, with neutrons a local control rate of 67% was obtained, whereas the rate for photons was 17%.

Chemotherapy

Chemotherapy has no part in the management of low-grade salivary tumours. More aggressive tumours including mucoepidermoid, adenoid cystic, and undifferentiated carcinomas appear initially to respond well but these responses are short-lived. The most commonly used drugs are:

• Cisplatin
• 5-fluorouracil

Table 24.4 Results of treatment of salivary gland tumours

Histology	5-yr survival (%)
Acinic cell	92
Mucoepidermoid (low-grade)	76
Adenocarcinoma	66
Adenoid cystic	50
Squamous cell	50
Mucoepidermoid (high-grade)	46
Undifferentiated	33

- Doxorubicin
- Cyclophosphamide

Adjuvant or neo-adjuvant therapy has not been fully evaluated.

Further reading

Ho, J.H. (1978) An epidemiologic and clinical study of nasopharynx carcinoma. *Int J Radiat Oncol Biol Phys* **4**, 182–98.

International Nasopharynx Cancer Study Group. (1996) Preliminary results of a randomized trial comparing neoadjuvant chemotherapy (cisplatin, epirubicin and bleomycin) plus radiotherapy vs. radiotherapy alone in Stage IV (> or = N_2, M_0) undifferentiated nasopharynx carcinoma. A positive effect on progression-free survival. *Int J Radiat Oncol Biol Phys* **35**, 463–9.

Teo, P., Tsao, S.Y., Shiu, W., *et al.* (1989) A clinical study of 407 cases of nasopharyngeal carcinoma in Hong Kong. *Int J Radiat Oncol Biol Phys* **17**, 515–30.

Chapter 25
Tumours of the central nervous system

Primary brain tumours

Aetiology

The majority of primary brain tumours are sporadic. Gliomas and meningiomas may be induced by radiation, and there is an association between primary CNS lymphoma and immunosuppression, including AIDS. There are other candidate aetiological agents, but none has been proven and all remain controversial:

- Industrial and agricultural chemicals
- Electro-magnetic fields
- Viruses
- Trauma

Epidemiology

The incidence worldwide is very uniform with a few exceptions such as a higher incidence of pineal tumours in Japan and CNS lymphoma in the AIDS population of the West coast of the US. Recent reports suggest the incidence of glioma and (non-AIDS) lymphoma is increasing in developed countries. Primary brain tumours occur at any age but display two peaks. One occurs in children, where they are the most common solid tumour, and the other in (late) middle age.

Pathology

Primary brain tumour pathology is extremely varied reflecting diverse histogenesis. The most widely used classification system is the WHO 1993 scheme. Gliomas are the most common tumours. Their behaviour and prognosis are strongly linked to histological subtype. Benign tumours (e.g. meningiomas) are not uncommon and some malignant non-glial tumours carry a good prognosis (medulloblastoma, pineal

Table 25.1 Syndromes associated with primary brain tumours

Predisposing syndrome	Tumour
Neurofibromatosis type 1	Glioma
Neurofibromatosis type 2	Glioma, meningioma, Schwannoma
Li–Fraumeni syndrome	Glioma
von Hippel–Lindau syndrome	Cerebellar haemangioblastoma
Gardener's syndrome	Glioma
Familial glioma	Glioma
Tuberose sclerosis	Subependymal giant cell astrocytoma

germinoma). Precise histological identification is therefore essential to appropriate management.

Primary brain tumours rarely metastasize outside the CNS but are highly infiltrative, with a tendency to spread along white matter tracts to more distant regions of the brain, a feature which contributes to their resistance to treatment. Spread through cerebrospinal fluid (CSF) to remote areas of the neuraxis is a feature of germ cell tumours, medulloblastoma, and other primitive neuroectodermal tumours. This has important implications for their treatment.

The dominant prognostic features for the majority of brain tumours are usually a combination of histological type and clinical features such as age and performance status. Therefore, staging systems that are commonly used for other tumour types are rarely used for brain tumours.

Molecular changes associated with glioblastoma are:

* Type 1—loss of tumour suppression (p53 mutation in 65%)
    —oncogene upregulation
    —chromosome changes
    —younger patients
    —may arise in pre-existing low-grade tumour
    —better prognosis
* Type 2—mainly chromosome changes
    —oncogene overexpression
    —older patients
    —poor prognosis

Presentation

Brain tumours present either with neurological dysfunction or with signs of raised intracranial pressure. Presentation with epilepsy or with slow onset of symptoms carries a relatively favourable prognosis.

Table 25.2 Abbreviated WHO (1993) classification of intracranial gliomas

Subgroup	Grade or type	Prognosis
Astrocytoma	Pilocytic	Excellent
	Low-grade	Good
	Anaplastic	Poor
	Glioblastoma	Very poor
Oligodendroglioma	Low-grade	Good
	Anaplastic	Poor
Ependymoma	Low-grade	Good
	Anaplastic	Poor

Table 25.3 Presenting symptom in patients with intracranial glioma

Symptom	Frequency as principle presenting symptom (%)	Overall frequency at presentation (%)
Epilepsy	30	53
Headache	25	71
Cognitive distance	12	52
Motor disturbance	8	43
Speech disturbance	5	27
Clouding of consciousness	4	25
Visual disturbance	4	25
Sensory change	2	14
Miscellaneous	10	

Investigation is dominated by brain imaging. Maximal tumour resolution in structural imaging involves full-sequence magnetic resonance scanning with gadolinium enhancement. Contrast-enhanced CT is more readily available and frequently adequate. Functional imaging with SPEC, PET, and MR are gaining importance both in diagnosis and assessment of response to treatment. The imaging agents [201]thallium and ^{123}I-tyrosine in SPECT scanning and [18]FDG glucose in PET give important insights into the functional activity of the tumour and can frequently aid differentiation between high- or low-grade neoplasms and treatment-induced necrosis. Tumours that spread via CSF pathways require whole neuraxis MRI.

Treatment options

Surgery alone is the treatment of choice for most benign lesions though additional radiotherapy is appropriate after incomplete resection in some (e.g. pituitary adenoma or meningioma). Low-grade astrocytomas presenting with epilepsy alone and without mass effect on scan can often be managed medically; the development of other neurological symptoms or imaging evidence of growth or transformation are indications for surgery. The role of radiotherapy for these tumours remains controversial though treatment is frequently given following partial resection.

Suspected high-grade gliomas require surgery for histological confirmation. This may be with stereotactic biopsy or, where possible, by craniotomy and debulking of tumour. Whilst resection is often valuable for relief of pressure symptoms its value in tumour control is more contentious. 'Blind' burr-hole biopsy carries a high risk of morbidity. Without further treatment the median survival for patients with anaplastic astrocytoma or glioblastoma is approximately one year and three months respectively. Radiotherapy improves median survival to three years for anaplastic tumours and one year for glioblastoma.

Post-operative radiotherapy is normally given, except in elderly patients or those with low performance status when the prognosis is too poor irrespective of treatment. The area irradiated is usually limited to tumour-bearing brain and doses of 30–60 Gy are given over 2–6 weeks depending on prognostic factors.

Chemotherapy adds little, if any, advantage in the adjuvant setting and is usually reserved for relapse. The nitrosoureas (BCNU, CCNU) are the most common agents used. Procarbazine and the platinum compounds and Temozolomide may also have some value.

Medulloblastoma is managed by resection followed by cranio-spinal radiotherapy; the role of chemotherapy is currently being explored. Overall, 50% of patients are disease-free at five years. Similar approaches are required for ependymomas and supratentorial primitive neuro-ectodermal tumours.

Patients with brain tumours suffer a wide variety of related physical, cognitive, and emotional problems. Prominent are:

• Movement disorders

• Tumour-associated epilepsy

• Pain (headache)

• Speech disorders

• Intellectual decline

These are best managed jointly by the GP and a specialized unit with access to a dedicated tumour surgeon, a neuro-oncologist, a neurologist, a nurse specialist, and rehabilitation team, whose intentions are to maximize the quality of life as well as delivering optimal therapy to improve survival. Early involvement of the palliative care team can be valuable.

Recent advances and future treatments

Surgery and radiotherapy remain the mainstays of treatment for these tumours and most advances involve applying these modalities more effectively to more precisely delineated tumours. Prominent in surgery is the use of neuro-navigation, where recently acquired images of the patient's brain and tumour are projected intra-operatively onto the operating field. Laser or ultrasound resection allows the identified tumour to be completely resected. The use of intra-operative, photo-activated, cytotoxic compounds to improve the tumour clearance further is being investigated. Following surgical clearance the application into the resection cavity of sustained-release chemotherapy (BCNU-Gliadel) has shown some survival benefit.

The availability of stereotactic localization and beam conformation allow an identified intracranial target to be more accurately delineated and irradiated with consequent sparing of normal brain tissue. This sparing in turn allows for an escalation of dose to the tumour with the possibility of greater tumour control. These techniques are currently being evaluated. Third generation radiation sensitizers such as the hypoxic cell cytotoxin, tirapazamine, have shown some early promise in glioblastoma. The rationale for using angiogenesis inhibitors in the brain is strong. The drug thalidomide has shown early activity and new generation drugs are in development.

Conventional chemotherapy has been disappointing in brain tumours. However, modification of the local environment with O-6-alkylguanine DNA alkyltransferase inhibitors or blood–brain barrier modifiers may improve the poor results seen with the nitrosoureas or platinum compounds. Some new compounds (e.g. temozolomide) have shown activity.

The brain has been an intensive research target in the use of gene therapy, much of it involving the HSVtk/Acyclovir suicide gene system. Many other therapeutic strategies are possible but the lack of effective vectors currently limits the applicability of this approach. The prospect of using adenovirus or herpes simplex virus might overcome the limitations inherent in the current retroviral approaches and represents the greatest hope currently for an improvement in the management of malignant gliomas.

Brain metastases

Incidence

Metastasis to the brain from an extracranial primary is common. Symptomatic metastases have an incidence of around 6 per 100 000, but autopsy studies have revealed an overall incidence in 24% of patients with known cancer. There is a slight male preponderance and the incidence increases with age.

Whilst brain metastases may arise from any primary site, the most common are from the respiratory tract (50%), breast (15%), and melanoma (10%). In (at least) 10% the primary site is unknown. Some cancers which commonly metastasize to other organs rarely involve the brain e.g. prostate, bladder, cervix, and ovary. The reason for this is not known. Rare tumours that have a predilection for the brain include choriocarcinoma and clear cell renal cancer. Carcinomatous meningitis is less common but may occur in:

- Leukaemia
- Lymphoma
- Cancers of the lung and breast

Pathology

- Site—80% in cerebral hemispheres
    —15% in cerebellum
    —5% in other sites e.g. basal ganglia
- Macroscopically—discrete
    —circumscribed
    —areas of bleeding, necrosis, cystic
    —50% are multiple
- Histology—similar to primary
    —vascular proliferation, tumour necrosis common
    —usually well demarcated from adjacent tissue

Presentation

The presentation of brain metastases is similar to that of primary brain tumours with the additional complication that the patient may be unwell with systemic disease. The most sensitive investigation is high-resolution contrast-enhanced MR scan.

Metastases most frequently appear as multiple, discrete, well-demarcated lesions that are hypo-intense on T1 and hyper-intense on T2 and with marked gadolinium enhancement. There is often copious surrounding vasogenic oedema. Up to 20% of lesions revealed in this way are not seen on CT scan where visible lesions again appear as discrete, enhancing masses.

Various reports have suggested that brain metastases are solitary in 20–50% of cases.

Management

Initial management requires control of the presenting symptoms, with anti-convulsants, analgesics, and other medication as appropriate. Dexamethasone is indicated in the majority of patients and frequently produces a reversal of symptoms. A starting dose of 8–16 mg daily is common and improvement can often be maintained with doses of 2–4 mg. The failure of a response to dexamethasone may be an argument against more aggressive therapy.

Since the outcome for patients with multiple adverse prognostic factors is so poor, irrespective of treatment, it is reasonable to manage those individuals with symptomatic therapy alone. For patients whose condition is improved following dexamethasone, treatment with radiotherapy can be offered. This approach may produce temporary tumour control, improve survival, and allow a reduction in the steroid dose. Typically, the whole brain is irradiated. A dose of 20 Gy in five fractions has been shown to be as effective as any of the more protracted fractionation schemes.

Solitary metastases should be considered differently in an otherwise fit patient, especially if originating from a primary with 'good prognosis' histology. Here, tumour resection, where possible, is the treatment of choice. The growth pattern of brain metastases often allows complete macroscopic removal to be achieved. Post-operatively, whole-brain radiotherapy is given (20 Gy in 5 fractions or 30 Gy in 10 fractions) with or without a local boost. An alternative approach is to offer stereotactic radiosurgery (20 Gy in a single fraction), again with whole-brain radiotherapy to follow. Although it is conventionally given, the value of additional whole-brain treatment is not determined.

Chemotherapy can be useful in patients with brain metastases from chemo-sensitive primaries. It should be used as first-line therapy (or following resection) in germ cell tumours or as an alternative to radiation in small cell lung cancer and lymphoma. It can also be used as second-line treatment in less chemo-sensitive tumours such as breast cancer. The disruption of the blood–brain barrier by the tumour means that agents normally used to treat systemic metastases in these diseases may be tried, with response in about 30%.

Outcome

Overall, the prognosis is poor for patients with brain metastases from the common cancers. For patients with poor prognostic features, the median survival may be only 6–8 weeks, irrespective of treatment. At the opposite end, patients with 'good prognosis', solitary metastases

Table 25.4 Prognostic factors for patients with brain metastases

Factor	Description	Influence
Age	Increasing age (>50)	Adverse
Performance status	Poor general condition	Adverse
	Fixed neurological deficit	Adverse
Histology	Adenocarcinoma	Favourable
	Squamous (esp. lung)	Adverse
	Germ cell	Very favourable
Number	Solitary	Favourable
	Multiple	Adverse
Size	Small	Favourable
	Large	Unfavourable
Operability	Resectable	Favourable

that are adequately treated with surgery and radiotherapy enjoy a much better outlook, with many surviving two years or more.

Further reading

Davies, E. and Hopkins, A. (ed.) (1997) Royal College of Physicians, *Improving care for patients with malignant glioma* London.

Kleihues, P. and Cavenee, W.K. (ed.) (1997) *Pathology and genetics: tumours of the nervous system.* International Agency for Research on Cancer, Lyon.

Chapter 26
Skin cancer

Primary cutaneous malignant melanoma

Definition

Primary cutaneous malignant melanoma arises from the melanocytes found in the basal layer of skin. These cells produce melanin pigment and are responsible for producing the tanning response after exposure to ultraviolet radiation.

Aetiology

• Excess exposure to UV radiation

• Genetic susceptibility—CDKN2A found on chromosome 9 (tumour suppressor gene)

• 33% of patients with familial melanoma have mutations of CDKN2A

Incidence

The incidence of melanoma in the UK is around 10 new cases per 100 000 per year—approximately 6000 patients annually.

Clinical presentation

Primary melanoma of the skin presents as a growing, irregular brown or black lesion on the skin. Important features to alert clinical suspicion include an irregular outline to the lesion; irregular pigmentation containing shades of brown, black, and red; and, occasionally, oozing or crusting. Most melanomas are around 5 mm in diameter when first recognized but a small number are identified at an earlier stage. They may arise on previously normal skin or on a previously apparently benign melanocytic naevus.

Pathology

Pathological examination shows neoplastic melanocytic cells invading beneath the basement membrane into the underlying dermis. The depth to which these cells have invaded can be measured accurately from the granular layer of the epidermis to the deepest invading cell. This is referred to as the tumour thickness or *Breslow thickness* and is the most important prognostic feature. For patients with tumours thinner than 1.5 mm, the five-year disease-free survival rate is over 90%, but those with tumours thicker than 3.5 mm have less than 50% chance of survival even after appropriate and adequate surgery.

Staging

The current UICC staging of melanoma divides the tumour into four stages.

- **Stage 1:** tumours less than 1.5 mm thick
- **Stage 2:** primary tumour thicker than 1.5 mm
- **Stage 3:** tumour spread to the local draining lymph nodes
- **Stage 4:** distant disease

Prognosis for patients with Stage 3 and 4 disease is poor, with only 25% disease-free two-year survival for Stage 3 and around 6% two-year survival for Stage 4.

Differential diagnosis

Growing pigmented lesions on the skin can be divided into benign and malignant. Benign lesions are more common, including benign melanocytic naevi in young adults and seborrhoeic keratoses in older adults. A small excision biopsy is frequently necessary to differentiate between these benign lesions and malignant melanoma.

Treatment

The treatment for primary malignant melanoma is complete excision of the lesion. There is still controversy and ongoing trials to establish the exact margin of excision of normal skin necessary around the lesion. This is generally tailored to the tumour thickness with tumours thinner than 1 mm requiring only 1 cm of normal skin; tumours between 1–2 mm thick are often excised with a margin of 2 cm of normal skin; and the largest margin recommended, even for very thick tumours, is 3 cm of normal skin. It is important that excision is adequate in depth as well as at the lateral margins.

Most patients with primary melanoma currently have the defect resulting from excision of the lesion closed directly, but a small number may require either a flap or a graft to achieve closure.

Patients with Stage 3 disease should have dissection of the regional lymph nodes. At present there is one study suggesting that adjuvant alpha interferon, given subcutaneously for one year after lymph node dissection, statistically improves survival for this group of patients. Confirmatory trials are in progress.

For patients with Stage 4 disease there is no current accepted proven chemotherapy or immunotherapy. All patients should be accurately staged with CT or MRI as appropriate. Limited additional surgical procedures to debulk the tumour will often improve the patient's quality of life. Chemotherapy regimes include DTIC and/or vindesine and produce around 30% response rate, but responses are short-lived and do not signficiantly increase survival time. A recent study suggesting that the addition of tamoxifen to combination chemotherapy for melanoma improved response rates has not been confirmed. Trials are concentrating on the use of biotherapy that includes the use of interleukin 2, often combined with melanoma-directed vaccines.

Melanoma is in general not responsive to radiotherapy, but good palliation can be achieved in the case of pain from skeletal metastases. Cerebral metastases are relatively common in long-term survivors from melanoma. If these are asymptomatic there is controversy as to whether or not they should be treated. In some centres neurosurgery to one or two isolated metastases is practised. If cerebral metastases are symptomatic, systemic corticosteroid therapy, with or without additional radiotherapy, may bring symptomatic relief.

Experimental surgical approaches

• Adjuvant limb perfusion—melphalan alone
  —melphalan + tumour necrosis factor
  —good palliation for recurrent melanoma
  —no survival advantage for primary melanoma
• Sentinel node biopsy—radio-labelled colloid
  —methylene Blue
  —if this node is clear then block dissection is not required

Non-melanoma skin cancers

Epidemiology

These cancers are the commonest malignancies in Western populations, occurring particularly in fair-skinned Caucasians exposed to
ultraviolet radiation (e.g. farmers, fishermen). The causes are:

+ Ultraviolet radiation
+ Ionizing radiation
+ Chronic inflammation
+ Human papillomavirus
+ Immunosuppression
+ Hereditary conditions (Xeroderma pigmentosum, basal cell naevus
  syndrome)

As well as these primary lesions, metastases to skin are fairly common
from carcinomas of the breast, lung, and GI tract.

Pathology

Basal cell carcinomas (75% of non-melanoma skin cancers) are lesions
which arise on sun-exposed areas—face, neck, ears, scalp, and arms.
They are normally confined to hair-bearing skin. They present as a slow-
growing, pink papule with telangiectasia. Variant lesions include:

+ Nodular
+ Ulcerative
+ Pigmented
+ Superficial
+ Cystic
+ Morphoeic
+ Multicentric

Metastases are rare and they are usually curable by either surgical excision or radiotherapy. The latter is preferred around the eyelids, nose,
lips, and ears. Other treatment strategies are cryosurgery and topical
5-fluorouracil.

Squamous cell carcinoma (20%): this malignant lesion also arises on
sun-exposed sites, but appears as a faster-growing, red papule which
may erupt on a background of actinic keratosis. Ulceration, bleeding,
and metastases to regional nodes may occur. Treatment is either
surgery or radiotherapy; chemotherapy has been used for disseminated disease (cisplatin, methotrexate, 5-fluorouracil, bleomycin are
active agents).

Merkel cell carcinoma is a rare but highly malignant neuroendocrine tumour of the skin. It presents as a dermal nodule on the head or neck of an elderly patient, rarely ulcerates, but commonly spreads to adjacent skin and regional nodes. Treatment is surgical but palliative radiotherapy is useful in controlling metastatic disease. Less than 50% survive three years.

Apocrine and eccrine gland cancers: a variety of these are described but all are rare and most are only locally invasive.

Other uncommon malignancies are:

- Cutaneous angiosarcoma
- Kaposi's sarcoma (HIV-associated or endemic)
- Other soft tissue malignancies

Further reading

Kirkwood, J.M., *et al.* (1996) Interferon alfa-2b adjuvant therapy of high risk resected cutaneous melanoma: the Eastern Cooperative Oncology Group Trial EST 1684. *J Clin. Oncol.* **14**, 7–17.

Chapter 27
Haematological malignancies

Acute leukaemia

Epidemiology

The incidence of acute leukaemia is 4–7 cases per 100 000. The peak incidence of acute lymphoblastic leukaemia (ALL) is 3–4 years and of acute myeloid leukaemia (AML) is over 60 years.

Aetiology

The cause of most cases is unknown. Some inherited diseases carry an increased risk:

- Fanconi's anaemia
- Bloom's syndrome
- Klinefelter's syndrome
- Ataxia telangiectasia

There is a 3–5 times increased risk in identical twins.

Environmental factors such as ionizing radiation, chemical carcinogens, or chemotherapeutic drugs, and infectious agents (e.g. T-cell leukaemia virus 1 in the Caribbean or Japan) or more subtle mechanisms such as exposure in the very young of naive immune systems to infections, have all been implicated as rare causes.

Diagnosis and classification

Peripheral blood pancytopenia is the commonest finding, but a minority have an elevated white blood cell count (WBC) which may be a clinical manifestation of anaemia, bleeding, or infection. There may be associated adenopathy or hepatosplenomegaly, which is more likely in lymphoid disease.

A marrow examination using morphology, immunophenotyping, and cytogenetics will allow classification into myeloid or lymphoid leukaemia, with morphological subtypes related to cell maturity (designated FAB 0–7 for myeloid and L1–3 for lymphoid disease). CNS infiltration can be a feature of ALL and requires a diagnostic lumbar puncture.

Acute lymphoblastic leukaemia (ALL)

ALL is the commonest cancer in children but is responsive to effective treatment, with a 70% cure rate. Adult disease responds less well, with only 30% long-term survivors.

Chemotherapy

Induction of remission is routinely achieved by combining vincristine, prednisolone, and L-asparaginase. Additional anthracycline is used in adults. Remission rates are 90–95% in children and a little less in adults. Initial response to treatment can predict outcome e.g. remission within two weeks has a favourable outlook whereas failure to gain remission by four weeks of chemotherapy predicts a poor prognosis. Such findings reflect the use of more sophisticated molecular methods.

Consolidation is a crucial phase during which exposure to new drugs (e.g. cyclophosphamide, thioguanine, cytosine arabinoside) is a key strategy as is clearance of the CNS as a sanctuary site. This may be achieved by CNS irradiation or MTX intra-thecally or in high-dose IV.

In high-risk cases there remains a 10% risk of CNS relapse and there are concerns about the long-term effects of different treatment modalities.

Maintenance

For about two years patients in remission continue on a cyclical schedule of methotrexate, 6 thioguanine, vincristine, and prednisolone.

Prognostic factors

- Adverse factors—male sex
  —older age
  —age <1 year
  —high blast count
  —hypodiploidy
  —Philadelphia chromosome positive
- Good prognostic factors—cure rate 50%
- Bad prognostic factors—cure rate 20%

Treatment of high-risk disease

Various approaches are in use for high-risk disease. Intensification in consolidation with cyclophosphamide or methotrexate in higher dosage has brought some success. Stem cell transplantation in first remission will cure 50% (allograft) or 30% (autograft)—but insufficient prospective comparisons with intensified conventional chemotherapy have been undertaken. When treatment fails, outcome depends on age and length of first remission. In children with long remissions, further chemotherapy may achieve salvage, for others stem cell transplant is indicated.

Acute myeloid leukaemia (AML)

In clinical practice, three factors will be taken into account in establishing the diagnosis:

- Acute promyelocytic leukaemia must be identified at diagnosis to ensure that retinoic acid is included in the treatment schedule.
- The patient's age.
- The clinical condition or performance score. It is now usual that patients under 60 years are given intensive treatment that may

include stem cell transplantation. Older patients constitute the majority, and some patients are not considered suitable for intensive treatment and are offered a palliative approach.

Chemotherapy

Anthracycline and cytosine arabinoside, given over 7–10 days, has been the backbone of treatment for 30 years. The addition of a third drug (thioguanine or etoposide) is widely used, but there is little evidence that one or other is superior. There is recent interest in giving higher ara-C doses in induction but without definite evidence of benefit.

Successful induction depends on patient age (90% in children, 75% 50–60 years, 65% 60–70 years)—70–80% of all patients achieve complete response with the first course. Three or four further intensive courses incorporating other drugs (e.g. amsacrine, etoposide, idarubicin, mitoxantrone, and araC at higher doses) are usually given. It is not at present clear how many courses of consolidation is optimum. Older patients seldom tolerate more than two.

Maintenance treatment has become unfashionable—but may become of renewed interest for the elderly.

Prognostic factors

A number of characteristics can identify different risks of relapse and therefore survival. Most powerful of these are cytogenetics, patient age, and initial response of marrow blasts to treatment. Other factors are also important:

- Male sex
- High WBC on presentation
- Greater age
- Less cellular differentiation
- Leukaemia secondary to prior chemotherapy
- Myelodysplasia

Favourable cytogenetics are t(8;21), t(15;17), inv(16) that tend to be associated with young age and comprise about 25% of patients under 60 years. Adverse cytogenetics are abnormalities of chs 5 or 7 3q- or more complex abnormalities that tend to be more frequent in older patients and are associated with therapy-related leukaemia and prior MDS. A chemoresistance phenotype of P-glycoprotein overexpression occurs particularly in the elderly and is associated with a lower rate of remission and higher relapse risk.

Stem cell transplantation

If the patient is under 45 years and has an HLA-matched sibling, allogeneic transplantation of blood or bone marrow stem cells will be considered. In good-risk patients this is only used when patients fail first-line treatment, but is given as consolidation in other groups.

Acute promyelocytic leukaemia

This is a separate entity having FAB-M3 morphology, the t(15:17) rearrangement creating the PML-RAR fusion gene. All-transretinoic acid (ATRA) used alone can induce remission by differentiation without hypoplasia but is not curative. Additional chemotherapy, either given with or subsequent to chemotherapy, remains essential. The level of the WBC at diagnosis is of key importance. Low count patients given ATRA and chemotherapy will have 80% survival. The 25% of patients who present with higher WBC have a high risk of early death and only 60% survival.

Autologous transplantation has been widely used to consolidate first remissions with results almost equivalent to allogeneic BMT. It is available to older patients (up to 60 years) and those without donors. It appears to be superior to chemotherapy, except in children, where it adds little.

Treatment outcome

Remission is achieved in 80% of patients under 60 years, and 60–65% of patients over 60 years. Survival is age-related and will depend on prognostic factors. Most patients will relapse, but the patient's age, length of first CR, and initial cytogenetic risk group will dictate outcome. If first remission is short and cytogenetics are not favourable in older patients, the outlook is grave.

Future prospects

AML is a heterogenous disease and it is likely that subtypes require risk-directed therapy. Arsenic compounds may find a role in AML; there will be refinements in the techniques of stem cell transplantation; and immunologically based approaches will be evaluated. The disease in the elderly remains a major challenge. It must be established which patients benefit from an intensive approach and improved non-intensive treatment is needed. Modulation of molecular resistance is theoretically possible and will be evaluated in the next few years.

Chronic lymphoid leukaemias

Heterogeneous group of conditions associated with accumulation of lymphoid cells in the peripheral blood. Classified by morphology, surface immunophenotype, cytogenetics, and molecular biology. Some lymphomas may present with lymphoid cells in the blood and bone marrow infiltration.

B-cell chronic lymphocytic leukaemia

Common leukaemia of late middle-age and old age with accumulation of small, mature-looking B lymphocytes in the peripheral blood, bone marrow, and lymphatic tissues.

Accounts for 30–40% of all leukaemias diagnosed in adults in Europe and North America. Annual incidence, 2.5 per 100 000; male to female ratio 2:1; median age at diagnosis 65–70 years; 79% of patients over 60 years of age at diagnosis; only 6% under 50 years.

Environmental associations:

- Farming (especially soya bean, cattle, diary, herbicide use)
- Rubber manufacture
- Abestos
- Tyre-repair
- Carbon tetrachloride exposure

Table 27.1 Chronic lymphoid leukaemias (CLL)

B-cell

B-cell chronic lymphocytic leukaemia/small lymphocytic lymphoma

B-cell prolymphocytic leukaemia

Hairy-cell leukaemia and variants

Splenic lymphoma with villous lympocytes

Leukaemic phase of mantle cell lymphoma

Leukaemic phase of follicle centre cell lymphoma

Leukaemic phase of lymphoplasmacytoid lymphoma

T-cell

T-cell chronic lymphocytic leukaemia (large granular lymphocytic leukaemia)

T-cell prolymphocytic leukaemia

Adult T-cell leukaemia/lymphoma

Leukaemic phase of mycosis fungoides/Sézary syndrome

Genetic factors may predominate—compare, for example, the low incidence of CLL in Japanese people both in Japan and after emigration.

Clone expansion is due to prolonged survival of CLL cells through failure to respond to apoptotic signals rather than through proliferative advantage; CLL cells constitutively express high levels of Bcl-2 protein, inhibiting apoptosis.

Pathology

Gradual accumulation of small lymphocytes in the lymph nodes, spleen, bone marrow, and blood causing slowly progressive enlargement of the lymph nodes and spleen and bone marrow infiltration with anaemia, thrombocytopenia, and neutropenia (important prognostic factors at diagnosis). Other features:

• Sometimes autoimmune haemolytic anaemia
• Evan's syndrome
• Hypogammaglobulinaemia
• Disorders of T-lymphocyte function are common

Clinical presentation

Variable but generally indolent clinical course. Now usually diagnosed early, often after routine blood count or presentation with painless lymphadenopathy, anaemia, or infection. Constitutional symptoms restricted to patients with advanced disease.

Lymphadenopathy is symmetrical, often generalized. Splenomegaly at presentation in 66%; hepatomegaly much less frequent at presentation but common in advanced disease; involvement of other organs infrequent at diagnosis.

Diagnosis

Clear criteria for the diagnosis of CLL. Surface antigen immunophenotyping is essential to exclude reactive causes (usually T-lymphocytosis) and lymphocytosis due to other lymphoid neoplasms.

Management

No evidence that treatment prolongs survival of patients with lymphocytosis or uncomplicated lymphadenopathy. Systemic therapy is indicated for advanced disease and those with diffuse infiltration on the trephine biopsy or a low lymphocyte doubling time (<12 months), irrespective of stage.

NCI Working Party guidelines are to initiate treatment if:

• Constitutional symptoms referable to CLL (weight loss >10% in 6 months, fatigue or performance score 2 or worse, fever without overt infection, night sweats)
• Symptomatic lymphadenopathy; symptomatic hepatosplenomegaly
• Progressive anaemia with haemoglobin <10 g/dl

Table 27.2 NCI Working Group revised criteria for diagnosis of CLL

Peripheral blood lymphocytosis:	(1) absolute lymphocyte count >5 × 10⁹/l
	(2) morphologically mature appearing cells
Characteristic phenotype:	(1) predominance of CD19+, CD20+, CD23+ and CD5+ B-cells
	(2) light chain restriction i.e. monoclonal — or λ expression
	(3) low-density surface immunoglobulin (sIg) expression
Bone marrow examination:	>30% lymphocytes in bone marrow if peripheral blood lymphocytosis is relatively low i.e. close to 5 × 10⁹/l

- Progressive thrombocytopenia with platelets <100 × 10⁹/l
- Progressive lymphocytosis >300 × 10⁹/l or rapid rate of increase
- Autoimmune disease refractory to prednisolone
- Repeated infections with or without hypogammaglobulinaemia

Chlorambucil

Remains first-line therapy. Generally produces a partial response: reduction in peripheral blood lymphocytosis and improvement in haemoglobin and platelet count, shrinking of lymphadenopathy and splenomegaly, and improvement in constitutional symptoms in >50% of patients. Complete responses rare.

Discontinue when normal lymphocyte count is achieved or continue as long as patient responds, usually some 6–12 months. Restart on progression.

Median survival in responding patients, four years.

Corticosteroids

Single-agent prednisolone (1 mg/kg/day) produces reduction in lymphocytic infiltration of bone marrow and can result in significant improvement in cytopenia and symptoms. Useful initial treatment (1–2 weeks) for patients with advanced disease and pancytopenia at diagnosis.

Combination chemotherapy

No survival advantage of COP[†] or CHOP[†] over chlorambucil. Higher response rate in advanced disease. Response rate low when resistant to chlorambucil. Purine analogues better second-line therapy.

[†] COP: Cyclophosphamide, Oncovin (vincristine); Prednisolone;
   CHOP: Cyclophosphamide, Adriamycin, Oncovin, Prednisolone.

Purine analogues

Effective treatment of CLL. Cause profound depletion of normal lymphocytes especially CD4+ T-cells and predispose to opportunistic infection, in particular *P. carinii, Listeria monocytogenes, M. tuberculosis, Norcardia* and herpes viruses.

Single-agent **fludarabine** produces higher response rate than chlorambucil—previously untreated patients (70 vs. 40%), CR rate (27 vs. 3%), and disease-free survival (33 vs. 17 months). Also effective in previously treated patients (31–57% response rate, 13% CRs). No evidence of improved overall survival. Generally administered at a dose of 25 mg/m^2 Intravenously for 5 days on a 4–6 week cycle until maximum response or 6 cycles. Complications include:

- Myelosuppression
- Prolonged CD4+ T-lymphocytopenia
- Infection
- Autoimmune haemolysis

Routine prophylaxis of *P. carinii* pneumonia with either co-trimoxazole or pentamidine advisable for one year after treatment, with or without acyclovir prophylaxis of *Herpes zoster* reactivation. Caution is needed in patients with previous history of autoimmune haemolysis.

Fludarabine is an option for first-line therapy and also an effective second-line therapy for alkylator-resistant CLL.

Radiotherapy

Effective local treatment for lymph nodes compromising vital organ function. Splenic irradiation is effective for painful splenomegaly, though splenectomy better for massive splenomegaly if patient is fit for surgery.

Splenectomy

Effective for massive splenomegaly, anaemia, or thrombocytopenia due to hypersplenism and for autoimmune haemolytic anaemia refractory to prednisolone and cytotoxic therapy

Hodgkin's disease

Epidemiology and aetiology

Hodgkin's disease (HD) is a rare malignancy, with an annual UK incidence of 1000–1500 new cases. The age distribution is bimodal, with a large peak in the 20–30 year age group, and a smaller peak at 50–60 years. The cause is unknown, and may differ between the various histological subtypes. An association between infection with Epstein–Barr virus and HD is well documented, although its precise aetiological role is unclear.

Pathology

The characteristic diagnostic feature is the binucleate Reed–Sternberg (RS) cell, seen in an appropriate cellular background of small lymphocytes, eosinophils, neutrophils, histiocytes, and plasma cells. The RS cell is the malignant cell in HD, and recent molecular studies have confirmed its B-cell lineage. The major subtypes are:

+ Nodular sclerosing (NS) (~50%)
+ Mixed cellularity (MC) (30-40%)
+ Lymphocyte/histiocyte predominant (LP, HP) (~10%)

Lymphocyte-depleted HD is very rare—studies have showed that cases previously diagnosed as lymphocyte-depleted HD were mostly B-cell non-Hodgkin's lymphoma (NHL). Lymphocyte/histiocyte-predominant HD is a distinct entity, characterized by 'L&H Hodgkin's cells' which are of B-cell lineage. A small proportion develop into diffuse, large, B-cell NHL. This subtype has a favourable prognosis, as does a recently described similar entity—lymphocyte-rich classical HD. Some subtypes of NHL, particularly anaplastic large-cell lymphoma, can be confused with HD. Expert review of the pathology is an essential component of management.

Presentation

+ Painless lymphadenopathy (cervical nodes especially)
+ May be generalized lymphadenopathy
+ Later spread to liver, lungs, marrow
+ 'B' symptoms—fever
        —night sweats
        —weight loss >10%
        —itch
        —alcohol-induced pain in nodes

Table 27.3 Ann Arbor staging system

Stage	Feature
I	Disease in a single lymph node region
II	Disease in two or more regions on the same side of the diaphragm
III	Disease in two or more regions on both sides of the diaphragm
IV	Diffuse or disseminated disease in extra lymphatic sites including liver and bone marrow
Various suffixes are added to each anatomical stage:	
	A No systemic symptoms
	B Systemic symptoms present
	E Extranodal disease

Staging

Spread of HD is typically to contiguous lymph node groups. As a result, anatomical staging using the Ann Arbor system has been the basis of treatment decisions in HD. However, the identification of other prognostic factors has refined treatment decisions, which are now rarely made on the basis of anatomical stage only.

Prognostic factors

Recent studies have identified various presenting factors that may influence outcome in HD. For patients with early stage (I and IIA) disease, several studies have identified prognostic groups based on histological subtype, age, sex, symptom status, number of nodal regions involved, and the presence of bulky mediastinal disease.

For patients with advanced (Stage IIB to IVB) disease, various prognostic factors have been identified in an analysis of over 5000 patients. The adverse factors are as follows:

- Albumin <4 g/l
- Haemoglobin <10.5 g/l
- Male gender

Table 27.4 EORTC prognostic groups in early-stage HD

Group	Prognostic factors
Very favourable	Stage I and age <40 or 'A' + ESR <50 or female and MT ratio* <0.35
Favourable	All other patients
Unfavourable	Age ≥40, or 'A' and ESR ≥50, or 'B' and ESR ≥30, or Stage II$_{4/5}$, or MT ratio ≥0.35

* MT ratio = size of mediastinal mass compared with transverse diameter of the chest on chest X-ray.

- Age 45 years or over
- Stage IV
- Leukocytosis $15 \times 10^9/l$
- Lymphocytopenia $<0.6 \times 10^9/l$

In the absence of any adverse factors, the five-year failure-free survival (FFS) rate is 84%. The presence of each of these factors reduces the expected five-year FFS by about 8%.

Treatment

Since HD predominantly affects young adults, potential long-term toxicities of therapy are of major importance. The recognition of the long-term toxicities of radiation therapy, particularly to the mediastinum (second malignancies, including lung and breast cancer; pulmonary fibrosis; coronary artery disease) and alkylating agent-based chemotherapy (secondary leukaemia and NHL; infertility; early ovarian failure) has had a major impact on therapy.

Early stage

The majority of patients with early-stage HD present with supradiaphragmatic disease. For these patients, treatment should be determined by prognostic factors that predict the likelihood of occult subdiaphragmatic disease not detected by routine clinical staging techniques.

Standard therapy for these patients comprises nodal irradiation with the classic mantle field (occipital, cervical, supraclavicular, axillary, mediastinal, and hilar nodes). In the US this is commonly extended to the upper abdomen to incorporate the coeliac nodes, splenic hilar nodes, and spleen (subtotal nodal irradiation—STNI). 70–80% of patients achieve long-term Disease Free Survival (DFS) with this approach. Although relapse occurs in up to 30% of patients, subsequent salvage with chemotherapy is very successful, in around 80–90% of patients.

In view of the long-term toxicity of extended field radiotherapy, the role of chemotherapy combined with limited (involved field) radiotherapy has been explored in many centres, and is currently being assessed in randomized clinical trials. Regimens such as VBM (vinblastine, bleomycin, methotrexate) and ABVD (doxorubicin, bleomycin, vinblastine, dacarbazine) combined with involved field radiotherapy can produce long-term DFS equivalent to STNI, with fewer relapses after initial therapy and less long-term toxicity.

Patients with very favourable prognostic features (e.g. female patients with LP or NS histology, low ESR, and presentation with high cervical nodes) are at very low risk of subdiaphragmatic relapse and are treated in some centres with involved field radiotherapy alone.

Advanced stage

MOPP (mustine, vincristine, procarbazine, and prednisone) and its variants have been considered standard chemotherapy for advanced HD until recently. However, doxorubicin-based chemotherapy, particularly ABVD, has now become widely accepted as standard therapy following the completion of a major trial by the CALGB.[1] This study compared MOPP, MOPP alternating with ABVD, and ABVD alone. The respective five-year failure-free survival (FFS) rates were 50%, 65%, and 61%, demonstrating that ABVD and MOPP/ABVD were equivalent, and both superior to MOPP alone.

More recently, brief-duration regimens such as Stanford V (mustine, doxorubicin, vinblastine, prednisone, vincristine, bleomycin, etoposide) and BEACOPP (bleomycin, etoposide, doxorubicin, cyclophosphamide, vincristine, procarbazine, prednisolone) have been introduced, on the basis of increased dose intensity but reduced total doses of therapy, with a lower potential for long-term toxicity. These regimens are combined with limited field radiotherapy to sites of disease bulk. Initial reports have shown high response and FFS rates. For example, Stanford V produced a three-year actuarial overall survival (OS) and FFS of 96% and 87% respectively in patients with advanced HD. Similar results have been reported for BEACOPP. These regimens are now being compared with standard regimens such as ABVD in randomized trials.

Salvage therapy

Patients with early-stage HD who relapse after radiotherapy have high response rates to subsequent chemotherapy, with most (80–90%) achieving long-term DFS. For patients who relapse after first-line chemotherapy, high response rates are seen with second-line conventional dose regimens, especially if the initial remission duration is greater than 12 months. However, only 20–25% of patients achieve long-term DFS with conventional-dose salvage therapy.

High-dose therapy and autologous stem cell transplantation (ASCT) can produce superior long-term DFS compared with conventional-dose salvage and are now generally regarded as standard salvage therapy in HD, producing long-term DFS in 40–50% of patients. Primary refractory HD is rare, and the role of high-dose therapy and ASCT in this setting is unknown.

Future directions

If adverse prognostic features, consider:

• High-dose therapy and ASCT as first-line
• Antibodies against CD30 antigen on R-S cell; some responses in Phase II trials

Reference

1. Canellos, G.P., *et al.* (1992) Chemotherapy of advanced Hodgkin's disease with MOPP, ABVD, or MOPP alternating with ABVD. *NEJM* **327**: 1478–84.

Non-Hodgkin's lymphomas

Definition and aetiology

Non-Hodgkin's lymphomas (NHL) are a group of malignant diseases arising from cells of the immune system (lymphocytes and their precursors). The spectrum of NHL ranges from indolent low-grade lymphomas which are incurable yet compatible with a number of years of survival, to aggressive high-grade lymphomas which, left untreated, are rapidly fatal, but which modern treatment can cure in a significant proportion of patients.

NHL is increasing in frequency, and in the USA this increase has been 3–4% per annum since the early 1970s, with a present incidence of approximately 15 per 100 000. The pathogenesis of the majority of NHL is unknown, but identified aetiological factors include:

- Longevity
- Prolonged immunosuppression e.g. congenital immunodeficiencies, HIV-associated NHL, and transplant-associated lymphoproliferative disease
- Epstein–Barr virus (EBV) infection in Burkitt's lymphoma, HIV- and transplant-related lymphomas, and HTLV-1 infection in adult T-cell leukaemia/lymphoma (ATLL)
- Helicobacter infection in gut lymphoma
- Lifetime accumulation of genetic changes to immune cells.

Classification of NHL

Immunological identification of lymphocytes and molecular analysis of immunoglobulin and T-cell receptor gene rearrangements has allowed improved classification of NHL based on the biology of the cells rather than just morphological description. The majority of cases of NHL are B-cell type.

The pathological classification presently employed is the Revised European and American Lymphoma (REAL) classification. This is based on whether lymphoma cells are B-lymphocytes or T-lymphocytes, the perceived original cell of origin of the lymphoma, and whether or not a group of expert pathologists agree that the lymphoma can be reproducibly identified as a distinct entity.

In day-to-day practice the clinical behaviour of NHL (grade) is the most useful parameter, and treatment strategies are still based on classification systems which divide NHL into indolent (low-grade) and aggressive (high-grade) diseases. The general differences between low- and high-grade NHL are summarized in the table.

Table 27.5 Outline of Revised European and American Lymphoma (REAL) classification, with examples of disease entities in each group

B-cell lymphoma

Stage I	Precursor B-cell neoplasms
	Precursor B-lymphoblastic leukaemia/lymphoma
Stage II	Peripheral B-cell lymphomas
	Follicle centre cell lymphoma
	Diffuse large B-cell lymphoma

T-cell and putative NK-cell lymphoma

Stage I	Precursor T-cell neoplasm
	Precursor T-lymphoblastic lymphoma/leukaemia
Stage II	Peripheral T-cell and NK-cell neoplasm
	Mycosis fungoides/Sézary syndrome
	Peripheral T-cell lymphomas, unspecified

Table 27.6 Differences between low-grade and high-grade NHL

Low-grade NHL	High-grade NHL
Indolent clinical course with relatively long survival	Aggressive clinical course and rapidly fatal without treatment
Incurable with present therapy	Curable in a significant proportion of patients
Non-destructive growth patterns	Destructive growth pattern
CNS involvement rare	CNS and extranodal involvement common

Clinical features and staging of NHL

The majority of adult patients (60–70%) present with nodal disease, whereas the majority of children present with extranodal disease. One or more areas of lymph nodes are painlessly enlarged, and may remain unchanged or slowly increase in size in low-grade NHL, or rapidly increase in size in high-grade lymphomas. Hepatosplenomegaly is common and extranodal sites are protean and include the gut, testes, thyroid gland, bone, muscle, lung, CNS, facial sinuses, and skin. Systemic symptoms include drenching night sweats, loss of weight, and culture-negative fever.

Medical emergencies associated with NHL include mediastinal obstruction, obstructive nephropathy, spinal cord compression, hypercalcaemia, and metabolic derangement. Ascites and pleural effusions (sometimes chylous) are common end stage features, especially in high-grade NHL. Patients may develop bone marrow failure from lymphomatous involvement, and low-grade NHL can cause immune-mediated haemolysis or thrombocytopenia.

Diagnosis requires a lymph node biopsy or, in the absence of lymphadenopathy, biopsy of an involved extranodal site. Morphological diagnosis is aided by immunohistochemistry and cytogenetic and molecular techniques.

The extent or stage of the disease should be determined by clinical rather than pathological (surgical) staging. This involves:

- CXR
- CT scanning of the chest, abdomen, and pelvis to define areas of nodal and extranodal involvement
- Blood count and blood film for leukaemic involvement
- Bone marrow aspiration and trephine biopsy for morphology, immunophenotyping, and cytogenetic analysis
- Renal biochemistry, liver function, calcium, and uric acid
- Markers of tumour burden: serum LDH and α2-microglobulin
- Others, depending on circumstances e.g. CT head scan, MRI of spine, lumbar puncture, bone scan

Clinical staging is based on a modification of the Ann Arbour classification of Hodgkin's disease.

Low-grade NHL

The low-grade lymphomas comprise 20–45% of NHL. They tend to be disseminated at the time of presentation with widespread lymphadenopathy, hepatosplenomegaly, and, often, blood and marrow involvement.

B-cell follicle centre cell NHL (follicular NHL)

This is the archetypal low-grade NHL. It typically presents in older age, though is also seen in young people. Rarely, it presents as an apparent true Stage I, when it may be cured by radiotherapy. More commonly, it presents as Stage III or IV, when it remains incurable with present treatments.

This lymphoma can transform to high-grade NHL. The lymphoma cells contain a reciprocal chromosomal translocation—t(14; 18) (q32; q21). This leads to the oncogene *Bcl-2*, from chromosome 18, coming under the regulation of the immunoglobulin heavy chain gene (IgH) on chromosome 14. The increased production of *Bcl-2* protects the lymphoma cell from apoptosis (programmed cell death) and, as such, follicle centre cell lymphoma represents a relentless accumulation of malignant cells.

- Indolent disease
- Fatal in 10 years
- No active treatment until significant symptoms

- Local radiotherapy to bulky disease sites
- Single-agent chemotherapy—chlorambucil
- Combination chemotherapy—CHOP
- Initial remission; relapse inevitable
- New treatments—purine analogues: fludarabine and 2-CDA
  - —autologous transplant
  - —α interferon
  - —palliation with anti-CD20 antibody (rituximab)
  - —antisense therapy to suppress *Bcl*-2 protein

High-grade NHL

High-grade NHLs are best considered as those with a strong tendency to involve the CNS—lymphoblastic, Burkitt's, ATLL, primary CNS lymphoma (PCL), and those others with a lesser tendency to do so. However, these latter histological types have an increased risk of CNS disease if they involve marrow, testes, or facial sinuses, and such patients require CNS examination and prophylaxis.

Burkitt's lymphoma

- Endemic
  - —endemic in equatorial Africa
  - —90% associated with EBV infection
  - —young adults/children, present with head/neck tumours
- Non-endemic
  - —NHL associated with EBV in 20%
  - —abdominal disease more common
  - —associated with HIV infection
- Treatment
  - —intensive chemotherapy with methotrexate, cyclophosamide, ifosamide, with intrathecal therapy

Lymphoblastic lymphoma

Presents with or without leukaemia, is commoner in children than adults, and is most often T-cell type; typically featuring a mediastinal mass and pleural effusion. Treatment includes emergency management of mediastinal obstruction and prevention of the tumour lysis syndrome. Intensive combination chemotherapy schedules similar to those used in ALL and including CNS-directed therapy have improved the outlook in children, but results in adults remain less good.

Poor prognostic features include bone marrow and/or CNS involvement, LDH > 300 iu/l, age > 30 years, and delayed achievement of CR. Allogeneic and autologous progenitor cell transplantation may improve survival in these cases.

Diffuse large B-cell NHL

This, the commonest high-grade NHL, presents as nodal or extra-nodal disease. Radiotherapy can cure 90% of non-bulky Stage IA disease. For other stages, CHOP chemotherapy with radiotherapy to bulk disease remains the gold standard treatment with 40–50% cure. Relapsed patients who respond to salvage chemotherapy have been shown to have a survival benefit with autologous progenitor cell transplantation.

Myeloma

Myeloma (multiple myeloma, myelomatosis) is due to the unregulated proliferation of monoclonal plasma cells in the bone marrow. Their accumulation leads to marrow failure and, indirectly, to bone resorption resulting in osteoporosis and fracture. The cell of origin has not been conclusively identified but may be a memory B lymphocyte. The cause is unknown. An important mechanism is local production of interleukin 6, which stimulates plasma cell proliferation. Both paracrine and autocrine sources of the cytokine have been demonstrated.

The overall incidence of the disease is 4 per 100 000 in the UK, but over 30 per 100 000 in subjects over 80 years of age. It is higher amongst African–Americans and much lower in Chinese and Japanese–Asian populations. It is rare under the age of 40, the median age at presentation being 70 years.

The clonal plasma cells in myeloma synthesize, and usually secrete, a monoclonal protein (M protein, paraprotein). This is most commonly intact immunoglobulin, but may be immunoglobulin together with free light chain, or free light chain only. IgG is secreted in 60% of cases, IgA in 20%, and free light chain only in 20%. Light chains can pass through the glomerular filter and appear in the urine as Bence–Jones protein. In rare cases there is synthesis of monoclonal IgD, IgE, or IgM, or of two clonal proteins. Also uncommon are non-secretory and non-synthesizing variants of the disease.

Pathology

Monoclonal gammopathy associated pathology:

* Monoclonal gammopathy of uncertain significance (MGUS)
* Solitary plasmacytoma
* Lymphoma
* Waldenstrom's macroglobulinaemia
* Chronic lymphatic leukaemia
* Amyloidosis

Clinical features

These are explained by the accumulation of plasma cells in bone marrow, induction of bone resorption, and paraprotein synthesis.

Marrow infiltration

Malignant plasma cells accumulate in the red marrow of the axial skeleton and flat bones. Anaemia and thrombocytopenia are common, and frequently present at diagnosis.

Bone resorption

There is abnormal bone remodelling with increased, cytokine-driven osteoclastic bone resorption and inhibition of osteoblastic bone formation. Interleukin 6 is a major stimulus to osteoclastic activity. Bone pain is the most common presenting complaint, especially severe back pain. There may be fractures. The increased bone resorption also leads to hypercalcaemia and associated symptoms of thirst, polyuria, nausea, constipation, drowsiness, and even coma. X-ray examination typically reveals osteoporosis and lytic lesions that are often visualized on skull films.

Secretion of paraprotein

Accumulation of M protein in the plasma may result in hyperviscosity with lethargy and confusion, progressing to fits and coma. There is a characteristic retinopathy in hyperviscosity syndrome, with distension of retinal veins and irregular vessel constrictions; haemorrhages and papilloedema may be present. IgA and IgG paraproteins are especially likely to induce hyperviscosity. Bence–Jones protein is deposited in the renal tubules and may lead to renal failure. Other factors contributing to renal failures are:

* Hypercalcaemia
* Amyloid deposition
* Infection

Paraproteinaemia is typically accompanied by immune paresis, which contributes to the infection risk. In non-secretory myeloma the only immunological abnormality may be immune paresis, giving rise to diagnostic confusion.

Other features

Plasmacytomas may be palpable and also cause pressure effects. Spinal cord compression is most frequent and constitutes a medical emergency with the need for urgent assessment and local radiotherapy and/or decompressive surgery. Amyloidosis is frequently present and may dominate the clinical picture: macroglossia, renal failure, peripheral neuropathy, and cardiac failure occur. A syndrome of high-output cardiac failure is an occasional feature, unrelated to cardiac amyloid.

Very occasionally the bone lesions appear sclerotic, and this variant of the disease is often accompanied by severe progressive peripheral neuropathy. This combination of sclerotic lesions and neuropathy may also occur as part of the 'POEMS' syndrome, where plasma cell dyscrasia is accompanied by:

* Sensorimotor Polyneuropathy
* Organomegaly (principally hepatomegaly)
* Endocrinopathy (diabetes mellitus, amenorrhoea, gynaecomastia)

- M protein
- Skin changes (predominantly pigmentation)

Diagnosis

The classic diagnostic triad consists of bone marrow infiltration with monoclonal plasma cells, osteolytic lesions on skeletal X-rays, and paraproteinaemia/Bence–Jones' proteinuria. The plasma cell count may be only 5–10% in marrow, but is often over 30%, usually with morphologically abnormal forms.

Cytogenetic abnormalities, most commonly on chromosomes 13 and 14, and aneuploidy, are usually present, although their demonstration is not necessary for diagnostic purposes. The myeloma cells tend to be positive for CD 19, 38, 56, and syndecan-1. Additional common features are:

- Raised ESR
- Normocytic anaemia
- Pancytopaenia
- Renal impairment (present in 20% of cases)

In approximately 30%, hypercalcaemia is present at diagnosis and, typically, the serum alkaline phosphatase concentration is normal and the isotope bone scan negative (due to suppressed osteoblastic activity). The serum albumin may be low.

The main differential diagnosis is 'monoclonal gammopathy of uncertain significance' (MGUS), defined as the presence of a serum paraprotein without the features of myeloma. Its prevalence is around 20 times higher than that of multiple myeloma and it is age-related—3% of subjects over 80 years of age have detectable paraprotein. The serum concentration of the M protein is usually less than 30 g/l of IgG (less than 20 g/l of IgA), with no immune paresis. The blood count is normal as are skeletal X-rays. An excess of clonal plasma cells may be detected in the marrow, but these total less than 5% of nucleated cells.

In **'smouldering' myeloma** there are more than 10% plasma cells in bone marrow and a serum paraprotein concentration greater than 30 g/l, but no bone symptoms, radiological skeletal abnormality, anaemia, or renal failure. It is associated with an initially stable course and relatively long survival.

In **plasma cell leukaemia** there are greater than 20% plasma cells in peripheral blood. It may be a presenting feature or develop late in the disease course and is typically poorly responsive to therapy.

Solitary plasmacytoma presents as a single bone lesion with normal bone marrow and absent, or only low titre, paraprotein in serum. The tumour is radio-sensitive, but myeloma subsequently develops in most cases.

Extramedullary plasmacytoma is a rare soft-tissue plasma cell tumour, most commonly affecting the head and neck areas, especially the nasopharynx, nasal sinuses, and tonsils. Again the bone marrow is normal and there is no paraprotein. The tumour is radio-sensitive. Multiple myeloma develops in up to 40% of cases.

Management

Untreated, death usually occurs within months, especially from infection and renal failure, and is often preceded by intractable bone pain. Initial therapy should include:

* Adequate analgesia, often necessitating the use of opiates, with radiotherapy to areas of persisting local bone pain.
* Rehydration and vigorous management of hypercalcaemia using intravenous bisphosphonate. Dialysis is occasionally necessary for management of renal impairment, and plasma exchange for rapid correction of hyperviscosity syndrome.

Chemotherapy

* Cures are rare
* Palliation to improve symptoms and reduce paraprotein
* Chemotherapy for 3 months is sufficient
* Maintenance chemotherapy is of no value
* Plateau phase lasts 3 months to 3 years
* Oral melphalan is best—4-day pulses every 4 weeks
  —50% of patients achieve 50% reduction in M protein
* Median survival, 3 months

A more intensive regimen—VAD (vincristine and adriamycin by IV infusion and oral dexamethasone)—may produce a rapid response, but this is often poorly sustained. Combination chemotherapy (e.g. doxorubicin, BCNU, cyclophosphamide, melphalan) has improved the response rate in some trials, at the expense of greater toxicity.

Complete remission is uncommon. High-dose (marrow ablative) melphalan with autologous stem cell transplantation induces complete remission in around 20% of recipients, and prolongs survival. It can be considered in younger patients. Long-term survival has been reported after allogeneic transplantation, but treatment-related mortality is high (up to 40%).

Additional therapy

Oral clodronate appears to reduce the fracture rate, when administered continuously. Pamidromate—a more potent bisphosphonate—administered by monthly IV infusion, reduces fracture rate, pain, and hypercalcaemia and improves quality of life. Interferon-α, administered as maintenance therapy, appears to extend the duration of the plateau phase. It is unclear whether survival is meaningfully prolonged. The therapy is associated with significant side-effects and is expensive. Erythropoietin can be used to reduce transfusion requirements in a minority of cases.

Further reading

Bartlett, N.L., Rosenberg, S.A., Hoppe, R.T., *et al.* (1995) Brief chemotherapy, Stanford V, and adjuvant radiotherapy for bulky or advanced stage Hodgkin's disease: a preliminary report. *J Clin Oncol* 13, 1080–8.

Canellos, G.P., Anderson, J.R., Propert, K.J. *et al.*(1992) Chemotherapy of advanced Hodgkin's disease with MOPP, ABVD or MOPP alternating with ABVD. *New Engl J Med* 327, 1478–84.

Hasenclever, D. and Diehl, V. (for the International Prognostic Factors Project on Advanced Hodgkin's Disease) (1998) A prognostic score for advanced Hodgkin's disease. *New Engl J Med* 339, 1506–14.

Chapter 28
Bone and soft tissue malignanicies

Osteosarcoma

Background

Malignant bone tumours are rare, accounting for only 0.2% of all new cancers. Osteosarcoma is the commonest primary bone tumour and occurs predominantly in adolescence with a peak incidence coinciding with the growth spurt. Cases occurring over the age of 40 years are usually associated with:

* Paget's disease
* Irradiated bone
* Multiple hereditary exostosis
* Polyostotic fibrous dysplasia

The majority of tumours arise in the region of the metaphysis, most commonly in the tibia close to the knee joint. Other long bones may be involved, but presentation in the axial skeleton is relatively rare. Pain at the site of the tumour, often with overlying erythema and tenderness, is the usual mode of presentation. More rarely, fracture through a tumour site can occur. Serum alkaline phosphatase is elevated in 50% of cases.

Pathology

Osteosarcomas are composed of malignant spindle cells and osteoblasts that produce osteoid or immature bone. The 'classic' subtype is a central medullary tumour but rarer types with a better prognosis exist— parosteal, periosteal, and low-grade intra-osseous osteosarcoma.

Radiological evaluation

Plain X-rays of the affected area are usually sufficient to make a diagnosis of osteosarcoma. The classic features of osteosarcoma are:

* Poorly delineated or absent margins around the bone lesion
* Bone destruction
* New bone formation with calcification of the matrix
* Periosteal reaction, usually non-continuous and thin, with multiple laminations

Note: histological confirmation of the radiological diagnosis must be deferred until the patient is assessed by a surgeon with expertise in the management of bone malignancies.

Staging

Bone tumours disseminate almost exclusively via the bloodstream. Lymph node metastasis is rare (less than 5% of patients) and, if present, represents a very poor prognosis. Metastases may be within the same bone (skip lesions) or to other organs, most commonly the lungs.

Several staging systems exist, the most commonly used being that described by Enneking. This stages patients from Ia–III. The stage is derived from a combination of the histological grade of the tumour, the presence or absence of distant metastases, and the extent of local spread of disease.

Management of patients with osteosarcoma

Surgical resection (usually amputation of a limb) alone was used to treat osteosarcomas until the 1970s. Overall survival was only 15–20%, largely because of the development of pulmonary metastases. Subsequent use of chemotherapy in the adjuvant (post-operative) or neo-adjuvant (pre- and post-operative) setting has improved the survival rate to 55–80%. Surgical management has also improved in the past 20 years, with amputation being replaced in the majority of patients by limb-sparing surgery.

Pre-operative assessment

When plain radiology suggests an osteosarcoma, staging should be performed prior to biopsy. Investigations include:

- **Bone scan**—determines multiple sites of involvement and provides a guide to the intra-osseous extension of disease.

- **CT scanning of bone**—this allows accurate determination of intra- and extra-osseous extension of disease. The entire bone and adjacent joint should be imaged and contrast used to identify vascular structures.

- **MRI of bone**—this provides excellent contrast discrimination and is particularly valuable for imaging the medullary marrow. It is the most useful method for detecting skip metastases.

- **Angiography**—this is used when limb-sparing procedures are planned to determine individual vascular patterns before resection. It is especially valuable in proximal tibial lesions.

- **Biopsy**—biopsies of suspected osteosarcomas must be performed by orthopaedic specialists with experience of this technique. Ideally, the biopsy should be performed by the surgeon who will undertake the definitive resection. Trephine or core biopsy is recommended. It must be assumed that there is potential tumour contamination of all tissue planes and compartments traversed by the biopsy needle. The site of biopsy must be carefully chosen as it will have to be removed *en bloc* during definitive resection. An incorrectly sited biopsy may necessitate amputation instead of limb-sparing surgery. Frozen section should be obtained during the biopsy to ensure that the tumour has been obtained. Clearance biopsies are normally taken during this procedure.

• **CT scan of the thorax**—to detect pulmonary metastases.

Surgery

Sarcomas grow radially and produce a pseudo-capsule. The tumour invariably spreads through the capsule and expert surgery is necessary to ensure an adequate resection margin to remove all locally viable tumour. While previously amputation was almost always necessary, approximately 80% of osteosarcomas are now treated successfully with limb-sparing techniques. A wide variety of endo-prosthetic devices are available including extendable prostheses for growing children.

Chemotherapy

The outcome for patients with osteosarcomas has been markedly improved with the addition of chemotherapy to surgery. The most active agents are doxorubicin, cisplatin, ifosfamide, and high-dose methotrexate. Chemotherapy may be given pre-operatively and post-operatively (neo-adjuvant treatment). This has several potential benefits:

• Treatment starts without delay before surgery (time is taken obtaining a customized endoprosthesis).

• The bulk of viable tumour is reduced and thus, perhaps, the risk of dissemination of tumour at surgery.

• Reduction of tumour volume makes surgery technically simpler.

• It allows assessment of the pathological response to chemotherapy when examining the definitive resection specimen.

On the other hand, this approach delays the time of resection in patients who do not respond to chemotherapy. Post-operative adjuvant chemotherapy may be used instead with the advantages that only microscopic disease, if any, remains, and definitive local treatment with surgery is not delayed.

Clearly, pathological response to chemotherapy cannot be assessed and alternative regimens cannot therefore be considered in those failing to respond to first-line chemotherapy. The optimum regimen has not been defined and, wherever possible, patients with this rare tumour are included in clinical trials.

Radiotherapy

Osteosarcomas are relatively radio-resistant. Radiotherapy is rarely used in the primary treatment of this disease. Its use is limited to the palliative care of patients who refuse surgery, have lesions in axial sites which are not resectable, or have bone metastases.

Metastatic osteosarcoma

The majority of patients developing recurrent disease will have pulmonary metastases. Up to 30% may be salvaged with surgical resection of the metastases. Metastasectomy may be considered on several occasions. Local recurrences are managed with surgical resection or palliative irradiation. The role of chemotherapy in relapsed disease is uncertain but patients with lung metastases at presentation undoubtedly benefit from combined modality treatment, and a few will be long-term survivors after chemotherapy and surgery for both the primary and residual metastases.

Ewing's sarcoma

Introduction

First described by James Ewing, New York pathologist, in 1926, this is one of the two common bone tumours occurring in young people, with a peak age of incidence of 15–18 years. It occurs with an annual incidence of 0.6 per million in most populations but is extremely rare in non-Caucasians.

Aetiology is unknown and is not generally associated with cancer 'syndromes'. Any bone in the body can be affected, with 55% in the axial skeleton and 45% in the limbs. Within the long bones, the tumour tends to be more centrally situated in the diaphysis rather than at the ends of the bone.

Clinical presentation is usually with a painful swelling that may be warm and/or red. Those occurring in central sites may present with severe pain, signs of abdominal organ or urinary tract compression, or nerve compression from those arising in the vertebral bodies. About 10% present with a hot, swollen bone, along with a substantial fever, and in this situation osteomyelitis is part of the differential diagnosis.

Diagnosis

- X-ray—destructive, osteolytic lesions
    - —elevation of periosteum
    - —onion skin appearance
- CT
- MRI
- Aspiration biopsy rarely sufficient
- Open biopsy—send to laboratory fresh
- Histology—small, blue, round cell tumour
    - —glycogen within cells (PAS, neural markers positive – S – 100, vimentin, NSE)
- EM—glycogen granules
- Cyogenetics—t(11,:22) translocation
    - —EWS/FL11 gene rearrangement
- Subtypes—typical Ewing's sarcoma
    - —atypical Ewing's sarcoma
    - —primitive neuroectodermal tumour of bone (PNET)

In practical terms, treatment and outcome are identical for all three subtypes. Other pre-treatment investigations that can be helpful are:

- Full blood count
- Alkaline phosphatase
- LDH
- Plasma creatinine

Prior to therapy, a test of renal function (e.g. $Cr^{51}EDTA$) and cardiac function (e.g. echocardiogram) should be undertaken. The most important prognostic factor is the presence of metastases at diagnosis and, in order to ascertain such lesions, it is important to undertake an isotope bone scan, a CT of the lungs, and a bone marrow aspirate/trephine from a bone not affected by the primary tumour.

The basic treatment plan is similar for all patients—but chemotherapy → definitive treatment of primary → chemotherapy → follow-up—needs to be individualized depending on the site of the primary tumour and the presence of metastatic disease.

This is a rare tumour and should be treated in a specialist centre.

Chemotherapy

There are six drugs that have substantial proven activity in this disease:

- Vincristine
- Doxorubicin
- Actinomycin D
- Etoposide
- Cyclophosphamide
- Ifosfamide

While there is some controversy as to whether maximally tolerable doses of cyclophosphamide are inferior to ifosfamide, the latter is usually used.

Treatment of the primary tumour

Surgery and/or radiotherapy may be used. Surgery should be considered in all cases and if it is possible to remove the tumour without undue mutilation, then it is the treatment of choice. Surgical developments mean that there are few bones in the body which are not amenable to surgery. Complete removal is recommended but if it is incomplete, radiotherapy should be given in addition. The latter should be given to the whole bone, but the most distant epiphysis may be spared in tumours arising at the end of the long bone.

Patients with metastases

Lung metastases should be treated with conventional chemotherapy as detailed, with whole-lung irradiation to any residual disease. However, those with bony metastases have a dismal prognosis and it may be worth considering megatherapy after conventional induction treatment. Either melphalan, busulphan, or TBI, or a combination, may be used as a conditioning regime.

Prognosis

The major prognostic factors are metastases at presentation and site and volume of the tumour. For those with small tumours (<100 cc), usually in the long bones, over 80% can be cured. Pelvic tumours and those with lung metastases have a 30% chance of survival. With conventional therapy, the majority of those with bone metastases die. Ewing's tumour may relapse up to 10 or more years after diagnosis.

Late effects

Cardiac and nephrotoxic late effects, as a result of chemotherapy, may occur, but these are not disease-specific. Second primary tumours, most often osteosarcomas, may occur in the irradiation field, and the late effects of major endoprosthetic surgery can be substantial.

Other primary bone tumours

Primary malignant spindle cell sarcoma of bone

Most often malignant fibrous histiocytoma, but other pathologies include:

- Liposarcoma
- Angiosarcoma
- Leiomyosarcoma
- Haemangiopericytoma

All are rare; they comprise less than 1% of all bone tumours. May arise in any bone (usually the metaphysis of a long bone) and tend to occur in middle age. Can occur after a previous insult to the bone, e.g. ionizing radiation, bone infarct, or fibrous dysplasia.

The treatment is surgical removal of all disease but, as with osteosarcoma, limb-sparing surgery and insertion of a customized prosthesis may be feasible. The role of chemotherapy is still being explored and comparison with historical controls does suggest some benefit.

Osteoclastoma

Account for 5% of primary bone tumours and are usually benign. Occur in young adults, often in an epiphysis around the knee. Are treated by curettage and bone packing or bone resection and insertion of an endoprosthesis. Local recurrence occurs in 30–50%, but radiotherapy carries a definite risk of malignant transformation and is only appropriate where the alternative local therapy is amputation. Rarely, these tumours can metastasize to the lung. Where possible, these should be dealt with surgically. Anecdotal responses to chemotherapy have been reported.

Chondrosarcoma

Slow-growing tumours of middle to late age and the second most common bone tumour (approximately 20%). Occur around the pelvis and shoulders. Grade is a good guide to behaviour, although about 10% of low-grade tumours transform to a higher grade. Treatment is surgical resection with radiotherapy for incomplete resection or palliation of advanced disease.

Mesenchymal chondrosarcoma is a high-grade tumour of adolescence frequently involving the mandible, ribs, or spine. Combined treatment with surgery, chemotherapy, and radiotherapy provide a 50% cure rate.

Chordoma

Slow-growing tumour that arises from notochord remnant cells in the sacrum/coccyx (50%), skull base/clivus (35%), or upper cervical vertebrae, in middle age. Presents with persistent pain and often only discovered on CT or MRI after 'normal' plain X-rays of the bone. Metastases are rare (lung or bone) and survival is determined by the success or failure of local control.

Surgery is the treatment of choice but may not be feasible because of the tumour site. Radiotherapy (55–60 Gy) is used after incomplete resection or as palliation. Particle therapy with protons has shown some promise. 30–50% survive five years but late recurrences are possible.

Solitary plasmacytoma

Isolated lytic lesion rich in plasma cells. The diagnosis depends on the exclusion of myeloma (no other skeletal lesions, no hypercalcaemia, no suppression of other immunoglobulins, and bone marrow contains <5% plasma cells). Paraproteinaemia is common.

Treatment is either surgical excision of the lesion or, more commonly, radiotherapy (45–50 Gy). Prognosis is good, with a median survival of over 5 years, but about a half will transform into myeloma.

Primary bone lymphoma

One of the differential diagnoses of malignant, small, round, dark cell tumours of bone (Ewing's neuroblastoma). Full staging with CT, bone scan, and bone marrow examination is required to exclude systemic lymphoma. Localized high-grade NHL is treated with initial chemotherapy (e.g. CHOP) followed by either radiotherapy or surgical excision and endoprosthesis (latter is preferred for long, weight-bearing bones, where there is otherwise a high risk of fracture). Multifocal disease is usually low-grade NHL. Treatment is with chlorambucil chemotherapy and radiotherapy.

Soft tissue sarcomas

Diagnosis and management of sarcomas

- Any enlarging mass, deep to deep fascia should be regarded as a potential sarcoma.
- Tissue for histology should be obtained by cutting needle (e.g. Trucut), not incisional biopsy. The biggest surgical problems are caused by injudicious incisions.
- Incision biopsy should never be performed—this disseminates the tumour and is never curative. Surgery should be preceded by appropriate CT or MRI.
- Multidisciplinary care of sarcomas is best carried out in centres with appropriate expertise—including surgery, pathology, radiotherapy, and chemotherapy.

Rhabdomyosarcoma (RMS)

The commonest soft tissue tumour in childhood and adolescence. More than half the cases occur in children under 10 years and is rare in adults over 40. Male to female ratio is approximately 1.3:1. Arises from primitive mesenchymal cells with the capacity for rhabdomyoblastic development. Commonest sites of origin are:

- Head and neck
- Genitourinary tract
- Retroperitoneum
- Extremities

Disease may spread locally (e.g. from the orbit to the meninges and central nervous system) and disseminates to lymph nodes, lungs, bones, marrow, and brain. An aggressive disease requiring multimodality treatment. Outlook depends on the disease site and histological subtype.

Pleomorphic RMS is a rather rare adult soft tissue tumour, which behaves in a similar fashion to other adult soft tissue tumours in that while it may be curable if localized it is not as chemosensitive as the childhood variety and carries a poor prognosis once metastatic.

Diagnosis

Presents with swelling or other local symptoms such as displacement of the eye, vaginal bleeding, dysuria, etc. In establishing a histological diagnosis it is currently advisable to obtain fresh tissue for chromosomal studies.

Embryonal RMS

Accounts for about 60% of cases. Occurs mainly in children under 15, most commonly affecting:

* Head and neck, including orbit
* Genitourinary tract
* Retroperitoneum

'Embryonal' refers to the spectrum of cell type, from primitive round cells to rhabdomyoblasts, which may be thought to mimic the stages in muscle embryogenesis. Botryoid RMS is a subtype characterized by polypoid growth, like a 'bunch of grapes', and is usually found in hollow organs such as the vagina, bladder, and nasopharyngeal sinuses.

Alveolar RMS

Characterized by poorly differentiated round or oval cells forming irregular spaces and separated by fibrous septae, giving the appearance of 'alveoli'. Sometimes this appearance is absent but the uniform appearance of the cells is distinct from that of the embryonal variety. Multinucleate giant cells may be observed. Alveolar RMS has a significantly worse prognosis than embryonal.

If fresh tissue is available, the diagnosis may be confirmed by the presence of a t(2;13) (q37;q14) or variant t(1;13) (p36;q14) chromosomal translocation. The result is fusion of PAX3 or PAX7 genes respectively with the FKHR gene, producing a chimeric protein. Translocation may be identified by fluorescence *in situ* hybridization (FISH) or reverse transcriptase polymerase chain reaction (RT-PCR) methods that require little tumour tissue. Translocation may be detected in about half of cases and, where present, reliably distinguishes alveolar from embryonal RMS.

Staging

Staging should include MRI or CT of the primary site, CT scan of the thorax, isotope bone scan, and bone marrow aspirate and trephine. The stage is usually assigned using the SIOP-UICC TNM (tumour, nodes, metastases) staging system which is useful in determining appropriate therapy.

Prognostic factors

The prognosis in RMS depends on site, size, extent of spread (i.e. stage, histology, sex, in that the outlook is somewhat worse in girls), and response to chemotherapy.

Treatment

Treatment usually begins with combination chemotherapy, followed by local treatment i.e. complete surgical resection where possible plus radiotherapy if excision incomplete, or radiotherapy alone if resection

Table 28.1 Prognostic factors in rhabdomyosarcoma

Good	Poor
Orbit, paratesticular, vagina extremities	Parameningeal, retroperitoneal,
Localized to tissue of origin	Contiguous spread, nodal or metastatic disease
Complete resection feasible	Unresectable
Embryonal histology	Alveolar histology
Infant or child	Adult
Complete response to chemotherapy	Poor response to chemotherapy

is not feasible. Patients with embryonal histology may be treated with vincristine plus actinomycin D; treatment is intensified with the addition of ifosfamide, doxorubicin, and other drugs for worse staging histology. Additional drugs such as etoposide and carboplatin and high-dose alkylating agent therapy, with peripheral blood progenitor cell rescue, may improve the outlook for some patients with metastatic disease, but the prognosis remains grave for alveolar RMS.

RMS is highly sensitive to radiotherapy. In combination with chemotherapy, doses of 40–50 Gy will usually ensure local disease control. However, there are serious long-term sequelae associated with the combined modality treatment in children. These include:

- Damage to sensitive organs, such as bladder, eye, brain, testis, ovary, and thyroid
- Risk of second malignancy
- Imbalanced bone growth, especially where epiphyses are included in the field

In infants and children with localized tumours and favourably histology, such as embryonal RMS of the orbit, it may be possible to omit radiotherapy. Extremity tumours, alveolar histology, and parameningeal tumours require radiotherapy.

Soft tissue Ewing's sarcoma and primitive neuroectodermal tumour (PNET)

Ewing's tumours are the second commonest bone malignancy in children. These are small round cell tumours of neuroectodermal origin and are characterized by chromosomal translocations involving the EWS gene, located at chromosome 22q12, fused with FL11 [t(11;22) (q24;q12)] or, more rarely, ERG [t(21;22) (a22;q12)]. Genetic analysis with FISH or RT-PCR methods may aid diagnosis. Soft tissue Ewing's sarcoma or PNET most commonly involves the extremities, chest wall (Askin's tumour), or pelvis.

In terms of treatment, much of the management of RMS applies to the Ewing's family of tumours. Prognosis with surgery alone is dismal (<10% cure) because of the frequency of systemic spread. Pre- and post-operative combination chemotherapy (doxorubicin, actinomycin D, ifosfamide, vincristine) is of crucial importance. Surgery is the preferred primary local treatment but radiotherapy is required after incomplete resection or where surgery is not feasible. Tumour bulk and response to chemotherapy are the two most important prognostic factors. The outlook is worse for those patients with tumours larger than 200 ml or with lung metastases, worse still in the case of bone metastases at diagnosis. Site is also important—axial primaries fare worse through a combination of late presentation and problems achieving local control of disease. Five-year survival rates are about 60% overall—80% for good-risk cases, falling to 20% in metastatic or larger tumours.

Adult sarcomas

Soft tissue sarcomas (STS) are rare tumours, accounting for 1% of adult malignancies and 6% of those in childhood. There are about 1200 new cases in the UK annually. Many histopathological varieties of STS are described, the most common being leiomyosarcoma, malignant fibrous histiocytoma, and liposarcoma. Classification of an individual tumour is based on morphology and immunohistochemistry.

Certain types of adult STS, such as clear cell, epithelioid, and synovial, always behave in an aggressive fashion. For those tumours that are more variable in their behaviour, such as liposarcoma, grade is more important than subtype since grade, tumour size, and resectability are key prognostic factors.

Low-grade, well-differentiated tumours may recur locally but rarely metastasize. Alveolar soft part sarcoma may behave in an indolent fashion but nevertheless does metastasize, and the prognosis is poor.

Disease pattern and prognosis

- 50% have high-grade sarcomas
- 50% of high-grade sarcomas die from metastases
- Metastases—rare with primary tumour <5 cms
  —common with primary tumour >15 cms
- Superficial tumours have better prognosis
- Extremity tumours spread to lung
- RMS, clear cell, epithelioid sarcomas spread to nodes
- Angiosarcomas, synovial sarcomas spread to bone
- Retroperitoneal sarcomas spread to liver
- Gynaecological sarcomas—diagnosed late, bad prognosis

- Older patients—worse prognosis
- Liposarcoma—better prognosis
- Synovial sarcoma is chemosensitive

Treatment

Radical surgery for the primary STS offers the only hope of cure. Complete compartmental resection for extremity tumours is no longer advocated since it is known that sarcomas rarely cross fascial boundaries. If possible, some muscle in the compartment should be spared. Sarcomas do, however, spread longitudinally. It is for this reason that careful pre-operative planning is required using MRI or CT scan to delineate the tumour extent and relationship to major vessels or nerves that may indicate the need for reconstructive surgery. If required, in the case of diagnostic difficulty the surgeon performing the definitive operation should carry out further biopsies. There needs to be close collaboration between surgeon and radiotherapist.

Preservation of function should be a priority, and amputation is rarely necessary. For high-grade tumours and any locally recurrent tumour, adjuvant radiotherapy is advised. This may be delivered pre- or post-operatively. Doses in the range of 55–65 Gy are recommended.

Retroperitoneal tumours are rarely radically resectable and recurrence is common, especially for higher-grade tumours. While radiotherapy may reduce local recurrence, it is likely to do little to influence prognosis, and the dose which can be safely delivered to the abdomen (40–50 Gy) will be insufficient to control the majority of STS.

Advanced disease

Metastases may be surgically removed in the case of limited relapse in the lungs. Any benefit increases with the relapse-free interval and if metastases are few in number. Chemotherapy for resectable locally recurrent or metastatic disease is palliative.

Ifosfamide and doxorubicin are the most active agents, but reported response rates are still disappointing (15–30%). There is clear evidence for a dose-response relationship with both drugs. Combination chemotherapy may produce higher response rates but is more toxic. Synovial sarcoma is chemosensitive and complete responses are observed. Low-grade tumours and especially gastrointestinal stromal tumours are generally unresponsive to conventional chemotherapy.

The role of adjuvant chemotherapy remains unclear but a recent meta-analysis of primary data from all published randomized trials showed significantly improved progression-free survival and a small improvement in overall survival, amounting to 4% at 10 years, which failed to reach statistical significance. There remains an urgent need for more effective systemic therapy in this group of diseases.

Cancer of unknown primary site

Such cancers are a common problem for oncologists, representing up to 15% of new referrals. Before accepting the diagnosis, it is important that the patient has:

- A thorough history
- Full clinical examination (including rectal, pelvic, and breast examination)
- Additional investigations

Aetiology/epidemiology/ pathology

A mixed group of cancers with a high metastatic potential. The reason the primary site remains undetected may be due to spontaneous regression (well recognized in melanoma) or mucosal sloughing, but in most cases is probably due to the unusual metastatic potential of the tumour. The pattern of metastatic disease is often very different from cases where the primary site is known e.g. lung cancer causes bone metastases 10 times more often when the primary site is known than when the lung cancer is occult.

Rare under the age of 40 years, this is the third commonest cancer presentation in patients over 70 years of age. The mean age at diagnosis is 60 years. It is a frequent cause of cancer death with a median survival of four months in most series. However, there are some patients with curable disease and some clinical scenarios are associated with a much longer survival. In about 20% the primary site is detected antemortem, but in 25% it remains undetected even after post mortem.

Four broad groups can be identified by light microscopy:

- Adenocarcinoma (60%)
- Poorly differentiated carcinoma (30%)
- Undifferentiated malignancy (5%)
- Squamous carcinoma (5%)

Appearances of adenocarcinoma and squamous carcinoma are similar irrespective of their site of origin and light microscopy rarely provides further clues. The diagnosis of undifferentiated malignancy should be made with caution as a high proportion will turn out to be lymphomas and further staining is essential. Poorly differentiated carcinoma may also be confused with seminoma, amelanotic melanoma, and epidermal carcinoma.

Immunohistochemical staining may be helpful, and is essential where lymphoma or germ cell tumour are possibilities. Unfortunately, few stains are specific to a primary site e.g. neuro-endocrine markers and chorionic gonadotrophin may be found on many tumours other than small cell lung cancer and germ cell cancer respectively. Electron microscopy can confirm a diagnosis of lymphoma but rarely distinguishes the primary site in other cancers.

Identification of specific genetic abnormalities is limited to a few tumours at present (lymphoma, Ewing's sarcoma, rhabdomyosarcoma) but holds promise for the future.

Table 29.1 Site-specific immunohistochemical stains

Stain	Tumour
Common leukocyte antigen (CLA)	Lymphoma
B & T cell gene rearrangement	Non-Hodgkin's lymphoma
Prostate specific antigen (PSA)	Prostate
Thyroglobulin	Thyroid

Clinical presentation

Presentation with lymphadenopathy is commoner than visceral or bone metastases. A wide variety of presentations may occur but the following are of clinical importance.

Axillary lymph nodes

A woman with metastatic adenocarcinoma in the axillary lymph nodes may have an occult breast cancer. This group has a longer survival than average. Negative mammography does not exclude the diagnosis. In the absence of distant metastatic disease, loco-regional therapy with surgical excision and radiation, with or without chemotherapy, should be given.

Cervical lymph nodes

Squamous or undifferentiated carcinoma in cervical lymph nodes must be referred for full ENT examination under anaesthetic with biopsy of the naso-, oro-, and hypo-pharynx. Radical loco-regional radiotherapy can result in median survival of several years especially if the nodes are high in the neck. Thyroid cancer can be excluded by staining for thyroglobulin. Supraclavicular lymph node metastases are usually associated with widespread malignancy and have a poorer prognosis.

Inguinal lymph nodes

A small anal cancer should be excluded by rectal examination and proctoscopy as this tumour may be curable with chemo-radiation. A thorough examination of the lower limbs may identify a primary skin cancer.

Positive PSA staining

Rectal examination may reveal an abnormality, but random transrectal biopsies may be indicated even with a normal prostate gland.

Peritoneal carcinomatosis in women

Ovarian cancer or a similarly behaving primary peritoneal carcinoma should be considered. Serum CA125, gynaecological examination, and pelvic ultrasound may be useful but are not specific. A mucin-secreting adenocarcinoma is more likely to be of gastrointestinal origin but can arise in the ovary. A trial of platinum-based chemotherapy may be pragmatic and good responses can be achieved.

Retroperitoneal or mediastinal lymph nodes in men

This pattern of disease in men—the extra-gonadal germ cell syndrome—is well recognized and associated with excellent responses to chemotherapy even in the absence of histological confirmation of germ cell cancer or serum tumour markers. Chemotherapy with bleomycin, etoposide, and cisplatin should be given.

Investigation

There is a tendency to over-investigate these patients. Only tests that are likely to alter treatment should be performed. Tumours that respond well to therapy, even in the presence of metastases, must be excluded (breast, prostate, thyroid, germ cell, lymphoma). Extensive investigation of the GI tract with barium and endoscopy is rarely useful. CT or MRI may identify an incurable cancer and avoid inappropriate treatment.

Treatment

Diagnosis and investigations are directed at classifying the patient in one of the following groups:

* Potentially curable
* Effective palliation available
* No active treatment indicated

The following cancers are potentially curable when presenting as cancers of unknown primary site:

* Germ cell tumors
* Lymphomas
* Thyroid cancer

Effective palliation with chemotherapy is indicated if the patient is fit and the tumour is chemo-responsive. There is no convincing evidence

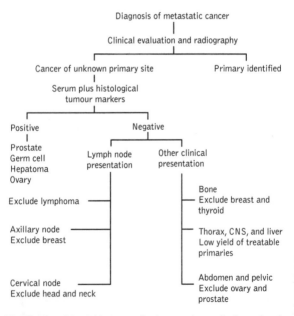

Identification of treatable cancer of unknown primary site (reproduced with permission from the *Oxford Textbook of Oncology*, 1995).

that combinations are better than single agents but there have been very few randomized trials. Hormone therapy is valuable in breast, prostate, endometrial cancer. Thyroidectomy and radioactive iodine therapy can provide long-term disease control in thyroid cancers. Radiotherapy can provide useful palliation for painful bone metastases, brain metastases, and troublesome lymph node masses.

Patients for whom no active treatment is indicated are often the most difficult to manage. The situation should be discussed with the general practitioner and, if appropriate, referral should be made to community or hospice-based palliative care teams.

Further reading

Hainsworth, J.D. and Greco, F.A. (1993) Treatment of patients with cancer of an unknown primary site. *N Engl J Med* **329**, 257–63.

Lindeman, G.J. and Tattershall, M. (1995) Tumours of unknown primary site. In *Oxford Textbook of Oncology* (ed. Peckham, M., Pinedo, H., and Veronesi, U.), pp. 2155–65. Oxford University Press, Oxford.

Chapter 30
Paraneoplastic syndromes

These pathological conditions are caused by a cancer but are not due to direct local infiltration or metastatic spread. Occurring in approximately 10% of cancer patients overall, they are most commonly associated with certain cancer types. They are important to recognize because they may be the presenting feature of an undiagnosed cancer. Paraneoplastic syndromes (PS) can also cause significant morbidity that may be treatable, and they may sometimes act as markers of disease activity.

Cancers commonly associated with paraneoplastic syndromes (PS):

- Lung: small cell (SCLC) and non-small cell (NSCLC)
- Pancreatic
- Lymphoma: non-Hodgkin's (NHL) and Hodgkin's Disease (HD)
- Breast
- Prostate
- Ovary

Although the mechanisms of PS are not fully understood, there appear to be two main causes:

- The inappropriate secretion of hormones and/or growth factors
- The production of anti-tumoural antibodies that cross-react with normal tissue antigens

Endocrine paraneoplastic syndromes (PS)

Syndrome of inappropriate ADH (SIADH)

The most common endocrine PS is due to inappropriate secretion of anti-diuretic hormone (arginine-vasopressin).

Cancer types SCLS (10% of patients), pancreatic, prostate, NHL, HD.

Presentation Often asymptomatic. CNS effects—fatigue, headaches; progressing to altered mental state, confusion, and seizures.

Diagnosis Exclude non-malignant causes e.g. CNS disease (infection, trauma, vascular), pulmonary disease (infections, cystic lesions, asthma), drug-induced (thiazides, cytotoxics, narcotics); clinically euvolaemic; laboratory studies.

Treatment Fluid restriction (0.5–1.0 L/day); democlocycline (150– 300 mg 8 hourly).

> **Laboratory criteria for diagnosis of SIADH**
> - Hyponatraemia Na+ <130 mmol/L
> - Normal serum albumin and glucose
> - Serum hypo-osmolarity <275 mmol/Kg
> - Urine osmolarity > serum osmolarity
> - Urinary sodium >25 mmol/L
> - Non-suppressed ADH

Cushing's syndrome

Inappropriate overproduction of adenocorticotrophic hormone (ACTH) precursors.

Cancer types SCLC, NSCLC, pancreatic, thymic, and carcinoid tumours.

Presentation Rapid onset, marked weakness secondary to proximal myopathy, hyper-pigmentation, metabolic disturbances (e.g. hyper-glycaemia, hypokalaemic alkalosis).

Diagnosis Clinical features, especially hyper-pigmentation, myopathy; hypokalaemia and metabolic alkalosis; high 24-hr urinary cortisol, high plasma ACTH/precursors, no response to high-dose dexamethasone suppression or corticotropin-releasing hormone stimulation.

Treatment Specific anti-tumour treatment. Decrease cortisol secretion either surgically (bilateral adrenalectomy) or medically (metyrapone, octreotide, ketoconazole).

Hypercalcaemia

A common problem that in many cases is due to bony metastases. True paraneoplastic hypercalcaemia is due to tumour production of parathyroid hormone-related protein. This syndrome is called Humoral Hypercalcaemia of Malignancy (HHM).

Cancer types NSCLC, head and neck, renal, other squamous cancers. (Rare in breast cancer where hypercalcaemia is usually due to bone metastases.)

Presentation Rapid onset of nausea, polyuria, polydipsia, dehydration, cardiac arrhythmias.

Diagnosis Serum Ca^{2+} >2.7 mmol/l, serum chloride low, hypercalcuria, high urinary phosphate, low/undetectable plasma parathyroid hormone.

Treatment Saline hydration, IV pamidronate (60–120 mg).

Hypocalcaemia

Associated with tumours with lytic bone metastases (breast, prostate, and lung); can also occur with calcitonin-secreting medullary carcinomas of the thyroid. Usually asymptomatic. Rarely develop tetany and neuromuscular irritability. Treatment with calcium infusions.

Hypoglycaemia

Rarely caused by non-islet cell pancreatic tumours; often associated with mesenchymal tumours of the mediastinum and retroperitoneum and with hepatic cancers. Most likely cause is tumour production of the precursor to insulin-like growth factor II. Treatment with glucose infusions, tumour debulking.

Neurological paraneoplastic syndromes

Common, occurring in up to 7% of cancer patients. Most common syndromes are:

• peripheral neuropathy
• proximal myopathy

Other major syndromes are relatively rare. Can affect any part of the neurological system and most are thought to be secondary to autoimmune mechanisms via production of anti-tumour antibodies that cross-react with nervous tissue e.g. anti-Hu, anti-Yo, anti-Ri. Treatment is based upon treatment of the cancer and decreasing antibody production by immune system suppression e.g. corticosteroids, IV immunoglobulin, and plasma exchange. In contrast to endocrine syndromes, response to treatment is often poor (except for Lambert-Eaton myasthenic syndrome (LEMS)).

Peripheral neuropathy (PN)

Asymptomatic PN is common; symptomatic PN less so. Usually occurs after diagnosis of cancer has been made and caused by axonal degeneration or demyelination. Many types of PN e.g. motor, sensory, autonomic, sensorimotor.

Cancer types SCLC, myeloma, HD, breast, GI cancers

Presentation Depends upon type and site.

Diagnosis Exclude non-paraneoplastic causes; nerve conduction studies, nerve biopsy—look for inflammatory infiltrates; serum anti-Hu antibodies in some cases.

Treatment Corticosteroids; treat underlying cancer.

Encephalomyelopathies

Perivascular inflammation and selective neuronal degeneration at several levels of the nervous system. Can affect the limbic system, brainstem, and spinal cord.

Cancer types SCLC (75% of cases), breast, ovary, NHL.

Presentation Slow, subacute onset; progressive

Diagnosis CSF—raised protein/IgG level, pleocytosis; serum—anti-Hu antibody; MRI.

Treatment Anti-tumour therapy.

Paraneoplastic cerebellar degeneration (PCD)

Cancer types Breast, SCLC, ovary, Hodgkin's disease (HD).

Presentation Rapid onset and progression; usually prior to cancer diagnosis; bilateral cerebellar signs; late diplopia and dementia.

Diagnosis CT—cerebellar atrophy (late); serum auto-antibodies—anti-Yo, -Tr, and -Hu.

Treatment Response to anti-tumour treatment, steroids, plasmapheresis.

Cancer-associated retinopathy (CAR)

Cancer types SCLC, breast, melanoma.

Presentation Visual defects i.e. blurred vision, episodic visual loss, impaired colour vision; leads to progressive painless visual loss; usually precedes cancer diagnosis.

Diagnosis Loss of acuity; scotomata; abnormal electroretinogram; anti-retinal ab's.

Treatment Corticosteroids.

Lambert–Eaton myasthenic syndrome (LEMS)

Disorder of the neuro-muscular junction; reduced pre-synaptic calcium-dependent acetylcholine release. About 60% of patients with LEMS have underlying cancer.

Cancer types SCLC (60–70%), breast, thymus, GIT cancers.

Presentation Proximal muscle weakness.

Diagnosis EMG—normal conduction velocity with low-amplitude compound muscle action potential that enhance to near normal following exercise.

Treatment Cancer treatment, corticosteroids, plasma exchange (high response rate).

Dermatomyositis/polymyositis

Inflammatory myopathies, often present prior to cancer diagnosis.

Cancer types NSCLC, SCLC, breast, ovary, GIT cancers

Presentation Proximal myopathy, skin changes, other systemic features; cardiopulmonary conditions, arthralgias, retinopathy.

Diagnosis Serum—high CK, LDH, aldolase; muscle biopsy—myositis; EMG—fibrillation, insertion irritability, short polyphasic motor units.

Treatment Search for and treat tumour; corticosteroids, azathioprine.

Haematological paraneoplastic syndromes

Red cell disorders

Erythrocytosis Common, often secondary to increased erythropoietin production e.g. renal cell carcinoma, hepatoma. Treat with phlebotomy if required.

Haemolytic anaemia

- Autoimmune—secondary to lymphoproliferative disorders (treatment—corticosteroids).
- Micro-angiopathic—secondary to vascular tumours, acute promyelocytic leukaemia, or widespread metastatic adenocarcinoma. Treat the tumour; replace coagulation factors; IV heparin.

Red cell aplasia Seen in thymoma, CLL; rare in solid tumours.

White cell disorders

Autoimmune neutropenia (rare)

- Granulocytosis—secondary to haemopoietic growth factor-secreting tumours (e.g. squamous cell cancers of lung, thyroid).
- Eosinophilia—in patients with HD.

Platelet disorders

- Thrombocytosis—($>450 \times 10^9$/L) is common and usually asymptomatic; in some cases may be secondary to IL-6 production.
- Idiopathic thrombocytopenia—is associated with leukaemias and lymphomas.

Coagulopathy

- Minor abnormalities of fibrin and fibrinogen degradation products are common.
- Overt disseminated intravascular coagulation is rare, associated with Acute Myelocytic Leukaemia and adenocarcinomas.
- Diagnosed by triad of thrombocytopenia, abnormal prothrombin time, and hypofibrinoginemia
- Treatment is controversial.

Dermatological paraneoplastic syndromes

Pruritus

Common; characteristic of HD, leukaemias, CNS tumours, NHL.

Pigmentation

Acanthosis nigricans   Itchy brown hyperkeratotic plaques, mainly in flexures; may precede cancers by many years; associated with GIT tumours e.g. gastric adenocarcinoma.

Vitiligo   Patchy depigmentation, especially face, neck, and hands; associated with malignant melanoma; possibility due to anti-melanoma immune response.

Erythematous

Necrolytic migratory erythema   Islet cell tumour.

Exfoliative dermatitis—cutaneous   T-cell lymphoma.

Bullous

Pemphigus Characteristic bullous lesions on skin and mucous membranes; associated with lymphoma, Kaposi's sarcoma, thymic tumours.

Dermatitis herpetiformis Chronic, intensely itchy vesicles over elbows, knees, and lower back; precede tumour by many years; associated with lymphomas e.g. NHL of the small intestine.

Other syndromes

Hypertrophic osteoarthropathy

Characterized by finger clubbing, periosteal new bone formation, and arthropathy.

Cancer types Lung cancer, especially NSCLC.

Presentation Painful, swollen joints.

Diagnosis Clinical—X-ray showing periosteal shadowing; bone scan—increased uptake.

Treatment Anti-tumour therapy, NSAIDS, corticosteroids, radiation.

Constitutional symptoms

Fever Can be presenting feature of lymphomas, hepatomas, renal cell carcinoma; mediated by IL-1; treat with NSAIDS, corticosteroids; exclude other causes.

Cachexia Very common, >10% loss of body weight is associated with poor prognosis; due to complex, multi-factorial metabolic derangements; treat with enteral caloric supplements and appetite stimulants e.g. corticosteroids, megesterol acetate.

Further reading

MacCaulay, V.M. and Smith, I.E. (1995) Paraneoplastic syndromes. *Oxford Textbook of Oncology*, p. 2228–53. Oxford University Press.

John, W.J., Patchell, R.A., and Foon, K.A. (1994) Paraneoplastic syndromes. In *Cancer—Principles and Practice of Oncology* (5th edn) (ed. V.T. DeVita *et al*) p. 2397–422.

Paraneoplastic syndromes (1997). *Seminars in Oncology* **24**, 265–381.

Chapter 31
AIDS-related malignancies

Patients with the acquired immune deficiency syndrome (AIDS) are at increased risk of developing certain malignant tumours. At present four malignancies define the onset of AIDS.

- Kaposi's sarcoma (KS)
- Non-Hodgkin's lymphoma (NHL)
- Primary CNS lymphoma
- Cervical cancer

Epidemiological research has identified other tumours, such as anal cancer and Hodgkin's disease, that also have an increased incidence in HIV-positive individuals.

Kaposi's sarcoma (KS)

Prior to the HIV epidemic, this tumour was seen in three clinical settings:

- The classical form affects predominantly the lower legs in men of East European or Jewish origin and often follows an indolent course, rarely requiring any specific treatment.

- An African variant, which has been endemic for many years. This can be indolent in nature or it may be more aggressive with widespread lymph node and visceral involvement.

- Patients receiving immunosuppressive therapy e.g. in organ transplant recipients. In this instance the tumour may regress when this treatment is reduced.

However, the commonest form of KS in the developing world is the epidemic form associated with AIDS. Due to the successful treatment and prophylaxis of opportunistic infections and effective antiretroviral therapy, AIDS patients are now surviving longer. Although the incidence of KS is declining, the morbidity and mortality ascribed to KS has increased. Visceral KS now accounts for the death of one in four HIV-positive homosexuals.

KS affects male homosexuals in particular and rarely affects other groups at risk of AIDS, such as infected blood recipients and intravenous drug abusers. In those developing AIDS in an African environment, KS can be seen frequently in heterosexuals. A sexually transmitted co-factor may play an important role in its development. Recent research has identified a virus—the Kaposi's sarcoma herpes virus (KSHV), also known as human herpes virus 8(HHV8). DNA from this virus has been identified in KS lesions in semen, blood, and bronchial washings from affected patients. However, its precise role in the development of KS is not yet fully understood.

KS is a multi-focal tumour and new lesions occur at various cutaneous and internal organ sites. The most likely cell of origin is mesenchymal with vascular or lymphatic cell markers and factor VIII antigen is often positive on immunocytochemistry staining. A diagnostic feature is the intradermal proliferation of abnormal vascular structures, lined with large, spindle-shaped endothelial cells. Frequent extravasation of red blood cells and mononuclear leukocytes occur.

Recent advances have identified that AIDS KS cells produce growth factors and cytokines, for example TNF and IL6, which appear to regulate their growth. This suggests an important role in the pathogenesis of KS, which may hold promise for the development of future treatments.

Presentation

* Cutaneous red purple multiple lesions
* Flat, then progress to plaques, nodules, with oedema
* Site—upper body, face, legs
* Diagnosis—skin biopsy
* Systemic lesions—presents with lung, GI tract
  * —pain, dyspnoea, haemoptysis, bowel obstruction
  * —diagnosis by endoscopy

Staging

Important prognostic factors relate not only to disease extent but to the patient's immune status and KS can occur as an early and late feature in AIDS patients. The Aids Clinical Trials Group (ACTG) has developed a staging classification.

Treatment

There is currently no cure for KS. Therefore, the primary goal of treatment is to prolong life, while maintaining quality. The treatment should be tailored to the form of the disease. Localized treatment options include:

* Camouflage with cosmetics
* Cryotherapy and laser, especially if lesions are <1 cm diameter
* Intra-lesional chemotherapy with vinblastine or interferon
* Radiotherapy

KS is responsive to radiation treatment. A 70% response rate, equal to intra-lesional chemotherapy, can be achieved with single fraction doses of 8 Gy. This can be repeated if there is recurrence or insufficient regression. Palatal lesions can also be irradiated using iridium wire moulds.

Systemic treatment is required if there is widespread cutaneous or visceral involvement. Immunotherapy using interferon is most

Table 31.1 ACTG guidelines

	Good prognosis—all of	Poor prognosis—any of
Tumour	Skin only ± lymph nodes and or minimal oral disease	Oedema/ulceration, extensive oral disease, visceral KS
Immunological	CD4 >200	CD4 <200
Symptoms	Nil, Karnofsky >70	Opportunistic infection or thrush, B symptoms, Karnofsky <70, other HIV-related illnesses

effective if the CD4 count is >200. This form of treatment results in less bone marrow suppression. The high doses required often result in fever, night sweats, and lethargy. If the CD4 count is below 200, treatment with vincristine and bleomycin can achieve response rates of 50–60%. Side-effects include some degree of bone marrow suppression, dose-related pulmonary fibrosis (in the case of bleomycin), and a peripheral neuropathy (with vincristine). The addition of doxorubicin may result in significant bone marrow suppression and alopecia.

Recent developments have led to liposomally packaged preparations that enable selective distribution to and retention in tumours, reducing uptake in unwanted sites such as the bone marrow. Response rates of 80% have been observed. Several new treatments are also being researched in clinical trials, including taxol, beta HCG, trans-retinoic acid, and anti-angiogenic agents such as thalidomide.

Table 31.2 Treatment options for KS

Local intervention	Systemic intervention
Cryotherapy/laser esp <1 cm	Interferon — if CD4 >200
Radiotherapy — 8 GY single fraction	Vincristine 2 mg and bleomycin 30 units every 3 weeks
Intra-lesional chemotherapy	Liposomal doxorubicin 20 mg/m² every 3 weeks
Brachytherapy — palate	Liposomal daunorubicin 40 mg/m² every 2 weeks

Non-Hodgkin's lymphoma

The second most common malignancy to affect those with AIDS. Almost half of these will already have a prior AIDS-defining illness. Unlike KS, its incidence is 3% within all risk groups—one hundred times higher than in the general population. NHL also has a higher incidence in other congenitally and iatrogenically immune-suppressed individuals.

A viral co-factor—the Epstein–Barr virus (EBV)—is closely linked to the development of lymphoma in AIDS. EBV proteins can be demonstrated in 50% of lymphomas in nodal or extra-nodal sites. It is thought that in the immune-deficient host the proliferation of EBV-infected cells may proceed unchecked. Oncogenic alterations, e.g. p53 and C-*myc*, have also been identified. 90% of HIV-related NHLS are of B-cell origin and are commonly high-grade. The most common sub-types are immunoblastic, centroblastic, lymphoblastic, and Burkitt-like lymphoma.

Presentation

- At advanced stage
- Usually involves marrow and CNS (extra-nodal)
- Frequently B symptoms
- Differential diagnosis TB, CMV
- Gland biopsy essential
- Investigations—chest X-ray, CT head, abdomen, pelvis
    —bone marrow biopsy
    —LDH level
    —lumbar puncture
- Poor prognosis—median survival 6 months
    —50% die from opportunistic infections
    —50% die from lymphoma

Prognosis

Poor prognostic factors include:
- Absolute CD4 count <200 ul
- Prior AIDS-defining diagnosis
- Karnofsky performance score <70
- Extra-nodal disease including bone marrow
- Raised LDH
- Immunoblastic subtype

Treatment

Systemic treatment with chemotherapy is usually the only available curative treatment. However, if the disease is truly localized, radiotherapy can result in long-term control and is invaluable for the palliation of local symptoms.

The standard treatment for more advanced disease is combination chemotherapy. CHOP (cyclophosphamide, doxorubicin, vincristine, prednisolone) is a typical chemotherapy regimen, given every three weeks. More intensive schedules can be used, but due to increased toxicity are often not well tolerated. In those at high risk of meningeal involvement, concomitant intrathecal chemotherapy of methotrexate and cytarabine is also used.

Recent studies suggest that more aggressive chemotherapy regimens result in an overall decrease in survival due to toxicity-related complications. Modified schedules including a 75% dose reduction may produce similar response and overall survival rates. Those who achieve a complete response with chemotherapy have a survival benefit ranging from 6–20 months.

Primary CNS lymphoma

Primary CNS lymphoma (PCNSL) affects 2–6% of HIV-positive individuals. It is usually a late manifestation of AIDS and the patients commonly have other serious opportunistic infections. The histology is similar to AIDS-related NHL, except almost all cases are associated with EBV. Patients often present with epileptic seizures, hemiparesis, or severe headaches. A CT or MRI is the investigation of choice. However, the scan appearances may be indistinguishable from cerebral toxoplasmosis and, for this reason, patients are often treated initially with a trial of toxoplasmosis treatment. A histological diagnosis is ideal but not often possible.

Treatment involves whole-brain radiotherapy in combination with steroids and, sometimes, intrathecal chemotherapy. There is little evidence to support the use of systemic chemotherapy. In good performance status patients, the median survival is 12 months. If no treatment is given, the survival rate falls significantly to just a few months. Patients usually die from the late complications of AIDS.

Other malignancies

Hodgkin's disease has an increased incidence in HIV-positive patients—5–9 times higher than the general population. It is seen more commonly in patients where transmission of HIV has been by intravenous drug use. The disease is often advanced at the time of presentation. Standard chemotherapy is with ABVD (adriamycin, bleomycin, vinblastine, dacarbazine). The median survival with chemotherapy is 12 months.

Cervical cancer in HIV-positive females became an AIDS-defining diagnosis in 1993. Its increased prevalence may be because both HIV virus and the human papillomavirus (HPV) are sexually transmissible. It is advisable to screen this group more frequently, (every 6–12 months).

Anal cancer is related to both HIV and HPV. It has an increased prevalence in homosexual men practising anal intercourse. However, the risk is higher for those who are also HIV-positive.

Spinal cord compression is a medical emergency. Treatment must begin within hours, not days.

Presentation

- Bone involvement from cancer—breast
  - —prostate
  - —lung   } all common
  - —myeloma
  - —lymphoma
  - —thyroid
  - —kidney
  - —bladder   } all less common
  - —bowel
  - —melanoma
- Initial presentation of malignancy—prostate, breast, myeloma.
- Crush fracture or tumour extension common.
- Occasional direct extension from retroperitoneal, mediastinal tumours e.g. lymphoma.
- Occasional extra-dural compression in absence of bone involvement.
- Occasional intra-medullary metastases.
- 66% of cases occur in the thoracic cord.

Table 32.1 Spinal cord compression syndromes

Complete compression

Sensory level just below level of lesion

Loss of all sensory modalities—may be variable at onset

Bilateral upper motor neurone weakness below lesion

Bladder and bowel dysfunction

Anterior compression

Partial loss of pain and temperature below lesion

Bilateral upper motor neurone weakness below lesion

Bladder and bowel dysfunction

Posterior compression

Loss of vibration and position below lesion

Relative sparing of pain, temperature, and touch

Band of dysthaesia at level of lesion

Lateral compression (Brown–Séquard syndrome)

Contralateral loss of pain and temperature (touch relatively spared)

Ipsilateral loss of vibration and position

Ipsilateral upper motor neurone weakness

Symptoms

Pain, characteristically with a nerve root or 'girdle' distribution, exacerbated by coughing or straining and not relieved by bed rest frequently precedes neurological symptoms or signs. Any patient with cancer who develops severe back pain with a root distribution should be considered at risk of spinal cord compression and urgently investigated.

Weakness of the legs (and arms if the lesion is high in the spine), retention, dribbling, or incontinence of urine or faeces, and constipation, may occur and are late symptoms.

Cauda equina syndrome

The spinal cord ends at the level of L1 or L2. Tumours below this level may produce cauda equina compression with sciatic pain (often bilateral), bladder dysfunction with retention and overflow incontinence, impotence, sacral (saddle) anaesthesia, loss of anal sphincter tone, and weakness and wasting of the gluteal muscles. The symptoms may be unclear and the diagnosis difficult to make without MRI.

Examination

The following may be present:

- Visible or palpable gibbus at the site of a wedged or collapsed verte-bra
- Pain and tenderness on palpation or percussion of the vertebra over the site of compression
- Band of hyperaesthesia at the level of the lesion
- Sensory and motor loss (with defects of power and sensation) at and below the level of the lesion

The lesion may be partial or complete and the nature of the defect may depend on the portion of the cord compressed. In a patient pre-senting with spinal cord compression without a history of malig-nancy, the examination and investigations should also be directed towards excluding an underlying malignancy.

Investigations

- Plain X-rays may demonstrate destruction and/or collapse of a vertebra. Changes are sometimes more subtle e.g. loss of a vertebral pedicle. Paravertebral masses may sometimes also be shown. In 15–20% of cases, plain films show no abnormality.

- MRI scanning is the investigation of choice. It will demonstrate the site and extent of the lesion and presence of multiple lesions in vertebrae and in the spinal canal. It is particularly useful in cases of cauda equina syndrome.

- MRI has largely superseded myelography. Where MRI is not available, myelography will show the anatomical location of a spinal cord lesion and whether a block is complete or not. However, if a complete block is present the upper limit of a lesion may not be demonstrated without cisternal myelography.

- CT scanning may provide useful information if MRI is not available. Simultaneous myelography may enhance the usefulness of the investigation. It will demonstrate an abnormality within a defined region of the cord but is not an ideal primary investigation if the site of compression cannot be accurately predicted from clinical and plain radiograph findings.

If radiotherapy or surgery is proposed, it is useful to ask the radiologist to mark the level(s) of the lesion(s) on the patient's skin, to aid localization.

Management

Speed is of the essence in the management of spinal cord compression since the degree of recovery is dependent on the pre-treatment status. Fewer than 10% of patients with established paraplegia from metastatic disease walk again.

If spinal cord compression is suspected, dexamethasone 16–20 mg should be given immediately. This relieves peritumoural oedema. Awaiting radiological confirmation of spinal cord compression before starting steroids is almost never warranted. If neurological improvement occurs, the steroid dose may be reduced to the lowest that will maintain that improvement. If immediate surgery is not contemplated, neurological status should be assessed at least daily so that deterioration may be detected early and surgical intervention considered.

For patients able to walk or whose paresis responds to steroids, radiotherapy is as successful as surgery and is therefore the treatment of choice. Radiation is usually delivered via a single posterior field, which should extend one or two vertebrae above and below the compressing lesion. Typical doses include 8 Gy in a single fraction, 20 Gy in 4–5 fractions, or 30 Gy in 10 fractions. Some prefer longer fractionation regimes for patients with hormone-responsive tumours (breast, prostate) that are newly diagnosed as metastatic.

Radiation-induced oedema may exacerbate symptoms: be prepared to increase the dose of steroids again during radiotherapy.

Indications for surgery include:

• Acute-onset paraplegia

• Fracture dislocation

• Failure to respond to steroids

• Tumours known to be radio-resistant or when spinal cord compression progresses during, or recurs after, irradiation

• No histological proof of malignancy

Patients with spinal instability, retropulsed bone fragments, or complete collapse of a vertebra with myelopathy do not benefit from radiotherapy alone. Since complete surgical clearance of tumour is not likely to be attempted or achieved, post-operative radiotherapy is usually necessary.

Patients with established paraplegia are extremely unlikely to recover after either surgery or radiotherapy. No treatment may therefore be appropriate, unless persistent pain is itself an indication for active intervention.

The overall condition and prognosis should also determine how active management should be. For example, complex spinal surgery, involving weeks or months of hospitalization, is inappropriate for someone whose underlying disease carries a very poor prognosis.

Chemotherapy has no role in the management of acute spinal cord compression.

General advice

Early involvement of a physiotherapist and occupational therapist will ensure optimal rehabilitation and remobilization. Discharge plans should be made as early as a realistic estimate of likely final function is possible. Bear in mind the risk of deep venous thrombosis and pressure sores in those patients who remain paraplegic.

The prognosis for cancer patients who develop spinal cord compression is poor—8–9 months for those who are ambulant after treatment and only one month for those who are not.

Chapter 33
Bone marrow suppression

Introduction

The major dose-limiting toxicity of cancer chemotherapy is bone marrow suppression, compromising the potential for cure in many patients with chemotherapy malignancies. The ability to cope with myelosuppression and its consequent morbidity is integral to an oncologist's skills and requires a thorough understanding of haemopoiesis and the bone marrow response to different chemotherapies. Manipulation of myelosuppression kinetics with haemopoietic growth factors is a new and exciting development in cancer treatment and, with the advent of stem cell technology, the dose intensity of cancer chemotherapy is being taken to previously unheard of limits.

The bone marrow is a complex organ system responsible for haemopoiesis. In adults it is predominantly situated in the vertebrae, sternum, ribs, skull, and proximal long bones. A single early stem cell is thought to be the progenitor for all blood cells, producing a lymphoid stem cell and a mixed myeloid progenitor cell that then undergo further differentiation before being released as formed elements into the peripheral circulation. Between 10^{10} and 10^{12} cells are produced by the bone marrow every hour in a carefully controlled manner. Bone marrow failure usually produces a pancytopaenia.

Since red blood cells survive about 120 days, platelets about 8 days, and neutrophils approximately 1–2 days, early problems relate mainly to neutropenia and trombocytopenia. Therapeutic interventions in cancer patients producing bone marrow compromise include cytotoxic chemotherapy, bone marrow transplantation, and wide-field irradiation.

Normal healthy bone marrow is capable of supplying the peripheral blood with mature cells for 7–10 days after precursor cell damage by cytotoxic agents; drug effects tend to manifest between days 7 and 14. This time-frame is variable, with different drugs producing different neutrophil and platelet suppression profiles depending on precursor populations affected. Myelosuppression related to chemotherapy can be graded using defined criteria—a process useful in clinical trials and in judging risk in dose-intensive therapy.

Table 33.1 NCIC–CTG expanded common toxicity criteria

Toxicity grade	0	1	2	3	4
Hb g/dl	WNL	10.0–normal	8.0–9.9	6.5–7.9	<6.5
Platelets × 10⁹/l	WNL	7.5–normal	50.0–74.9	25.0–49.9	<25.0
WBC × 10⁹/l	≥4.0	3.0–3.9	2.0–2.9	1.0–1.9	<1.0
Granulocytes	≥2.0	1.5–1.9	1.0–1.4	0.5–0.9	<0.5
Lymphocytes	≥2.0	1.5–1.9	1.0–1.4	0.5–0.9	<0.5

Causes of bone marrow failure

- Depletion of anatomical and physiological elements e.g. myelofibrosis, myelodysplasia
- Intrinsic stem cell/precursor cell failure e.g. aplastic anaemia, paroxysmal nocturnal haemoglobinuria
- Iatrogenic e.g. chemotherapy, irradiation
- Bone marrow infiltration e.g. malignancy
- Peripheral consumption e.g. hypersplenism
- Autoimmune diseases e.g. systemic lupus erythematosis
- Vitamin deficiency e.g. megaloblastic anaemia

Pancytopenia in the cancer patient

* Neutropenia—life-threatening bacterial infections
* Associated with—poor nutrition
    —mucosal barrier defects
    —abnormal host colonization
* Qualitative and quantitative defects
* Defects in chemotaxis, neutrophil degranulation

Table 33.2 Most common micro-organisms in neutropenic patients

Gram-negative bacilli	Gram-positive bacilli	Fungi
E. coli	Staphylococcus aureus	Candida spp
Klebsiella spp	Staphylococcus epidermidis	Aspergillus spp
Enterobacter spp	Streptococcus pneumoniae	Mucorales
Proteus spp	Viridans streptococci	
P. aeroginosa	Enterococci	
	Corynebacterium	

Management of fever in a neutropenic patient

Fever is common in patients with cancer. Although commonly caused by infection it can also be related to underlying malignancy, blood product transfusion, and pyrogenic medications. Careful evaluation of fever in a neutropenic patient should not take long. Untreated sepsis in a neutropenic patient can be rapidly fatal. Generally, antibiotics are administered after the following simple investigations:

- Blood cultures (peripheral and central, if line *in situ*)
- Sputum culture
- Urine analysis and culture
- Chest X-ray
- Swabs from Hickman line exit site
- Careful physical examination

Treatment should then be instituted, with empirical antibiotic therapy, particularly if the patient is toxic or haemodynamically compromised. The widespread adoption of this approach has reduced the mortality of neutropenic sepsis to less than 10%.

Careful observation of the febrile response to antibiotics, coupled with body fluid culture results, will determine adjustment of antibiotic therapy over the next few days. If the fever is unremitting at 48 hours, or there is any clinical deterioration, an empirical change of antibiotics to a second-line antibiotic regime should be performed.

Failure to resolve the fever within 5 days may suggest other opportunistic infections such as fungi or parasites such as *Pneumocystis carinii*. Careful consideration of these diagnoses, in close consultation with a microbiologist, is required before initiation of specific treatments, such as amphotericin B, for these infections, since the therapies themselves are potentially toxic.

Often, resolution of neutropenia results in resolution of refractory fever. This process can be accelerated by the use of haemopoietic growth factors.

Thrombocytopenia in the cancer patient

Thrombocytopenia is commonplace in patients receiving cytotoxic chemotherapy. The trigger level to transfuse platelets is not always absolute. Spontaneous bleeding is unlikely if platelets are $>20 \times 10^9$/l, but the risk of traumatic bleeding is greater if $<40 \times 10^9$/l. Most clinicians would transfuse when platelets are $<10 \times 10^9$/l. However, if there is active bleeding, many clinicians would transfuse if $<50 \times 10^9$/l.

Careful consideration of the patient's vascular status, clotting status, and disease risks (e.g. gastric carcinoma) will determine the threshold for transfusion in an individual patient. Cross-matching is not required since patients generally receive random, pooled, donor platelets.

Some patients may become refractory after repeated transfusions and HLA-matched platelets should be used. Four units of fresh platelets, (doubled if platelets greater than three days old), should raise the count to >24–40×10^9/l in an adult. Although frequently part of the differential diagnosis of refractoriness, HLA allo-immunization is only one of many causes. Others include the presence of:

- Anti-platelet antibodies
- Disseminated intravascular coagulation
- Concomitant drugs e.g. septrin
- Hypersplenism

Red cell transfusions in cancer patients

A low haemoglobin in a patient with cancer is also common and requires careful diagnostic evaluation. Elimination of obvious causes such as bleeding from a gastrointestinal malignancy are important before repeated red cell transfusions are given. A one-unit blood transfusion should raise the haemoglobin by approximately 1 g/dl. Transfusion may reduce the platelet count, so platelet transfusion may be required before or after blood transfusion.

Red cell transfusion should be based on clinical criteria rather than absolute trigger values. The use of erythropoietin to maintain haemoglobin values in patients with cancer, on or off treatment, is unproven.

Chapter 34
Superior vena cava obstruction

Aetiology

The superior vena cava can be obstructed by:
- External compression (primary tumour or lymph nodes)
- Thrombus (secondary to compression; also IV catheters)
- Combination of above

In cancer patients the commonest cause is external compression by either a primary tumour in the right paratracheal region or a secondary tumour in the paratracheal lymph nodes.

Lung cancer is the commonest tumour to cause superior vena cava obstruction (SVCO), but any tumour spreading to the mediastinal nodes (especially lymphomas) may do so. Other causes include ruptured thoracic aortic aneurysm and trauma.

Clinical features

Symptoms:

- Swelling of the neck, face, and arms, especially in the morning
- Headache
- Visual disturbance

SVCO itself does not impair respiration but it is commonly associated with dyspnoea due to tracheal or bronchial obstruction/compression

Examination:

- Fixed engorgement of external and internal jugular veins
- Collateral veins over anterior and lateral chest wall (which drain down)
- Papilloedema (late feature)

Differential diagnoses

Heart failure   Jugular veins pulsating not fixed; other cardiac signs; dependent oedema.

Tamponade   Characteristic symptoms/signs and CXR appearances.

External jugular vein compression   No facial oedema; no collaterals; usually supraclavicular fossa nodes.

Investigations

The clinical diagnosis of SVCO is usually obvious and investigation should be aimed at establishing the cause, especially if there is no pre-existing diagnosis of malignancy. Unless the patient has very severe and life-threatening symptoms (e.g. associated stridor) treatment should not start until a clear diagnosis (including pathology if possible) has been made.

Chest x-ray usually shows a right paratracheal mass or other indications of lung cancer or mediastinal lymphadenopathy. It is rarely normal.

CT thorax is required only if CXR findings are equivocal or if indicated for the normal investigation of the underlying tumour.

Venogram is needed if there is no obvious mass causing external compression, or if thrombolysis or stent insertion are planned.

FNA cytology samples should be taken from, for example, cervical lymphadenopathy.

Bronchoscopy is essential if the clinical picture and CXR suggest lung cancer and a histopathological diagnosis is not yet obtained.

Mediastinal biopsy (mediastinoscopy, mediastinotomy, mini-thoracotomy, or directed-needle biopsy) is essential if a pathological diagnosis has not been established any other way. There is an increased risk of haemorrhage from these procedures in patients with SVCO, but this is small in experienced hands.

Treatment

In the majority of cases the treatment is that of the underlying cause and it is important to establish a clear diagnosis (including pathology) before starting. It is unusual for the symptoms to be so severe as to require emergency treatment (unless there is coincident tracheal compression) and the gradual development of collateral circulation means that symptoms often stabilize.

• Treatment choices for commonest underlying tumours include:

—*Small cell lung cancer:* chemotherapy (unless physical state very poor); radiotherapy (at relapse following chemotherapy).

—*Non-small cell lung cancer:* surgery is very rarely possible because SVCO is usually associated with locally advanced tumour; radical radiotherapy may be possible if the tumour is central but localized; for most, palliative radiotherapy is appropriate.

—*Non-Hodgkin's lymphoma:* usually chemotherapy.

• *Corticosteroids* are frequently prescribed (e.g. Dexamethasone 4 mg qds) but there is no good evidence for their efficacy; anti-tumour effect in lymphoma and Hodgkin's disease; helpful if the patient has associated stridor.

• *Thrombolysis* is increasingly used as a prelude to stenting. Extensive thrombus in the SVC and tributary veins may lead to persistent or increasing symptoms and signs despite successful tumour treatment. Thrombolysis should only be considered after venography and if other measures are unlikely to be successful. Where thrombus has formed around a Hickman line (often in association with continuous infusion chemotherapy) removal of the line will usually lead to resolution of SVCO.

• *Stenting:* an expanding metal stent can be manoeuvred into the SVC at the point of stricture. If an interventional cardiologist with experience can provide a rapid service, this is now treatment of choice for patients with severe symptoms.

Prognosis

The prognosis is that of the underlying tumour and its staging. SVCO does not *per se* imply a worse prognosis, even for patients with lung cancer.

Chapter 35
Raised intracranial pressure

The rigid bony skull surrounding the brain is resistant to any increase in the volume of its contents, with any such change readily leading to a rise in intra-cranial pressure and displacement of structures. Elevated intra-cranial pressure is characterized in its early stages by headache and vomiting, often worse in the morning. With increasing pressure there is drowsiness, heralding a more rapid neurological deterioration. Changes in pressure can sometimes be more gradual with memory loss and behavioural difficulties.

Clinical signs

In addition to any focal neurological deficit, clinical signs suggesting a rise in intracranial pressure include bradycardia, systemic hypertension, and papilloedema. The latter may be difficult to identify in its early stages and may be suggested by optic nerve head swelling, blurring of disc margins, and loss of the normal retinal venous pulsation. Specific neurological localizing features should be sought—Parinaud's syndrome, (paralysis of conjugate upward gaze), for example, is suggestive of a lesion in the pineal region.

The three commonest causes of increased intracranial pressure are:

• A space-occupying lesion (tumour, abscess, haematoma)

• Hydrocephalus (due to obstruction of cerebrospinal fluid (CSF) circulation)

• Benign intra-cranial hypertension

It should be remembered that patients with malignancy are at risk of developing non-malignant space-occupying lesions (abscesses, haematoma) as a consequence of treatment. Of neoplastic brain disorder processes, approximately 50% are due to secondary metastases, the remainder encompassing the range of primary brain tumours, of which gliomas are the commonest.

Brain tumours can produce a rise in intracranial pressure either through mass effect or by the production of hydrocephalus. Hydrocephalus as a consequence of malignancy is seen more commonly in primary brain tumours, notably pineal tumours and medulloblastoma.

Diagnosis

- Clinical
- Contrast-enhanced CT scan—mass effect
—ventricular dilatation

Management

Early management:
- High-dose steroids—dexamethasone, 16 mg daily
- IV mannitol (100 ml 20% solution over 1–2 hours)

Further management:
- Steroids if poor prognosis
- Palliative whole-brain radiotherapy—little evidence of benefit
- Hormone manipulation—breast and prostate cancers
- If solitary, consider surgical resection

Treatment

Primary CNS tumours presenting with raised intracranial pressure require a tissue diagnosis. Ventricular shunting may be used in patients with hydrocephalus due to lesions situated in areas difficult to access surgically. However, if at all possible histological confirmation should be sought, as it has a major bearing on the therapeutic approach.

High-grade gliomas may occasionally have a substantial cystic component that, even in the setting of recurrent disease, may be drained, leading to rapid resolution of elevated intra-cranial pressure.

Patients with malignant meningitis can present with features suggesting raised intracranial pressure and often have associated cranial nerve palsies. This is often an ominous development in epithelial tumours, but may also occur in some primary CNS tumours, especially medulloblastoma and pineal region tumours; MRI may demonstrate meningeal tumour deposits. The diagnosis can otherwise be confirmed by lumbar puncture, seeking malignant cells in the CSF, although this must be preceded by CT scan to exclude hydrocephalus.

Chapter 36
Stridor

Stridor is the term applied to the high pitched musical noise produced by turbulent airflow through narrowed upper airways. It is caused by partial obstruction of the airway either in the region of the larynx or inferiorly in the trachea or major bronchi. Because of the anatomy of the larynx, obstruction above or at the level of the vocal cords produces predominantly inspiratory stridor, whereas obstruction in the subglottis or trachea causes biphasic stridor.

Aetiology

Stridor can be due to benign or malignant causes. Non-malignant causes may include inhaled foreign body, tracheal stenosis (e.g. post-tracheostomy), or bilateral vocal cord palsy (e.g. post-thyroid surgery). Malignant causes may be:

- *Intrinsic* Bulky or extensive primary tumours of the upper airway, larynx, hypopharynx, subglottis, and trachea. Bronchial tumours arising in a proximal bronchus invading the carina will produce similar symptoms.
- *Extrinsic* Thyroid tumours, especially anaplastic thyroid carcinoma; any tumour causing mediastinal lymphadenopathy e.g. Hodgkin's disease, non-Hodgkin's lymphoma, or metastatic carcinoma.

Diagnosis

- Clinical
- Features of underlying malignancy e.g. goitre, clubbing, weight loss
- Chest X-ray—widening of mediastinum (lymphadenopathy)
            —primary lung cancer
- Indirect laryngoscopy (mobility of cords)
- Fibreoptic nasoendoscopy
- Bronchoscopy—biopsy/cytology
- CT scan
- Mediastinoscopy

Treatment

Treatment is dependant upon the underlying cause. However, in most cases of malignant stridor (particularly if severe) high-dose steroids (e.g. dexamethasone 12–16 mg) should be given in an attempt to reduce peri-tumoural oedema and relieve airway obstruction. The need for supplemental oxygen may be assessed using pulse oximetry.

In severe cases of laryngeal obstruction due to an upper airway tumour or anaplastic thyroid carcinoma, emergency tracheostomy may be required to preserve the airway before appropriate treatment is initiated. Tumour debulking using laser may be helpful in bulky exophytic laryngeal tumours before treatment commences.

Treatment of stridor due to mediastinal lymph node compression is dependant on the nature of the underlying tumour type. Patients with non-small cell lung cancer should receive urgent palliative radiotherapy. There is anecdotal concern that radiotherapy may worsen peri-tumoural oedema initially, and all such patients should receive steroids. Those with small cell lung cancer or lymphoid malignancies will usually respond to chemotherapy. There may be little gained in utilizing radiotherapy initially in such patients. However, in urgent circumstances, with severe respiratory distress, radiotherapy may be initiated in the absence of histology.

In cases of recurrent malignancy affecting the trachea, laser fulguration, endoluminal stenting, or high dose-rate endoluminal brachytherapy may provide useful palliation.

Chapter 37
Acute blood loss

Massive blood loss (haemoptysis) is often a rapidly terminal event in patients with lung cancer, usually caused by erosion of major intrathoracic blood vessels by the primary tumour. Other causes include pulmonary or endobronchial metastases. Non-malignant causes, such as pulmonary embolism or pulmonary infection, should also be considered in a patient suffering from neoplasia.

Assessment

The first thought should be whether active resuscitation is indicated. For the patient in the terminal phase of illness, adequate sedation may be more appropriate. Should resuscitation be deemed appropriate, an immediate assessment of haemodynamic stability should be made and evidence of coagulopathy sought. A low platelet and fibrinogen level with elevated fibrinogen degradation products (FDPs) is indicative of disseminated intravascular coagulation. CXR and bronchoscopy will help to localize lesions within the major airways and pulmonary parenchyma.

An assessment of the patient's general condition and fitness should be made to dictate the extent of resuscitation that is appropriate.

Treatment

Adequate volume replacement with crystalloids, followed by blood, should be given. In patients with cardio-respiratory impairment, titration against central venous pressure may be necessary. Replacement of platelets and clotting factors will be needed in some patients. Specific therapy will be dictated by the individual situation. Radiation therapy can be effective in stopping bleeding from most tumour sites. A short fractionated course, such as 20 Gy in five fractions, or even a single fraction of 8 Gy, can be given.

Endoscopic brachytherapy can be a useful tool, especially in patients previously treated by radiation. Bleeding can also be treated endoscopically in accessible sites. Endoscopic sclerotherapy can sometimes be useful for bleeding from larger vessels; smaller vessel bleeding may respond to laser treatment with the Nd: YAG laser. In severe, recalcitrant cases, bronchial angiography and selective arterial embolization may be necessary.

Gynaecological haemorrhage

Primary or recurrent neoplasms of the uterus, cervix, vagina, or vulva may present with recurrent small bleeds or with massive life-threatening haemorrhage. Haemorrhagic metastases may also cause varying degrees of bleeding. Massive haemorrhage may be the terminal event in patients with end-stage disease.

Vaginal packing can be a useful holding measure while more definitive treatment is decided. Bleeding originating from the uterus or cervix is best treated with brachytherapy. A central tube is inserted into the uterine cavity and two ovoids are inserted into the vaginal fornices. The applicators are then loaded with caesium 137. External-beam radiotherapy can be integrated at a later date if indicated.

Vaginal bleeding more commonly arises from haemorrhagic metastases. A vaginal tube can be inserted and subsequently loaded with caesium or external-beam radiotherapy can be offered, usually to a dose of 20 Gy in four or five fractions. In severe cases, surgical ligation of the branches of the internal iliac artery may be required.

Head and neck haemorrhage

Bleeding in head and neck cancer can vary from small recurrent bleeds of no haemodynamic importance to the so-called 'carotid blow out' caused by erosion of the internal carotid artery. The latter is fatal in a matter of minutes. A warning 'herald bleed' can sometimes occur prior to such an event.

Recurrent small bleeds arise as a result of degradation of small intra-tumoural blood vessels. This symptom can sometimes be the presenting complaint. Bleeding can arise from the mucosal surfaces, from skin ulceration, or can be stomal following surgical treatment.

Significant bleeds arise from major vessel erosion (arterial or venous). This can occur in recurrent disease, often following surgery to the neck or in the advanced neglected primary. Significant bleeds from the neck most often arise following malignant infiltration of major neck vessels by metastatic lymphadenopathy.

Treatment

Recurrent small bleeds can sometimes be managed by CO_2 laser. Only vessels smaller than 0.5 mm will respond to such treatment. Slightly larger vessels will coagulate in response to Nd: YAG laser treatment. Should active resuscitation be appropriate, volume replacement with crystalloids and blood will be necessary.

Radiation treatment is the mainstay of palliative therapy in these cases: it often stops bleeding within a matter of days. Occasional patients presenting with haemodynamically significant haemorrhage may be candidates for more aggressive therapy. Even patients with T3/T4 lesions can attain a five-year survival rate of up to 25%.

Gastrointestinal haemorrhage

Acute blood loss in gastrointestinal cancers is less common than chronic bleeding resulting in iron deficiency. It can occur as the presenting feature or in the terminal phase of illness in the heavily pretreated patient. Haemorrhage occurs most often from the primary tumour or as a result of its local extension. Previous chemotherapy and clotting factor deficiency, in the case of hepatic impairment, may exacerbate bleeding. Endoluminal metastases are a rare cause of acute blood loss and metastases to the small bowel can occur in malignant melanoma.

Presentation may be with haematemesis, melaena, or fresh rectal bleeding, depending on the site of the lesion.

Treatment

Specific therapy will be dictated by the individual situation. Radiation therapy can be effective in stopping bleeding from most sites in the GI tract, although mobile organs (stomach or small bowel) are more difficult to irradiate.

Occasional patients presenting with an acute GI bleed from a localized cancer may be treated surgically.

Chapter 38
Obstruction

Intestinal obstruction

Aetiology

Predominantly associated with pelvic cancers and most commonly found in ovarian (6–42%), cervical (5%), and colonic cancers (10–30%). Cause is either intra-luminal disease (more common in colonic cancer) or extra-mural compression. In ovarian and cervical cancers there are often multiple levels of obstruction. Obstruction in a patient with previous cancer may also be due to non-malignant causes (such as adhesions or gross constipation).

Obstruction may be complete, subacute, or functional; it may be intermittent. Functional obstruction may be caused by a cancer-related or drug-related (vincristine) autonomic neuropathy, by direct involvement of the mesenteric plexus, or through ileus (e.g. due to perforation).

Presentation

- Symptoms—nausea, vomiting, colicky pain, constipation, increased bowel sounds
- Signs—distension, dehydration, splash, bowel sounds variable
    —gastric outlet obstruction
    —large volume projectile vomiting
    —large bowel obstruction; faeculent vomiting

Investigation

Erect and supine plain abdominal views may confirm the diagnosis and will show constipation if present. Where the diagnosis is not clear, contrast barium studies may be indicated. If surgery is a possibility and there is doubt about the number of levels of obstruction or the site of the lesion, MRI can be helpful. Appropriate resuscitation will be guided by clinical and biochemical assessment of dehydration and electrolyte disturbance.

Treatment options

First-line therapy is surgical if active treatment is appropriate. Intravenous fluids and nasogastric suction are usually instigated but are not normally necessary if surgery is not an option. The patient may not wish surgery or, due to the extent of disease, surgery may not be appropriate. Laser therapy may be useful to debulk obstructing oesophageal, gastric, and rectal carcinomas. However, this approach requires repeated treatments. Plastic tubes or expandable metal stents can also be considered and are generally of use in oesophageal or oesophago-gastric lesions.

Medical management

Inoperable intestinal obstruction can be managed medically. This may permit the patient to be cared for at home. The patient can eat and drink small amounts. Treatment approaches vary dependent upon whether subacute obstruction or complete obstruction is present. The aim is to remove the debilitating feeling of nausea and to reduce the frequency of vomiting to a level acceptable to the patient.

The symptoms to be palliated are nausea, vomiting, pain, and constipation. Oral medication is poorly absorbed in gastro-intestinal obstruction and the subcutaneous or rectal route should be used.

Pain

For colic, an anti-spasmodic—buscopan 80–120 mg over 24 hours via continuous subcutaneous infusion—is usually effective. Avoid prokinetic antiemetics (metoclopramide) if colic a problem. Pain from cancer or metastases usually requires parenteral analgesics (e.g. diamorphine given subcutaneously over 24 hours via a syringe driver, or transdermal fentanyl).

Nausea and vomiting

If partial obstruction without colic is present, metoclopramide, 80–120 mg over 24 hours sc, may stimulate effective bowel motility. This can be combined with high-dose dexamethasone, 16 mg/24 hours, to reduce peri-tumour oedema and to also serve as an antiemetic. As vomiting is controlled, introduce oral laxatives as tolerated.

If obstruction is complete or if colic is present, cyclizine, 100–150 mg/24 hours sc, is given with buscopan. Haloperidol, 5–15 mg/24 hours, is a suitable alternative. Haloperidol, cyclizine, and hyoscine are all miscible with diamorphine in a driver syringe.

Methotrimeprazine is a highly specific $5HT_2$ antagonist and has inhibitory effects on other emetic pathway receptors. It is a useful alternative to the aforementioned antiemetics and is also miscible with diamorphine. If vomiting persists then octreotide, 300–600 mg/24 hrs via continuous sc infusion—a somatostatin analogue—can be used. This drug is antisecretory and promotes reabsorption of electrolytes and, hence, water from the bowel. Effectively this decompresses the dilated bowel.

In difficult cases a nasogastric tube should be considered for short-term use. If all else fails to control the vomiting and it is distressing to the patient, then a venting gastrostomy must be considered, taking into account the patient's prognosis, current condition, and, above all, their own wishes. With a gastrostomy *in situ*, the patient can take oral liquids which can be drawn off via the gastrostomy, as needed.

Urinary tract obstruction

Aetiology

The following are the most common causes of urinary obstruction in patients with cancer:

- Carcinoma of the prostate or bladder when the urethra or ureteric orifices become occluded
- Carcinoma of the cervix or other carcinoma involving the pelvis obstructing the lower ureter
- Para-aortic nodes or retroperitoneal tumour compressing the ureters
- Transitional cell carcinoma of one or both ureters
- Fibrosis following surgery, chemotherapy, or radiotherapy

Symptoms

The gradual onset of unilateral ureteric obstruction is often asymptomatic, only diagnosed radiographically as hydronephrosis. Acute ureteric obstruction may cause painful spasm or dull aching in the flank, and the pain may radiate in the distribution of the L1 nerve root. Bilateral gradual obstruction becomes symptomatic as the serum urea rises above 25 mmol/l, ultimately leading to anuria and renal failure, with lethargy, drowsiness, confusion, nausea, and twitching.

Investigations

Selective use of abdominal ultrasound, IVU (contraindicated in uraemic patient), cystoscopy and retrograde ureteric studies, isotope renogram (assesses function of each kidney), and CT scan of the abdomen are helpful. CT of the abdomen with IV contrast as a single modality provides most information by defining any extra-ureteric pathology.

Treatment options

Bladder outlet obstruction causes symptoms of acute urinary retention or chronic obstruction, with overflow incontinence relieved by urethral or suprapubic catheterization. Palliative transurethral resection of a prostate or bladder tumour may be necessary to provide symptomatic relief.

Ureteric decompression can be accomplished by:

- Percutaneous nephrostomy with or without antegrade stenting
- Cystoscopy and retrograde placement of an internal ureteric stent

Percutaneous nephrostomy is a temporary measure, appropriate in the following specific circumstances:

- Undiagnosed malignant disease
- Prostatic or cervical primary, with an available treatment modality with reasonable chance of response

Patients with advanced cancer can gain symptomatic benefit from nephrostomy/ureteric stent insertion. However, since a nephrostomy drain may remain *in situ* for several months, it is prone to dislodgement, infection, and leakage around the site. Double pigtail ureteric stents can be inserted in preference to a long-term nephrostomy. Complications of these include transient bacteremia, urosepsis, haemorrhage, and obstructive encrustations.

Chapter 39
Biochemical crises

Introduction

Cancer and its treatment can cause a wide range of metabolic problems:

- Hypercalcaemia
- Hyponatraemia
- Hyperkalaemia
- Renal tubular dysfunction
- Hyperglycaemia
- Hypoglycaemia

The early symptoms of biochemical abnormalities may be subtle and easily confused with those of the underlying disease process. However, they undoubtedly adversely affect quality of life and, when severe, may be life-threatening and present as an oncological emergency.

Malignant hypercalcaemia

* Complicates 5–10% of all cancers
* Especially associated with breast, myeloma, and squamous cell carcinoma of lung
* If filtered, calcium load increases five-fold; kidney cannot excrete and hypercalcaemia occurs
* Calcium above 3.0 mmol/L leads to dysfunctional GI tract, CNS, and kidneys
* Effective treatment improves quality of life

Pathophysiology

Mechanisms involved in the pathogenesis of malignant hypercalcaemia include increased bone resorption (osteolysis) and systemic release of humoral hypercalcaemic factors, with or without evidence of metastatic bone disease. Local osteolytic hypercalcaemia is attributed to tumour cell production of cytokines, particularly interleukins and tumour necrosis factors (TNF), prostaglandins, and growth factors, which stimulate prostaglandin function, while parathyroid hormone-related peptide (PTHrP) is the best characterized humoral mediator of hypercalcaemia.

In some tumours, such as squamous cell cancers, humoral mechanisms are dominant, while in others, for example multiple myeloma and lymphoma, osteolysis predominates. In breast cancer, both osteolysis and humoral mechanisms appear to be important. Dehydration is also an important contributory factor; calcium is a potent diuretic causing salt and water loss.

In myeloma, renal impairment may also develop from deposition of Bence–Jones proteins. Some lymphomas produce active metabolites of vitamin D that increases the intestinal absorption of calcium.

Clinical features

* Renal failure
* Cardiac arhythmias
* Non-malignant causes—measure PTH: inappropriately high in hyperparathyroidism, undetectable in malignancy

Management

The basic principles of management involve rehydration to restore glomerular function and the use of drugs to inhibit osteoclastic bone

Table 39.1 Symptoms and signs of hypercalcaemia

Symptoms	Signs
Gastrointestinal	
Nausea	
Vomiting	
Anorexia	
Constipation	
Renal	
Polyuria	Dehydration
Thirst	Uraemia
Hypercalciuria	
Nephrocalcinosis	
Neurological	
Lethargy	Muscular weakness
Drowsiness	Stupor
Weakness	Confusion
Disorientation	Dysarthria
Visual disturbance	Diminished reflexes
Pain	

resorption. Where possible, specific anti-tumour therapy should be instituted. Occasionally, the secretion of humoral factors by a primary tumour results in hypercalcaemia, and in such cases the serum level may be corrected by surgical removal of the tumour. Typically however, the malignancy is advanced and treatment is palliative.

Absorption of calcium from the gut is usually reduced in patients with malignant hypercalcaemia and, except for the rare patient with lymphoma (usually T cell) associated with raised levels of vitamin D metabolites. They should be encouraged to eat what they like, when they like, irrespective of the food's calcium content. Immobilization should be avoided where possible as this may precipitate hypercalcaemia, since the lack of weight-bearing induces increased osteoclastic activity while reducing bone formation.

Dehydration is an inevitable feature of symptomatic hypercalcaemia and it is essential to rehydrate with 3–4 litres of 0.9% normal saline to restore glomerular function and increase urinary excretion of calcium. Rehydration will relieve many of the symptoms of hypercalcaemia but will rarely achieve total control.

Prior to the 1990s, specific treatment of hypercalcaemia relied mainly on the use of calcitonin and mithramycin as inhibitors of osteoclast action, but these have largely been superceded by bisphosphonates.

Corticosteroids have been widely used in the treatment of hyper-calcaemia but, except in steroid-responsive tumours, add little to the response achieved by intravenous rehydration.

• Selective inhibitors of osteoclast activity
• Agent of choice in hypercalcaemia—pamidronate, clodronate
• Highly effective (90% normocalcaemia)
• Usually normocalaemic in 3–7 days
• Side-effects—transient fever, hypocalcaemia
• IV route needed in acute situation
• Later, oral maintenance therapy.

Hyponatraemia

A fall in the serum sodium to less than 130 mmol/l is associated with weakness, confusion, headache, drowsiness, and seizures. In cancer, the likely reason for hyponatraemia is the ectopic tumour production of antidiuretic hormone (ADH). Small cell lung cancer is the most commonly associated malignancy, but carcinoid tumours, lymphoma, leukaemia, and pancreatic cancers may also be responsible. Cytotoxic drugs used in the treatment of cancer, particularly ifosfamide, vincristine, and high-dose cyclophosphamide, may also stimulate ADH production. Other causes for hyponatraemia include pneumonia and raised intracranial pressure.

Investigation will reveal continued renal excretion of sodium with an inappropriately high urinary sodium concentration, with the urinary osmolality exceeding that of the plasma.

Treatments include a restricted fluid intake of around 500–700 mls per day, demeclocycline (which inhibits the action of ADH on the renal tubule), and, rarely, for severe life-threatening situations, the slow and closely monitored infusion of hypertonic (3%) saline.

Hyperkalaemia

Renal failure is probably the most frequent cause of hyperkalaemia, but in cancer management other causes should be considered. Most important, and usually preventable, is the tumour lysis syndrome that accompanies the rapid breakdown of malignant cells in response to effective chemotherapy. Tumour lysis is most likely in the management of high-grade lymphomas, leukaemia, and trophoblastic and germ cell tumours, where the lysis of many millions of cells results in release of intracellular products, notably potassium and phosphate, into the circulation, along with urate generated by the breakdown of cellular proteins. Urate crystals may precipitate in the renal tubules causing acute urate nephropathy if appropriate precautions are not taken.

Prevention of tumour lysis is the key to management and patients who are predicted to respond rapidly to chemotherapy should be vigorously hydrated intravenously, urinary pH should be maintained in the alkaline range by administration of sodium bicarbonate, and urate nephropathy prevented by pre-treatment of the patient with allopurinol.

Severe, and particularly acute, hyperkalaemia may cause cardiac dysrhythmias and cardiac arrest. Emergency management is required and this should include intravenous rehydration with glucose, insulin, and sodium bicarbonate to correct acidosis and drive potassium into the intracellular space, and intravenous administration of 10% calcium gluconate. In occasional situations, haemodialysis may be necessary.

Other causes of hyperkalaemia in cancer patients include septicaemia, adrenal insufficiency (usually secondary to glucocorticoid withdrawal or adrenal destruction by a tumour), acute graft versus host disease following allogeneic bone marrow transplantation, and drugs (particularly diuretics such as spirinolactone).

Renal tubular dysfunction

The kidney is normally very efficient in ensuring that electrolyte concentrations are maintained. However, this can be severely disrupted by cytotoxic drugs, particularly cisplatin and ifosfamide, which may cause tubular dysfunction and excessive loss of calcium, magnesium, potassium, and sodium in the urine. Electrolyte loss results in lethargy, constipation, confusion, and, in severe cases, seizures. Patients receiving these drugs require regular monitoring of electrolyte concentrations and replacement where necessary.

Oral calcium and vitamin D may be required to maintain serum calcium levels and, for chronic treatment of hypomagnasaemia, oral magnesium glycerophosphate is preferred to other oral magnesium preparations as diarrhoea is less of a problem with this formulation.

Hyperglycaemia and hypoglycaemia

Disturbances in glucose metabolism may complicate cancer management. Administration of corticosteroids to patients with diabetes mellitus will increase glucose levels and increase insulin requirements, while loss of appetite, nausea, and vomiting may predispose the diabetic patient to hypoglycaemia.

Inappropriate insulin production may occur from islet cell tumours and pancreatic APUDomas, while, rarely, large metastatic tumours, particularly in the liver, may produce insulin-like growth factors (IGF) which are released into the circulation, especially in response to treatment.

Summary

Metabolic problems in cancer may present as a biochemical crisis. A high index of suspicion, understanding of the pathophysiological processes involved, and knowledge of the prevention and treatment of these problems is an important component of good cancer medicine.

Part 6
The way forward

Chapter 40
Novel therapeutic strategies

New drug discovery

Introduction

The process of drug discovery and development is undergoing a series of revolutionary changes. This is due to three factors:-

- The view that conventional, mainly cytotoxic approaches have been successful in the past, but have reached a plateau of effectiveness and therapeutic index with respect to activity in human solid tumours.
- The opportunities for novel molecular targets opened up by our new understanding of the molecular biology of cancer.
- The range of new technologies that are available today to increase the quality of candidate drugs and to accelerate their discovery and development.

Earlier approaches to drug discovery

The main approach used over the past 50 years has been to screen libraries of compounds (both chemically synthesized and natural products) either for cytotoxic activity against tumour cells in cell culture or for anti-cancer activity in tumour-bearing animals (e.g. inhibition of tumour growth or increase in life span of the host). This has been successful in that it has led to the discovery and clinical use of many of the major classes of established anti-cancer drugs e.g. alkylating agents, anthracyclines, topoisomerase inhibitors, and microtubule binders.

Historical developments in screening are best illustrated by the evolution of methodologies used by the influential National Cancer Institute in the US. In the early days, screening was commonly carried out against a mouse leukaemia, either the P338 or L1210 models. But success in identifying drugs with activity in leukaemias and lymphoproliferative malignancies did not translate well to the major solid tumours. Hence, in the mid-1970s, transplantable mouse solid tumours, and then human tumour xenografts, were included as a secondary panel. A decade later the need for an even greater focus on human cancer led to the introduction of a 60-cell line *in vivo* tumour panel as the primary screen. Promising activities arising from this were followed up in animal studies.

In some cases, the compound discovered in the screen was developed through preclinical and clinical testing. In others, a range of chemical analogues of the parent compound, already available or newly synthesized, were evaluated for improved performance.

These earlier approaches were very pragmatic. Studies of mode of action were commonly only conducted late in the development of a cytotoxic. Exceptions to this were the antimetabolite and anti-hormonal approaches. In these cases, compounds were usually designed rationally to inhibit a target enzyme (e.g. dihydrofolate reductase, thymidylate synthetase, aromatase) or to antagonize a receptor (e.g. for oestrogen or androgen). Thus, the primary screen was frequently for the biochemical mode of action, and studies to check for compliance with the desired mechanism could be included in subsequent *in vitro* and *in vivo* tests (e.g. thymidine reversal for thymidylate synthetase, oestrogen levels for aromatase).

Contemporary approaches to drug discovery

Over the last few years the increasing trend has been for a given drug discovery project to be aimed at a particular molecular target (e.g. a specific oncogene product), with which pharmacological intervention might deliver a particular desired biological or phenotypic effect (e.g. inhibition of proliferation, cell cycle progression, motility, invasion, angiogenesis, and metastasis; or the induction of apoptosis or differentiation) rather than a more general cytotoxic or cytostatic effect.

This new molecular target orientated approach is now dominant in the pharmaceutical industry and in biotechnology companies. Contemporary mechanism-based drug discovery can be divided into the following several phases.

Target identification and validation

The objective is to identify genes and their cognate proteins that are directly responsible for cancer causation and progression. Having identified a gene that is either mutated or shows deregulated expression, a variety of experiments can be carried out to validate the target—that is, to provide evidence that it is indeed involved in the disease process and to increase the level of confidence that pharmacological manipulations of the target would lead to an anti-tumour effect.

The identification of new molecular targets in cancer has been revolutionized by human and other genome projects. All 30 000 human genes were published in *Science* and *Nature* in February 2001. Determining the specific involvement of various genes in human tumours requires molecular studies on familial and sporadic cancers to reveal the natural history of various malignant diseases at the genetic level. A leading example of this has been colorectal cancer, where it is now clear that genes such as APC, *ras*, p53, and the mismatch repair proteins play key roles.

Various techniques can be used for target validation. These include transfection, gene knock-out and knock-in, micro-injection of inhibitory antibodies, dominant negative constructs, anti-sense constructs and oligonucleotides, inhibitory peptides, and pharmacological agents, through to clinical data linking gene mutation or deregulation to clinical outcome (e.g. overexpression of EGF and erbB2 receptors in ovarian and breast cancer).

The choice of molecular target will relate to the strengths of the validation package, together with the incidence of the abnormalities in human cancer and the technical feasibility of achieving pharmacological manipulation. For example, enzymes such as kinases and proteases are more readily inhibited by drugs than are protein-protein interactions.

Lead identification

The objective of this phase is to identify a chemical structure that has some activity against the molecular target. This may be done in two ways. The first way involves large, chemically diverse libraries being screened in automated, high-throughput assays. Here, both chemical diversity and speed can be increased by combinatorial chemistry, which uses robotic synthesis. The second way involves rational design based on a known substrate or ligand, or alternatively an X-ray crystallographic or NMR structure of the target itself.

Lead optimization

In this phase, the objective is to improve and refine the desired properties of the lead (e.g. solubility, potency, and selectivity) and eliminate undesirable features. This is done by making chemical derivatives or analogues of the lead, based on emerging biological results on the target structure. It involves an iterative process of 'making and testing' that leads to an understanding of structure–activity relationships. Robotics may be used to make a series of analogues very quickly.

Test cascade

The key to successful lead identification and optimization is the test cascade. This is a series of hierarchically arranged tests or screens (usually biological) which allow the progressive optimization of chemical structure, via the iterative 'making and testing' approach, to give the desired performance. In industry, the desired performance will normally be defined by a target profile listing the essential and desirable features of the prospective drug. This will define the mechanism of action and biological effect, as well as provide measures of physico-chemical properties, potency, selectivity, pharmacokinetics, and therapeutic index. A test cascade must be robust, rapid, and efficient.

The primary screen is usually a biochemical test using the recombinant protein target or a genetically engineered cell line. A selectivity screen will usually follow, together with an assay to confirm the biological effect or a surrogate thereof in intact cells. Ideally, an assay should be available to confirm that this effect is achieved by the desired molecular mode of action. Activity against tumour cells in culture is normally sought.

The transition from activity in cell culture to pharmacological effect in the intact animal is a challenging one. The latter requires the compound to display robust, 'drug-like' character, and inadequate pharmacokinetic/ADME (absorption, distribution, metabolism, and excretion) properties are often limiting. Hence a screen for blood levels, often using mixtures of compounds administered in cassette or cocktail dosing for higher throughput, can be useful.

Currently under evaluation by the NCI and others is the hollow fibre assay that has elements of an *in vitro–in vivo* hybrid test and gives an indication of the achievement of concentrations *in vivo* sufficient for at least minimal activity against human tumour cells.

The final stage of testing will involve seeking evidence of regression or growth arrest/delay in a human tumour xenograft. Depending on the biological effect sought, more complex tests such as orthoptic or

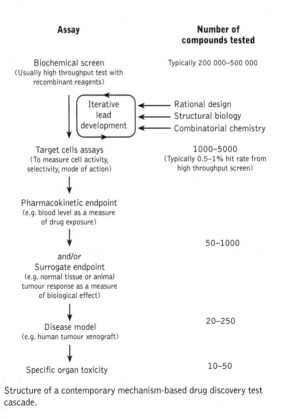

Assay	Number of compounds tested
Biochemical screen (Usually high throughput test with recombinant reagents)	Typically 200 000–500 000
Iterative lead development ← Rational design ← Structural biology ← Combinatorial chemistry	
Target cells assays (To measure cell activity, selectivity, mode of action)	1000–5000 (Typically 0.5–1% hit rate from high throughput screen)
Pharmacokinetic endpoint (e.g. blood level as a measure of drug exposure)	50–1000
and/or Surrogate endpoint (e.g. normal tissue or animal tumour response as a measure of biological effect)	
Disease model (e.g. human tumour xenograft)	20–250
Specific organ toxicity	10–50

Structure of a contemporary mechanism-based drug discovery test cascade.

metastatic models may be useful. Transgenic mouse models can be valuable, as can surrogate non-tumour endpoints.

Usually, activity will be sought in at least a small panel of tumours, including human xenografts. Ideally, these would be characterized for the molecular target and pathway involved, together with any other relevant features. Such a panel can be especially useful in selecting from a shortlist of potential clinical development candidates that may all display the target profile. An alternative to this scheme is a modification to the NCI *in vitro* cell panel approach, whereby compounds are selected based on correlation of sensitivity with molecular parameters.

Preclinical drug development

Following selection of a potential clinical candidate, a number of preclinical development activities must be carried out.

Formulation   Choice of formulation is influenced by solubility, stability, and dosage requirements (e.g. acute or intermittent oral administration versus chronic oral dosing). Approaches involve the use of various mixed solvent systems as well as more novel delivery methods such as liposomes.

Preclinical pharmacology   More detailed pharmacokinetic/ADME studies will be carried out. These will define drug distribution in the body (usually rodents) and the rate and means of drug elimination, including identification of major metabolites.

Preclinical toxicology   Usually the final step before Phase I trial in man, the objectives of preclinical toxicology are to define:

- Qualitative and quantitative organ toxicities
- The reversibility of the effects
- The initial safe starting dose

Conditions for the preclinical toxicology should reflect as closely as possible the formulation, schedule, route of administration, and dose/concentration features that will apply in patients. Precise requirements vary between countries and regulatory authorities, but in general there is a two-step approach to define the acute maximum tolerated dose or LD10 (dose giving 10% lethality) in a rodent species usually the mouse and either the rat or dog, followed by a more extensive phase. Organ-specific toxicities are often poorly predicted between species and the main objective is to define a safe starting dose in man.

Conclusion

Despite major advances in methodology, the drug discovery and development process is still likely to take around seven years from new target to regulatory approval. Success requires close co-operation of talented multidisciplinary teams. With the trend away from empirical screening for anti-cancer activity to new mechanism-based approaches targeted to specific molecular abnormalities responsible for cancer, we are now screening a range of exciting new agents emerging for clinical evaluation.

New drug development

Once a novel anti-cancer agent has been discovered, its structure and pharmacological and pharmaceutical properties optimized, and a decision made to test it in humans, a number of well-defined stages must be passed before the compound can enter clinical trials. The drug development process is very closely regulated to ensure the quality of preclinical and clinical data and to protect the safety and the rights of the human subjects participating in the trials. Therefore, the requirements of the regulatory authority in the country where the trials are to be performed must be considered.

The drug

The ideal candidate will have potent activity against its target (e.g. VEGF receptor tyrosine kinase), minimal against other targets, be water soluble, and be physically and chemically stable both in powder form and in solution. The specification should ensure the material is of adequate quality and conforms to current requirements (i.e. ICH guidelines). Methods should be developed with indicate stability and will detect and quantify, with sufficient sensitivity and accuracy, the drug, its degradation products, and the intermediates involved in its synthesis.

Ideally, several batches should be made to confirm that the synthetic route is robust and that consistency of material with respect to purity of drug substance and levels of contaminants (including solvents, synthetic intermediates, and degradation products) can be achieved. However, if several batches are not to be made, the batch produced initially should be large enough for all preclinical testing and early clinical trials.

Formulation

Formulation is the process by which the raw drug is converted into a form that can be administered to patients (e.g. an ampoule or vial for intravenous, intramuscular, or subcutaneous administration, or a capsule or tablet for oral administration). The route of administration selected must be appropriate for the biological and physico-chemical properties of the compound, and the agent must be shown to be active when given by that route. For example, for intravenous administration, the compound must be soluble in a pharmaceutically acceptable solvent at biological pH, whereas for oral administration, the product must be stable in acid. In some cases, it may be necessary to add excipients (other inert materials) to aid solubility, stability, etc. Once a putative formulation has been developed, the stability of the product in the excipients must be confirmed for a minimum of three months (one month for a solution in saline).

Batches of both the raw drug and the final product should be assessed for stability under a variety of environmental conditions for up to three years. These data will be used to attach a shelf life to the product when it is sent to the hospitals for clinical trials. The stability of the compound once reconstituted and compatibility with the giving sets (e.g. stickiness to plastic) should also be investigated so that clear instructions can be provided for the appropriate administration of the drug (e.g. use within two hours of reconstitution, or protect from light).

Pharmacology

Before undertaking a Phase I clinical trial, the pharmacological properties of the drug need to be established. This is to ensure that adequate levels of drug can be delivered for it to have its desired effect and that the drug is working by the mechanism postulated.

Preclinical toxicology

Before clinical trials can begin, preclinical toxicology studies must be undertaken. This is to investigate the safety of the compound, to define its toxicity profile (side-effects), to investigate the reversibility of the toxic effects, and to determine a safe starting dose for the first Phase I trial. These studies are generally undertaken in two species, often one rodent species (mouse or rat) and one non-rodent (dog). The Cancer Research Campaign in the UK are, however, based on extensive experience, pioneering the use of only rodent species for preclinical toxicology of anti-cancer agents.

The exact design of the studies undertaken should be appropriate for the drug in question. The route and schedule of administration should mimic that proposed for the Phase I clinical trial and the drug should be administered using the clinical formulation.

The initial studies should determine the maximum tolerated dose (MTD) of the drug, or if the compound is not very toxic, the maximum administerable dose (MAD). This is used to calculate the starting dose of the clinical trial which is generally one tenth of the MTD (or MAD) in the most sensitive of the two species, when the dose is related to body surface area (i.e. mg/m^2).

The toxicity profile of the drug is established by treating groups of animals at two or three doses (MTD and fractions of the MTD) or vehicle alone. Half of the animals in each group are then subject to haematology, clinical chemistry, and histopathology studies within 1–2 days of dosing. The other half are tested similarly after a 28-day recovery period to assess the reversibility of any toxicities seen. If there is any indication from its properties or its analogues that a particular drug may potentially have a particular toxicity (e.g. nephrotoxicity), specific tests should be undertaken during the toxicology studies to investigate this. Data from the toxicology studies should be used to design the Phase I trial.

Clinical trials

The primary aim of the Phase I trials is to establish the safety and tolerability of the compound being tested and to define an optimum dose and schedule for further (Phase II) studies. Other, secondary objectives may be to investigate the pharmacokinetics of the drug in humans and study the efficacy of the drug in the patients.

Because of the toxicity of anti-cancer agents, Phase I trials of these compounds are generally performed in cancer patients and not healthy volunteers. Moreover, unless the drug is designed to treat a particular type of cancer, patients with advanced cancer of any type may be treated in Phase I trials. These patients will often be those who have already received, and their disease progressed through, the standard treatments for their particular condition.

Patients entering all trials must be fully informed about the study and give their consent to participating. The details of the treatment, the patients to be entered, the doses, and the measurements to be made should all be detailed in the protocol that must be approved by the hospital ethics committee before the trial can begin.

Phase I

Phase I studies are generally dose escalation trials, where the initial dose level is calculated from the preclinical toxicology studies. This starting dose aims to be low enough to ensure the safety of the patients, but high enough to minimize the number of patients treated at ineffective (too low) doses.

Patients are generally treated in cohorts, with a number of patients all being treated at one dose level before the dose is escalated in the next cohort of patients. Traditionally, three patients are treated per dose level; however, increasingly trials are being designed where only one patient is treated at a particular level if no toxicity is seen.

The dose escalation scheme may vary (e.g. modified Fibonnaci scheme, pharmacokinetically guided dose escalation), although the principle is the same—to increase the dose rapidly at ineffective, non-toxic doses (thus minimizing the numbers of patients at these levels) and to reduce the rate of increase as effective and/or toxic doses are approached.

The endpoint of the Phase I trial is normally toxicity (MTD and dose-limiting toxicity (DLT) will be defined in the protocol), except for non-cytotoxic agents, when the endpoint may be the optimum activity of the drug as defined by its mechanism of action, unless unacceptable toxicity is observed first. For example, this may be inhibition of an enzyme or reduction of plasma levels of a hormone.

On completion of the Phase I trial, the basic toxicity profile of the agent in question should be known and an appropriate dose for further trials identified.

Phase II and III

Unless the drug has proved to be unacceptably toxic, it will then be subject to Phase II, and if successful, Phase III testing. The aim of Phase II trials is to assess the efficacy of the drug. Each Phase II trial will be undertaken in patients with one particular tumour type and they will all be treated with the same dose and schedule. Whist toxicity will continue to be monitored, the patients' disease will also be assessed for response. The aim of Phase III trials is to compare the new agent with existing best treatment for the disease in question.

If a new drug is proven to have an acceptable toxicity profile, efficacy in one or a number of disease types, and to compare favourably against existing standard treatments for the particular disease setting, then the compound may be submitted to regulatory authorities to register it as a product—the culmination of a costly process which can take in the region of ten years to complete.

Novel radiotherapeutic approaches

Radiotherapy is an effective anti-cancer treatment modality. Increasing the dose delivered to the tumour while sparing the surrounding normal tissue will commonly improve local tumour control. Novel radiotherapeutic approaches aim to:

- Increase the dose delivered to tumours, by more effectively targeting the tumour volume (but not at the expense of normal tissue damage).

- Increase the biological effectiveness of radiation by affecting the radiosensitization of the tumour (but not of normal tissue).

- Use different forms of radiation which have improved biological effects.
- Use changed schedules of radiation delivery in order to increase the differential between tumour kill and normal tissue damage.

Targeted radiotherapy

The biological properties of the tumour itself provide the basis for selective irradiation. In principle, this strategy should be capable of eradicating tumour cells anywhere in the body, but it is currently at an early stage of development for many sites.

- Iodine (well differentiated thyroid carcinomas)
- Monoclonal antibodies to cancer cell surface antigens (B-cell lymphoma)
- Catecholamine precursor analogue meta-iodo-benzl-guanine (MIBG) (neuroblastoma)
- Somatostatin (neuroendocrine tumours)

Until recently, the nuclides used in targeted radiotherapy were selected because of their availability and low cost rather than on account of their physical or radiobiological properties. Considerable experience has been gained with β emitters such as iodine-131 and yttrium-90, but short lived α emitters (e.g. astatine-211 or bismuth-212) or Auger-emitting radionuclides (e.g. iodine-125) are more potent cell killers and may find a clinical role.

Targeting strategies to improve clinical results include:

- Improving the specificity of the existing targeting agents
- Regional targeting (e.g. intraperitoneal therapy)
- Multiple treatments
- Decreasing side-effects (myelosuppression due to a radiation of bone marrow is the most important) by using peripheral blood stem cell support or haemopoietic growth factors
- Combination of targeted radiotherapy with other treatments

The effectiveness of targeted radiotherapy is strongly dependent on the extent to which a sufficient dose may be delivered to critical clusters of tumour clonogens, and micodosimetric studies have shown that fluctuations in dose uniformity can adversely affect treatment outcome. The optimal strategy may be to use 'cocktails' of radionuclides, or to supplement targeted radiotherapy with external-beam irradiation.

Boron neutron capture therapy is a specialized approach to targeted therapy in which non-radioactive boron atoms are selectively incorporated into tumour cells. When exposed to a beam of 'slow' neutrons the boron emits α particles locally within the tumour, causing dense ionizations and DNA damage. So far, clinical experience in brain tumours has produced controversial results.

Improvements in external-beam radiotherapy delivery

Improvements in focusing the external radiotherapy beam on the tumour and avoiding normal tissue should allow a safe increase in the dose of radiotherapy delivered.

Conformal therapy

This multi-step technique uses 3D image reconstruction and treatment planning, combined with sophisticated treatment verification, to conform a high dose of radiotherapy to the target volume (often irregularly shaped) but maintain a low dose to the non-target tissues of the patients. The commercial development of multi-leaf collimators for linear accelerators and megavoltage imaging systems has made this treatment available in a number of large radiotherapy treatment centres. Early clinical results suggest that normal tissue side-effects can be reduced and dose escalation is possible e.g. in the treatment of localized prostate cancer.

Intensity-modulated radiation therapy (IMRT)

Here the intensity of the radiotherapy beam is varied across the treatment field to ensure that a uniform dose can be achieved in a regular or irregular shape target while avoiding delivery of a high dose to the surrounding structures. Essentially, this may add to conformal therapy by further reducing the dose to sensitive structures.

Currently, 14 institutions worldwide specialize in this technology, prioritizing treatment of intracranial tumours and cancer of the head and neck and prostate. The beam can be produced by a modulatory accelerator or with the addition of a special collimator, but the technique is computationally complex.

Intra-operative radiotherapy

Radiotherapy can be delivered to a tumour volume under direct visual localization during an open operation within a designated radiotherapy suite. A large single dose is delivered at the one procedure. The potential advantage of a targeted boost (given in addition to external-beam fractionated therapy) is balanced by the theoretical limitations of the biological effects of the single large dose.

A few centers in the world currently use this technique and some results suggest a survival benefit. There remains controversy over the difficult logistics of delivery and further larger clinical studies are needed to define and quantify any benefit.

Improvements in radiotherapy fractionation

In general, tumours and critical normal tissues (those which limit the dose which may safely be delivered in a course of radiotherapy) are associated with different fractionation sensitivities. Thus, reducing the daily dose per fraction will allow a greater total dose to be delivered to the tumour without exceeding the normal tissue tolerance and the therapeutic index may be favourably altered.

Studies have demonstrated fast rates of growth in certain tumours (e.g. squamous cell carcinomas of the head and neck region) such that clonogens have potential doubling times of less than five days. This implies that the time taken to deliver a radical course of conventionally fractionated radiotherapy should not be extended. Indeed, clinical trials have demonstrated benefits with treatment acceleration where a radical course of treatment may be completed in two weeks (with thrice daily fractions), rather than the more usual 4–6 weeks.

Although the potential benefits of acceleration and changed fractionation are clear, the impact of their adoption on overall survival is likely to be modest and only on subgroups of patients. Even amongst tumours of common histology, there are wide variations in the radiobiological parameters such as potential doubling time.

There is interest in the development of predictive assays, from which it may be possible to tailor a schedule of radiotherapy to the individual tumour.

Particle beams

Conventional radiotherapy uses uncharged electromagnetic radiation of sufficient energy to ionize molecules in tissues—so-called 'ionizing radiation'. Particle radiation has a greater ionizing effect per unit dose and charged particles also have favourable dose-absorption profiles.

Neutron therapy

Neutrons are the commonest type of particle beam used for radiotherapy but the clinical results obtained are controversial. With a high LET (linear energy transfer) they produce more cell killing per dose than megavoltage X-rays. This may be particularly advantageous in hypoxic areas of tumour. Clinical trials have been carried out for salivary gland tumours, prostrate adenocarcinomas, soft tissue sarcomas, paranasal sinuses, and melanomas. The main problems have been the severity of the normal tissue reactions and lack of a clear clinical advantage.

The poor dose distribution and beam delivery systems of the early experimental neutron facilities may have hampered the clinical results.

Proton beam therapy

These heavily charged particles are produced by a cyclotron and deliver their energy and therefore biological effects in a small-defined area at the end of their range (often millimetres)—the so-called 'Bragg peak'. This reduces the dose to underlying normal tissue. Complex multiple beams can be used to deliver a high dose to a small area. So far their use has been limited to superficial tumours such as uveal melanomas. Higher-energy beams now allow deeper-seated tumours to be treated e.g. chordoma of the clivus.

Approximately 2000–3000 patients are treated worldwide each year and most of the treatment centres are still based in physics laboratories. Improvements may be made by better tumour selection and technical advances in treatment delivery.

Radiosensitization

If tumour cells can be made more sensitive to the delivered radiotherapy, improvements in local control can be gained only if radiosensitization is selective for the tumour.

Hypoxic cell sensitizers

Hypoxic tumour cells are resistant to radiation. The delivery of hypoxic cell sensitizers should theoretically improve tumour cell kill. Many international randomized clinical trials have been negative, perhaps due to the inability to stratify and select for hypoxic tumours. More recently, trials with, for example tirapazamine, have demonstrated benefit, but these agents are still under evaluation.

Synchronous chemotherapy

Chemotherapy delivered with radiotherapy may provide benefit over and above the addition of more cell kill. This may be due to the inhibition of DNA repair by the agent or some other mechanism of tumour radiosensitization. More clinical studies are required to define the optimal combination of chemotherapy and radiotherapy and to ensure this is a selective improvement for the tumour and does not just produce additive toxicity. The approach of targeted delivery of radiosensitizing agents selectively to tumours (e.g. via liposomes) may provide therapeutic gain.

Hyperthermia

Hyperthermia enhances the effect of radiotherapy by direct cell killing and radiosensitization. This interaction is time-dependent, maximum with simultaneous treatment. It is considered an experimental therapy, as clinical studies are ongoing, and one major limitation is the necessary equipment needed to deliver heat above 41°C.

Targeted radiotherapy

Introduction

Targeted radiotherapy means the selective irradiation of tumour cells by radionuclides that are conjugated to tumour-seeking molecules (targeting agents). Ideally, the targeting agent should be perfectly efficient in finding every tumour cell in the body and should be absolutely discriminatory in finding only tumour cells. Real agents fall well short of this ideal. In practice, a targeting agent has therapeutic potential if it can be stably conjugated to an appropriate radionuclide and allows significantly higher radiation doses to be delivered to tumour masses than to critical tissues. This is a 'therapeutic ratio' criterion similar to that which applies to most forms of cancer treatment. However, targeted radiotherapy also possesses unique features.

Targeting agents

Tumour targeting depends on the existence of biological differences between normal and tumour cells. Several categories of targeting agent have been used, or are under development:

- Monoclonal antibodies—limited discriminatory ability
  - epitopes are heterogenous and unstable in tumour cell population
  - poor penetration of tumour mass
  - murine antibodies provoke host response
  - used in cancer of ovary, colon, brain with modest response
  - best response in B-cell lymphoma
- MIBG—taken up by catecholamine-synthesizing cells of sympathetic nervous system
  - taken up by neuroblastoma, phaeochromocytoma
  - diagnostic and therapeutic
- Future—melanoma
  - glioma, squamous cell carcinoma: overexpressed cell receptor epidermal growth factor (EGF)

Radionuclides for therapy

Radionuclides which have potential for targeted therapy are the α, β, and Auger particle emitters. Though particle-emitting radionuclides

Table 40.1 Targeting agents for targeted radiotherapy

Biological differential	Targeting agent	Target tumour
Epitope	Antibodies	Various
Noradrenaline transporter	MIBG	Neuroblastoma
Melanin synthetic pathway	Methylene blue	Melanoma
EGF receptor overexpression	EGF	Squamous carcinoma, glioma
Proliferative differential	IUDR	Brain tumours
Oestrogen nuclear receptor	Oestrogen	Breast cancer
Genomic aberration	Oligonucleotide	?

usually produce some γ-ray photons as well, the photons make little contribution to the therapeutic effect.

The physical half-life of a targeting radionuclide must be long enough to allow radiochemical conjugation and the homing of the conjugate to its target tumour cells. However, it is not optimal to use radionuclides with half-lives longer than the time scale over which the conjugate will maintain its biochemical integrity and therefore targeting specificity.

In practice, clinical experience with targeted radiotherapy is largely confined to β-emitters, particularly ^{131}I and, to a lesser extent, [90]Y. The advantages of ^{131}I are its availability, ease of conjugation, and clinical familiarity. [90]Y has some physical advantages but is unfamiliar and the conjugates are less stable.

α-emitters have high radiobiological effectiveness and short-range emissions but are difficult to obtain and have inconveniently short half-lives. Experience with α-emitters is so far confined to the laboratory, but encouraging clinical potential has been demonstrated.

Auger electron emitters have been little used for targeted therapy because the short range of the Auger electron requires a DNA-targeting agent.

Radiobiological considerations

Targeted radiotherapy differs from conventional irradiation in its lower dose rate, dependence on the biodistribution and pharmacokinetics of the radioconjugate, particle range effects, and the role of tumour heterogeneity. The effects of particle range have been studied by mathematical modelling and in experimental tumour models and have produced therapeutic results of potential clinical importance.

Combined modalities

Targeted radiotherapy using β-emitters inevitably results in a whole-body radiation dose because of limited targeting specificities (cross-

Table 40.2 Radionuclides for targeted radiotherapy

Radionuclide	Half-life	Emitted particles	Particle range
[90]Y	2.7 days	β	5mm
[131]I	8 days	β	0.8 mm
[67]Cu	2.5 days	β	0.6 mm
[199]Au	3.1 days	β	0.3 mm
[211]At	7 hours	α	0.05 mm
[212]Bi	1 hour	α	0.05 mm
[125]I	60 days	Auger electrons	~1 μm
[123]I	15 hours	Auger electrons	~1 μm

targeting to normal tissues) and because of radionuclide in the general circulation. Radiobiological modelling suggested that systemic targeted radiotherapy might best be regarded as a kind of non-uniform TBI—with higher doses being given to tumour cells than to normal tissues. Therefore, systemic targeted radiotherapy might be most appropriate for patients for whom conventional TBI, with marrow rescue (or other forms of haematological support), was already an option.

These considerations suggest the possible advantages of a combined modality regime incorporating targeted radiotherapy, TBI, and marrow rescue. Computer simulation studies of the effect of combined modality treatment have suggested that disseminated tumours of differing size may be optimally treated by different components of the combination. For example, distributed single cells and very small micrometastases are effectively treated by TBI (and by chemotherapy), targeted ^{131}I is ideal for treatment of larger micrometastases, whilst macroscopic tumours are best dealt with by local modalities (radiotherapy, surgery).

These concepts are now being applied in the targeted radiotherapy of neuroblastoma using ^{131}I-MIBG in combination with TBI or with high-dose chemotherapy. Combined modality treatment of B-cell lymphoma using radio-labelled antibodies, TBI, or systemic chemotherapy and haemopoetic rescue may be an appropriate next step.

Regional treatment

+ Higher concentration of targeting agent
+ Higher radiation dose to tumour deposit
+ Cancer of the ovary—intraperitoneal ^{131}I or ^{90}Y conjugated antibodies
+ Cancer of the bladder—intravesical radio-labelled antibody
+ Brain tumours—intrathecal or intraventricular administration; CSF
+ Injection of radiolabelled agent directly into macroscopic tumour e.g. cystic glioma

Gene therapy for cancer

Gene therapy is the transfer and expression of genetic material into human cells for a therapeutic purpose. New insights into the control and growth of human cells and their deregulation in cancer have co-incided with advances in recombinant DNA technology. Novel methods of introducing 'therapeutic' DNA into cancer cells have allowed gene therapy to progress to clinical trials.

New anti-cancer strategies are urgently needed as most cancers are still ultimately resistant to conventional treatment modalities. Germ-line gene therapy has been deemed unethical, so current developments involve introducing foreign genes into somatic (non-sex) cells only. In the UK, clinical gene therapy trials are currently regulated by the Gene Therapy Advisory Committee (GTAC).

Table 41.1 Strategies for cancer gene therapy

Somatic correction of gene defect
Antisense to mutant oncogene
Expression of tumour suppressor gene
Genetic pro-drug activation
Genetic immunomodulation
Polynucleotide vaccination
Cancer vaccines
Vectoring of biotherapeutic genes to tumours and T cells
Dendritic cell immunity
Gene marking
Increased normal tissue tolerance

Gene delivery

The addition, substitution, or ablation of DNA sequences may be achieved by any of the following:

- Injection of naked DNA into skeletal muscle by simple needle and syringe.
- DNA transfer by liposomes (delivered by the intravascular, intra-tracheal, intraperitoneal, or intracolonic routes).
- DNA coated on the surface of gold pellets that are air-propelled into the epidermis (the 'gene gun').
- Biological vehicles (vectors) such as viruses and bacteria. Viruses are genetically engineered not to replicate once inside the host. They are currently the most efficient means of gene transfer.

Other techniques involve fusion of whole cells or viral envelopes, electroporation, micro-injection, or chemical precipitation of DNA into cells.

The efficiency of transfer of therapeutic DNA required (dictated by the nature of the genetic defect) influences the choice of vector e.g. for gene replacement, high-efficiency viral vectors are desirable, whereas short-term gene expression to prime an immune response or sensitize cells to radiotherapy may be achieved by liposomal delivery.

Some of these strategies can be achieved *ex vivo* by transfer of a therapeutic gene into isolated cancer or non-cancer cells that are then reimplanted into the host. Others require delivery and expression of genes to target cancer cells *in vivo* (at much lower efficiency than *ex vivo* transfer) by exploiting transcriptional differences of specific genes between cancer and normal cells. The efficiency of gene transfer also varies greatly according to cell type targeted (low in neural and haemopoietic cells; high in myocytes, fibroblasts, hepatocytes; and variable among different tumours).

Tumour-suppressor and drug-resistance genes

The inactivation of tumour suppressor genes such as retinoblastoma (Rb1), p53, Nm23, p16, or E-cadherin may result in the initiation or the progression of a cancer. Replacement with normal copies of these genes using viral vectors has resulted in suppression and/or reversal of the malignant phenotype in *in vivo* tumour models. Furthermore, combining successful restoration of genes such as wild type p53 and sequential administration chemotherapy (such as cisplatin) appears to be synergistic in reducing the malignant expression in these cell lines.

The clinical efficacy of intra-tumoural adenoviral delivery of wild type p53 into p53-mutant squamous cell head and neck tumours is currently being evaluated.

The MDRI multiple drug-resistance gene has been transduced *ex vivo* into normal marrow and blood-derived stem cells to produce a selectable population of cells resistant to high doses of chemotherapy, which could then be re-infused into the patient. This has allowed higher doses of taxol to be administered in breast and ovarian cancer patients.

Table 41.2 Viral vectors for gene therapy

	Retrovirus	Adenovirus	Adeno-associated virus	Herpes virus
Advantages				
	Small genome	High viral titres	Small genome	High viral titres
	Carries 10 kb insert	Carries 8–30 kb insert	Carries 4–5 kb insert	Carries up to 15 kb insert
	Stable co-linear integration			
	Efficient gene transfer	Highly efficient gene transfer	Efficient gene transfer.	Highly efficient gene transfer
			Can infect non-dividing cells	Can infect non-dividing cells
			Naturally replication-incompetent	Neural tropism
Disadvantages				
	Immunogenicity	Immunogenicity.	Immunogenicity.	Immunogenicity
	Requires actively dividing cells	Transient expression	Not well studied	Large genome
	Small DNA sequences only carried	Small DNA sequences only carried	Small DNA sequences only carried	Lytic virus
	Low titre, transient expression			
	Random integration			
	Insertional mutagenesis			

Genetic pro-drug activation therapy

The fundamental problem with current chemotherapy is its lack of selectivity. If drug-activating genes could be inserted that would be expressed only in cancer cells, then giving an appropriate pro-drug could be highly selective. There are many examples of genes preferentially expressed in tumours. In some cases their promotors have been isolated and coupled to drug-activating enzymes (suicide genes). Genetic pro-drug activation therapy (GPAT, also known as GDEPT and VDEPT) exploits differences in gene expression between cancer cells in this way to increase the specificity of cell destruction.

Two targeting strategies may be used independently or in combination to keep suicide gene expression limited to malignant tissue:

* *Transcriptional targeting* exploits regulatory sequences of genes overexpressed in cancer cells to drive the expression of a suicide gene selectively within tumour cells e.g. ERBB2 in breast cancer, tyrosinase in melanoma.

* *Transduction targeting* relies on preferential delivery of vectors constitutively expressing a suicide gene into actively dividing cells only e.g. glioma cells and not into normal neighbouring central nervous system cells.

Improvements in the efficacy of GPAT have resulted from successfully modifying both retroviral and adenoviral tropism, and the use of chimaeric transcriptional elements combining strong tissue-specific promoters with tissue-specific enhancers to improve targeting further e.g. combining the ERBB2/MUC-1 transcriptional elements to drive the HSV-tk gene in breast cancer cells increases their sensitivity to pro-drug activation compared with the use of single elements to drive the same suicide gene expression.

An important additional feature of GPAT systems is the 'bystander effect'. This is the process whereby non-transduced cells in a mixed population die in the presence of a given pro-drug due to diffusion, active transport, or recruitment of a local immune response. This effect varies in magnitude with the GPAT system and tumour cell line studied, but as little as 2% transduction of a colorectal tumour cell line results in almost complete cell kill upon exposure to a pro-drug. This may indicate that sustained high efficiency gene transfer may not necessarily be required.

Current clinical trials consist of transductional targeting of gliomas and mesotheliomas, transcriptional targeting of ovarian and breast carcinomas, and melanomas using adenoviral or retroviral transduction or direct intralesional injection of plasmid DNA.

Table 41.3 Prototype systems used for genetic pro-drug activation therapy

Enzyme	Pro-drug	Active drug
Viral thymidine kinase triphosphate	Ganciclovir	Ganciclovir
Cytosinedeaminase	5-fluorocytosine	5-flourouracil
Linamarase	Amygdalin	Cyanide
Nitroreductase	CB1954	Nitrobenzamidine
Cyp1A2	Paracetamol	Toxic metabolites
Superoxide dismutase	Radiation	DNA damage

Table 41.4 Cloned genes and their promoters that may be coupled to drug-activating enzymes for tumour-selective expression

Selective gene	Tumour(s)
α-fetoprotein	Hepatoma, germ cell tumours
Prostate-specific antigen	Prostate cancer
Thyroglobulin	Thyroid carcinoma
Tyrosinase	Melanoma
Carcinoembryonic antigen	Gastrointestinal and other cancers
Polymorphic epithelial mucin	Breast cancer
Neurone specific enolase	Small cell lung cancer
c-erbB2	Breast and gastrointestinal cancers

Genetic immunotherapy

Attempts at enhancing the naturally weak immunogenicity to tumours have resulted from a clearer understanding of antigen recognition, processing and presentation at the molecular level, and in particular, the nature of effector (T cell) responses to antigenic stimulation.

A number of approaches are currently being evaluated:

- *Systemic immunotherapy* for cancer with recombinant cytokine therapy is associated with low response rates at the expense of high systemic toxicity. Small doses of cytokines are delivered at the tumour site by inserting cytokine genes into cultured tumour-infiltrating lymphocytes (TILs) *ex-vivo*, then re-infusing the cells. Anti-tumour efficacy of this subset of T cells has been shown to improve with the transfer of the genes for tumour necrosis factor and interleukin-2 (IL-2).

♦ *Transducing tumour cells ex-vivo* with the same cytokine, allogeneic HLA (human leucocyte antigen), or genes encoding costimulatory molecules, such as the B7 family of genes, prior to re-infusion (after irradiation of eliminate malignant activity) so that T-cell recognition of tumour antigens is enhanced. CTLs recognize tumour-specific antigens presented on the surface of these cells. They are induced by the local secretion of the transferred cytokine gene product to expand, target, and destroy cancer cells.

♦ *Polynucleotide (naked DNA) vaccinations* (as opposed to previous vaccinations consisting of peptides, whole tumour cells, or tumour cell lysates) have great therapeutic potential in that delivery of genes that express unique oncoproteins (such as KRAS or lymphoma idiotypic protein) endogenously within a cell, may then result in an MHC class I CD8+ response and proliferate activation of CTLs, rather than a less effective class II CD4+ response induced by exogenous peptides. This may be a further means of breaking down immunotolerance to tumours and lead to the generation of tumour-specific responses. Targets for DNA therapy are shown in the table.

The limitation to this approach is the paucity of truly tumour-specific antigens which may be exploited as molecular targets. Most target antigens are tumour-associated (i.e. normal cellular genes inappropriately expressed in cancer) and lack epitopes to activate T cells. However, delivery of genes encoding the E6 and E7 proteins of HPV 16 and 18, in patients with advanced cervical cancer, resulted in antibody and HPV-specific T-cell responses.

♦ *Dendritic cells* (DCs) are potent antigen-processing and antigen-presenting cells which are critical to the development of primary MHC-restricted T-cell immunity to infectious agents, in auto-immune diseases and anti-tumour immunity. Recent technological advances have allowed their expansion *in vitro* from peripheral blood precursors and marrow using cytokines. Cultured DCs are able to take up exogenous antigen (as tumour protein, peptide, or RNA), or may be transduced with genes encoding tumour antigen using physical or viral methods of gene transfer, and then present it to T cells to induce a measurable anti-tumour effect.

Early clinical trials have involved DCs pulsed with idiotypic protein for relapsed B-cell lymphoma or whole tumour lysates for melanoma; in both cases antigen-specific immunity has been demonstrated.

Table 41.5 Targets for DNA vaccination strategies

Target	Class of antigen	Associated cancer(s)
p53	Mutated tumour suppressor	>50% all human cancers
RAS	Mutated oncogene product	>10% all human cancers; >80% pancreatic, colorectal
ERBB2	Growth factor receptor	Breast, ovary, stomach, pancreas
Igidiotypes	Idiotypicepitope	B-cell lymphoma
HPVE6, E7	Viral gene products	Cervical cancer
P210$^{BCR/ABL}$	Mutated oncogene product	Chronic myeloid leukaemia
MAGE-1	Embryonic gene product	Melanoma, breast
Tyrosinase	Normal differentiation antigen	>50% melanomas

Anti-sense DNA oligomer treatment: blocking oncogene expression

- Short (10–50 base), synthetic, nucleotide sequence
- Complementary to specific DNA or RNA sequences
- Enter all cells easily
- Specific to target individual oncogenes
- May produce downregulation
- Can inhibit transcription/translation of single gene
- Inhibition can be caused by triggering RNase H
  —degradation of target RNA
  —interferes with processing of pre-mRNA
- Examples include—pancreatic carcinoma (HRAS)
  —prostate cancer cell lines (Block bcl-2 expression)
- BUT—poor efficiency
  —poor specificity
  —may be increased cell invasiveness
- Initial trial results encouraging in AML and lymphoma patients

Genetic tagging

The insertion of a foreign marker gene into cells during a tumour biopsy, and replacing the marked cells prior to treatment can provide a sensitive new indicator of minimal residual disease after chemotherapy. Neomycin phosphotransferase (NeoR)—an enzyme that metabolizes the aminoglycoside, G418—has been retrovirally transduced *ex vivo* into purged marrow from AML and neuroblastoma patients prior to re-infusion. In those individuals with relapsed disease, as few as one in 10^6 cells expressing the NeoR gene has been detected by PCR, indicating failure of the purging process.

Future directions

Initial clinical studies indicate that gene therapy for cancer is safe and feasible, but hampered by inefficiency of current gene transfer technology. The precise role for gene therapy in the treatment of cancer may be limited to an adjuvant or palliative role rather than attempting to eliminate bulk disease. It may also serve as an efficient genetic marker or enhance tumour sensitivity to chemotherapy or radiotherapy.

Rapid progress in this field has to be tempered by appreciation of potential new toxicities. Transfer of DNA may initiate anti-DNA antibody responses similar to those associated with autoimmune diseases. The use of viral vectors may be associated with insertional mutagenesis and activation of oncogenes leading to neoplasia, antiviral immunity, and propagation of replication-competent viruses.

Further reading

Crystal, R.G. (2001) Adenoviral vectors in the gene therapy of cancer. *Clin Can Res* 7, W 836A Suppl 5.

Huber, B., Austin, E., Davis, S., Richards, B. and Good, S. (1994) Metabolism of 5-fluorocytosine to 5-fluorouracil in human colorectal tumour cells transduced with the cytosine deaminase gene: significant antitumour effects when only a small percentage of tumour cells express cytosine deaminase. *Proc Nat Acad Sci USA* **91**, 8302–6.

Xu, G., McLeod, H.L. (2001) Strategies for enzyme/prodrug cancer therapy. *Clin Can Res* 7, 3314–24.

Part 7
Appendices

Appendix 1:
NCIC common toxicity criteria (CTC) grading system (May 1991, revised)

	Grade 0	Grade 1 (Mild)	Grade 2 (Moderate)	Grade 3 (Severe)	Grade 4 (Life-threatening)
Allergy	None	Transient rash, fever <38°C, 100.4°F	Urticaria, fever = 38°C, 100.4°F, mild bronchospasm	Serum sickness, bronchospasm, req parenteral meds	Anaphylaxis

BLOOD/BONE MARROW

	Grade 0	Grade 1 (Mild)	Grade 2 (Moderate)	Grade 3 (Severe)	Grade 4 (Life-threatening)
White blood cells (10^9/l)	≥ 4.0	3.0–3.9	2.0–2.9	1.0–1.9	<1.0
Platelets (10^9/l)	WNL	75.0–normal	50.0–74.9	25.0–49.9	<25.0
Haemoglobin (g/dl)	WNL	10.0–normal	8.0–9.9	6.5–7.9	<6.5
Granulocytes (10^9/l) (i.e. neuts.+baso.+eosin)	≥ 2.0	1.5–1.9	1.0–1.4	0.5–0.9	<0.5
Lymphocytes (10^9/l)	≥ 2.0	1.5–1.9	1.0–1.4	0.5–0.9	<0.5
Haemorrhage (clinical) (includes nosebleeds, menorrhagia, etc.)	None	Mild, no transfusion (includes bruise/ haematoma, petachiae)	Gross, 1–2 units transfusion per episode	Gross, 3–4 units transfusion per episode	Massive, >4 units transfusion per episode

CARDIOVASCULAR

	Grade 0	Grade 1 (Mild)	Grade 2 (Moderate)	Grade 3 (Severe)	Grade 4 (Life-threatening)
Arterial	None	–	–	Transient events	Permanent event
Venous	None	Superficial (excludes IV site reaction—code under skin	Deep vein thrombosis not requiring anticoagulant therapy	Deep vein thrombosis req anticoagulant therapy	Pulmonary embolism

WNL = within normal limits

	Grade 0	Grade 1 (Mild)	Grade 2 (Moderate)	Grade 3 (Severe)	Grade 4 (Life-threatening)
Dysrhythmias	None	Asymptomatic, transient, req no therapy	Recurrent or persistent, no therapy req	Req trt	Req monitoring, or hypotension, or ventricular tachycardia, or fibrillation
Oedema	None	1+ or dependent in evening only	2+ or dependent throughout day	3+	4+, generalized anasarca
Function	None	Asymptomatic, decline of resting ejection fraction by <20% of baseline value	Asymptomatic, decline of resting ejection fraction by >20% of baseline value	Mild CHF, responsive to therapy	Severe or refractory CHF
Hypertension	None or no change	Asymptomatic, transient increase by >20 mm Hg or to >150/100 if previously WNL. No trt req	Recurrent or persistent increase by >20 mm Hg or to >150/100 if previously WNL. No trt req	Req therapy	Hypertensive crisis
Hypotension	None or no change	Changes req no therapy (incl transient orthostatic hypotension)	Req fluid replacement or other therapy but not hospitalization	Req therapy & hospitalisation; resolves within 48 hrs of stopping agent	Req therapy & hospitalisation for 48 hrs after stopping agent

	Grade 0	Grade 1 (Mild)	Grade 2 (Moderate)	Grade 3 (Severe)	Grade 4 (Life-threatening)
Ischaemia	None or no change	Non-specific T wave flattening	Asymptomatic, ST & T wave changes suggesting ischaemia	Angina without evidence for infarction	Acute myocardial infarction
Pain (chest)	None	Mild	Moderate	Severe	Life-threatening
Pericardial	None	Asymptomatic, effusion, no intervention req	Pericarditis (rub, chest pain, ECG changes)	Symptomatic effusion, drainage req	Tamponade, drainage urgently req, or constrictive pericarditis req surgery

COAGULATION

	Grade 0	Grade 1 (Mild)	Grade 2 (Moderate)	Grade 3 (Severe)	Grade 4 (Life-threatening)
Fibrinogin	WNL	$0.99-0.75 \times N$	$0.74-0.5 \times N$	$0.49-0.25 \times N$	$\leq 0.24 \times N$
Prothrombin time	WNL	$1.01-1.25 \times N$	$1.26-1.5 \times N$	$1.51-2.00 \times N$	$>2.00 \times N$
Partial thromboplastin time	WNL	$1.01-1.66 \times N$	$1.67-2.33 \times N$	$2.34-3.00 \times N$	$>3.00 \times N$

ENDOCRINE

	Grade 0	Grade 1 (Mild)	Grade 2 (Moderate)	Grade 3 (Severe)	Grade 4 (Life-threatening)
Amenorrhoea	No	Yes ≥3 months	—	—	—
Cushingoid	Normal	Mild	Pronounced	—	—
Hot-flushes	None	Mild or <1/day	Moderate & ≥ 1/day	Frequent & interferes with normal function	—

	Grade 0	Grade 1 (Mild)	Grade 2 (Moderate)	Grade 3 (Severe)	Grade 4 (Life-threatening)
Gynaecomastia	Normal	Mild	Pronounced or painful	–	–
Impotence/libido	Normal	Decrease in normal function	–	Absence of function	–

FLU-LIKE SYMPTOMS

	Grade 0	Grade 1 (Mild)	Grade 2 (Moderate)	Grade 3 (Severe)	Grade 4 (Life-threatening)
Arthralgia (joint pain)	None	Mild	Moderate	Severe	–
Diaphoresis (sweating)	None	Mild	Moderate	Severe	–
Fever in absence of infection (including drug fever)	None	37.1–38.0°C 98.7–100.4°F	38.1–40.0°C 100.5–104.5°F	>40.0°C >104.0°F For <24 hrs	>40.0°C (104.0°F) For >24 hrs or fever accompanied by hypotension

Fever felt to be caused by *drug allergy* should be coded as ALLERGY. *Non-allergic drug fever* (e.g. as from biologics) should be coded under FLU-LIKE SYMPTOMS. If fever is due to *infection*, code INFECTION only.

	Grade 0	Grade 1 (Mild)	Grade 2 (Moderate)	Grade 3 (Severe)	Grade 4 (Life-threatening)
Hayfever (includes sneezing, nasal stuffiness, post-nasal drip)	None	Mild	Moderate	Severe	–
Lethargy (fatigue, malaise)	None	Mild, fall of 1 level in performance status	Moderate, fall of 2 levels in performance status	Severe, fall of 3 levels in performance status	–
Myalgia (muscle ache)	None	Mild	Moderate	Severe	–
Rigors/chills (Gr 3 incl cyanosis)	None	Mild or brief	Pronounced and/or prolonged	Cyanosis	–

	Grade 0	Grade 1 (Mild)	Grade 2 (Moderate)	Grade 3 (Severe)	Grade 4 (Life-threatening)
GASTROINTESTINAL					
Anorexia	None	Mild	Moderate	Severe	–
Appetite-increased	None	Mild	Moderate	–	–
Diarrhoea	None	Increase of 2–3 stools/day over pre-trt	Increase of 4–6 stools/day, or nocturnal stools	Increase of 7–9 stools/day, or incontinence, malabsorption	Increase of ≥ 10 stools/day or grossly bloody diarrhoea, or need for parenteral support
Oesophagitis/dysphagia /odynophagia	None	Dys. or odyn. not req trt, or painless ulcers on esophagoscopy	Dys. or odyn. req trt	Dys. or odyn. lasting >14 days despite trt	Dys. or odyn. with 10% loss of body wt. dehydration, hosp. req
Mouth dryness	None	Mild	Moderate	Severe	–
Intestinal fistula	No	–	–	Req intervention	Req operation
Heartburn (includes dyspepsia)	None	Mild	Moderate	Severe	–
Nausea	None	Able to eat reasonable intake	Intake significantly decreased but can eat	No significant intake	–
Small bowel obstruction	No	–	Intermittent, no intervention	Req intervention	Req operation

	Grade 0	Grade 1 (Mild)	Grade 2 (Moderate)	Grade 3 (Severe)	Grade 4 (Life-threatening)
Pain/cramping (abdominal)(includes rectal pain)	None	Mild	Moderate	Severe	–
Proctitis (rectal)	None	–	Tenesmus or ulcerations relieved with therapy	Tenesmus or ulcerations or other symptoms not relieved	Mucosal necrosis with haemorrhage or other life-threatening
Stomatitis/oral	None	Painless, ulcers, erythema, or mild soreness	Painful erythema, oedema, or ulcers but can eat	With therapy painful erythema, oedema, or ulcers, and cannot eat	Proctitis, mucosal necrosis, and/or req parenteral or enteral support
Taste altered	None	Mild	Moderate	Severe	
Gastritis/ulcer	No	Antacid	Req vigorous medical management or non-surgical trt	Uncontrolled by medical management; req surgery for GI ulceration	Perforation of bleeding
Vomiting	None	1 episode in 24 hrs	2–5 episodes in 24 hrs	6–10 episodes in 24 hrs	>10 episodes in 24 hrs or req parenteral

	Grade 0	Grade 1 (Mild)	Grade 2 (Moderate)	Grade 3 (Severe)	Grade 4 (Life-threatening)
GENITOURINARY					
Bladder changes	None	Light, epithelial atrophy or minor telangiectasia	Generalized telangiectasia	Severe generalized telangiectasia (often with petechiae) or reduction in bladder capacity (<15 ml)	Necrosis, or contracted bladder (capacity <100 ml), or fibrosis/fistulae
Creatinine	WNL	<1.5 × N	1.5–3.0 × N	3.1–6.0 × N	>6.0 × N
Cystitis (non-bacterial)	None	Mild symptoms req no intervention	Symptoms relieved completely with therapy	Symptoms not relieved despite therapy	Severe (life-threatening) cystitis
		Urinary tract infection should be coded under infection, not genitourinary.			
Dysuria	None	Dysuria not req trt	Dysuria req trt	–	–
Fistula	None	–	–	Yes	–
Frequency	None	Freq of urination or nocturia twice pre-trt habit	Freq of urination or nocturia < hourly	Freq with urgency and nocturia ≥ hourly	–
Haematuria	Neg	Micro only	Gross, no clots	Gross + clots	Req transfusion
		Haematuria resulting from thrombocytopenia should be coded under haemorrhage, not genitourinary.			
Urethral obstruction	None	Unilateral, no surgery req	Bilateral, no surgery req	Not complete bilateral but stents, nephrostomy tubes or surgery req	Complete bilateral obstruction surgery req

	Grade 0	Grade 1 (Mild)	Grade 2 (Moderate)	Grade 3 (Severe)	Grade 4 (Life-threatening)
Proteinuria	No change	1 + or <0.3 g % or < 3 g/L	2–3 + or 0.3–1.0 g % or 3–10 g/L	4 + or > 1.0 g % or > 10 g/L	Nephrotic syndrome
HEPATIC					
Alk Phos or 5′ nucleotidase	WNL	≤ 2.5 × N	2.6–5.0 × N	5.1–20.0 × N	>20.0 × N
Transaminase ALAT (SGPT)	WNL	≤ 2.5 × N	2.6–5.0 × N	5.1–20.0 × N	> 20.0 × N
Transaminase ASAT (SGOT)	WNL	≤ 2.5 × N	2.6–5.0 × N	5.1–20.0 × N	> 20.0 × N
Bilirubin	WNL	–	<1.5 × N	1.5–3.0 × N	>3.0 × N
Liver (clinical)	No change from baseline	–	–	Precoma	Hepatic coma
LDH	WNL	<2.5 × N	2.6–5.0 × N	5.1–20.0 × N	> 20.0 × N
INFECTIONS					
Infections	None	Mild, no active trt	Moderate, localized infect req active trt	Severe, systemic infect req parenteral trt, specify site	Life-threatening sepsis, specify site

	Grade 0	Grade 1 (Mild)	Grade 2 (Moderate)	Grade 3 (Severe)	Grade 4 (Life-threatening)
Febrile neutropenia	None Fever felt to be caused by *drug allergy* should be coded as ALLERGY. *Non-allergic drug fever* (e.g. as from biologics) should be coded under FLUE-LIKE SYMPTOMS. If fever is due to infection, code INFECTION only.	–	–	Present	–

METABOLIC (SI UNITS)

	Grade 0	Grade 1 (Mild)	Grade 2 (Moderate)	Grade 3 (Severe)	Grade 4 (Life-threatening)
Amylase	WNL	$<1.5 \times N$	$1.5–2.0 \times N$	$2.1–5.0 \times N$	$>5.1 \times N$
Hypercalcaemia	<2.64 mmol/L	2.64–2.88	2.89–3.12	3.13–3.37	≥ 3.37
Hypocalcaemia	>2.10 mmol/L	2.10–1.93	1.92–1.74	1.73–1.51	≤ 1.50
Hyperglycaemia	<6.44 mmol/L	6.44–8.90	8.91–13.8	13.9–27.8	>27.8 or ketoacidosis
Hypoglycaemia	>3.55 mmol/L	3.03–3.55	2.19–3.02	1.66–2.18	<1.66
Hypokalaemia	No change or > 3.5 mmol/L	3.1–3.5	2.6–3.0	2.1–2.5	≤ 2.0
Hypomagnesaemia	> 0.70 mmol/L	0.70–0.58	0.57–0.38	0.37–0.30	≤ 0.29
Hyponatraemia	No change or >135 mmol/L	131–135	126–130	121–125	≤ 120

NEUROLOGICAL

	Grade 0	Grade 1 (Mild)	Grade 2 (Moderate)	Grade 3 (Severe)	Grade 4 (Life-threatening)
Cerebellar	None	Slight inco-ordination dysdiadochokinesis	Intention tremor, dysmetria, slurred speech, nystagmus	Locomotor ataxia	Cerebellar necrosis

	Grade 0	Grade 1 (Mild)	Grade 2 (Moderate)	Grade 3 (Severe)	Grade 4 (Life-threatening)
Constipation	None or no change	Mild	Moderate	Severe	Ileus > 96 hrs
Cortical (includes drowsiness)	None	Mild somnolence	Moderate somnolence	Severe somnolence, confusion, disorientation, hallucinations	Coma, seizures, toxic psychosis
Dizziness (includes lightheadedness)	None	Mild	Moderate	Severe (includes fainting)	–
Extra pyramidal/involuntary movement	None	Mild agitation (includes restlessness)	Moderate agitation	Torticollis, oculogyric crisis, severe agitation	–
Headache	None	Mild	Moderate or severe but transient	Unrelenting & severe	–
Hearing	None or no change	Asymptomatic, hearing loss on audiometry only	Tinnitus	Hearing loss interfering with function but correctable with bearing aid	Deafness not correctable
Insomnia	None	Mild	Moderate	Severe	–
Mood	No change	Mild anxiety or depression	Moderate anxiety or depression	Severe anxiety or depression	Suicidal ideation

	Grade 0	Grade 1 (Mild)	Grade 2 (Moderate)	Grade 3 (Severe)	Grade 4 (Life-threatening)
Motor	None or no change	Subjective weakness, no objective findings	Mild objective weakness without significant impairment of function	Objective weakness with impairment of function	Paralysis
Personality change	No change	Change, not disruptive to pt or family	Disruptive to pt or family	Harmful to others or self	Psychosis
Sensory	None or no change	Mild paresthesias, loss of deep tendon reflexes (incl. tingling)	Mild or moderate Objective sensory loss, moderate paresthesias	Sensory loss or paresthesias that interfere with function	—
Vision	None or no change	Blurred vision	—	Symptomatic subtotal loss of vision	Blindness
OCULAR					
Conjunctivitis/keratitis	None	Erythema or chemosis not req steroids or antibiotics	Req trt with steroids or antibiotics	Corneal ulceration or visible opacification	—
Dry eye	Normal	Mild	Req artificial tears	Severe	Req enucleation
Glaucoma	No change	—	—	Yes	—
PULMONARY					
Carbon Monoxide diffusion capacity (DLCO)	> 90% of pre-treatment value	Decrease to 76–90% of pre-trt	Decrease to 51–75% of pre-trt	Decrease to 26–50% of pre-trt	Decrease to ≤ 25% of pre-trt

	Grade 0	Grade 1 (Mild)	Grade 2 (Moderate)	Grade 3 (Severe)	Grade 4 (Life-threatening)
Cough	None	Mild	Moderate	Severe	
Pulmonary oedema	None	–	Out-pt management	In-pt management	Req intubation
Pulmonary fibrosis	Normal	Radiographic changes, no symptoms	–	Changes with symptoms –	
Pneumonitis (non-infectious)	Normal	Radiographic changes, symptoms do not req steroids	Steroids req	Oxygen req	Req assisted ventilation
SOB (dyspnoea)(includes wheezing)	None or no change	Asymptomatic, with abnormality in PFTs	Dyspnoea no significant exertion	Dyspnoea at normal level of activity	Dyspnoea at rest
SKIN					
Alopecia	No loss	Mild hair loss	Pronounced or total head hair loss	Total body hair loss	–
Skin changes	None	Hyperpigmentation	Atrophy	Subcut fibrosis	–
Desquamation	None	Dry desquamation	Moist desquamation	Confluent moist desquamation	Ulceration or necrosis
Flushing-facial	None	Mild	Moderate	Severe	–
Local toxicity (reaction at IV site)	None	Pain	Pain & swelling, with inflammation or phlebitis	Ulceration	Plastic surgery indicated

	Grade 0	Grade 1 (Mild)	Grade 2 (Moderate)	Grade 3 (Severe)	Grade 4 (Life-threatening)
Rash/itch (not due to allergy) (includes recall reaction)	None or no change	Scattered macular or papular eruption or erythema that is asymptomatic	Scattered macular or papular eruption or erythema with pruritus or other associated symptoms	Generalized symptomatic macular, papular, or vesicular eruption	Exfoliative dermatitis or ulceration dermatitis
WEIGHT					
Weight gain	<5.0%	5.0–9.9%	10.0–19.9%	≥ 20.0%	—
Weight loss	<5.0%	5.0–9.9%	10.0–19.9%	≥ 20.0%	—

Appendix 2:
Nomogram for determination of body surface area

Nomogram for determination of body surface from height and mass

Appendix 2: Nomogram for determination of body surface area.
(Reproduced with permission from Geigy Scientific Tables (8th edn)
(ed. Lentner, C.). Ciba Geigy Ltd., Switzerland, 1981.

Index